Contributors

Editor

Suzanne M. Mahon, RN, DNSc, AOCN®, APNG
Clinical Professor
Department of Internal Medicine and Adult Nursing, School of Nursing
Saint Louis University
St. Louis, Missouri
Chapter 1. Introduction; Chapter 2. Risk Factors; Chapter 6. Breast Restoration With Prostheses

Authors

Michelle Casey, CFA
Patient Care Coordinator
Medical West Healthcare Center
St. Louis, Missouri
Chapter 6. Breast Restoration With Prostheses

Dianne D. Chapman, ND, APRN,BC
Nurse Practitioner—Division of Hematology/Oncology
Geneticist—Rush Inherited Susceptibility to Cancer (RISC)
    Program
Rush University Medical Center
Chicago, Illinois
*Chapter 3. Prevention and Detection of Breast Cancer;
    Chapter 5. Local and Regional Control*

Ellen Giarelli, EdD, RN, CRNP
Research Associate Professor
School of Nursing
University of Pennsylvania
Philadelphia, Pennsylvania
*Chapter 10. Breast Cancer Research in the United States:
    Nursing Contributions 2000–2005*

Katina Kirby, MS, OTR/L, CLT-LANA
Manager, ENH Lymphedema Treatment Center
Evanston Northwestern Healthcare
Evanston, Illinois
Chapter 8. Symptom Management in Breast Cancer

Carole H. Martz, RN, MS, AOCN®
Clinical Coordinator
Living in the Future (LIFE) Cancer Survivorship Program
Evanston Northwestern Healthcare
Highland Park, Illinois
Chapter 8. Symptom Management in Breast Cancer

Gail Osterman, PhD
Assistant Professor
Northwestern Memorial Hospital
Bluhm Cardiovascular Institute
Chicago, Illinois
Chapter 9. Psychosocial Issues

Susan G. Yackzan, RN, MSN, AOCN®
Oncology Clinical Nurse Specialist
Central Baptist Hospital
Lexington, Kentucky
*Chapter 4. Pathophysiology and Staging of Breast Cancer;
    Chapter 7. Systemic Treatment*

Contents

Foreword

A vast amount of information is available about breast cancer. A PubMed search of the words "breast cancer" produces the titles of more than 92,000 published articles, and a Google search produces links to nearly 40 million Internet sites. Few healthcare providers have the time or resources to obtain, review, and continually evaluate the latest scientific data on breast cancer, yet they regularly care for patients with this disease.

Experts in breast cancer prevention, detection, treatment, and related areas closely examined the literature and other information sources to provide the up-to-date comprehensive information found in this book. This information can be used by healthcare providers to guide evidence-based practice and patient-focused care.

Highlighted in this book is the critical role of the nurse in caring for people at risk for, or experiencing, breast cancer. The nurse's role encompasses the spectrum of breast cancer, from prevention to treatment outcome and beyond, and includes related areas, such as breast restoration and patients' psychosocial concerns. Nurses also have been instrumental in conducting or participating in research on breast cancer, and a chapter of this book details the significant contributions of nurses in this role.

Suzanne M. Mahon, RN, DNSc, AOCN®, APNG, editor of this book, has compiled a definitive nursing-focused resource on breast cancer. She and the other contributors are to be commended for transforming the overwhelming body of knowledge about breast cancer into an easy-to-read informative text. Nurses and other healthcare providers will find the information contained in this book to be essential to practice and beneficial to the patients they care for.

Lisa Schulmeister, RN, MN, CS, OCN®, FAAN
Oncology Nursing Consultant
New Orleans, LA

CHAPTER 1

Introduction

Suzanne M. Mahon, RN, DNSc, AOCN®, APNG

Overview

The very term *breast cancer* sends a message of fear to many, if not all, women. With an estimated 180,510 new cases of invasive breast cancer and an additional 62,030 cases of in situ breast cancer diagnosed in 2007, it is not surprising that women and their loved ones fear the disease (American Cancer Society [ACS], 2007). Unfortunately, an estimated 40,460 women will die from breast cancer in 2007 (ACS, 2007). Most people know someone who has been affected by the diagnosis. Excluding skin cancer, breast cancer is the most common cancer among U.S. women, accounting for one out of every three cancers diagnosed in women (ACS, 2005, 2007).

The cultural and psychological significance of the breast in modern society, in addition to the large number of people affected by the disease, may explain much of the fear associated with the diagnosis. The female breast plays a significant role in nurturing and motherhood. Symbolically, it often is associated with femininity and sexuality. Threats to the health of the breast potentially influence a woman's perceptions of her body and her role in society.

Although breast cancer primarily affects women, an estimated 2,030 men are diagnosed each year. This accounts for about 1% of all cases of breast cancer diagnosed (ACS, 2007). The needs of this special population cannot be ignored. Although this text focuses on breast cancer in women, with regard to diagnostic, surgical, and adjuvant therapy, many of the strategies used to treat male breast cancer are similar to those used in women. For many men diagnosed with breast cancer, the psychosocial issues are complex and require much sensitivity and care from oncology health professionals.

Every October, numerous groups promote breast cancer awareness, including Susan G. Komen for the Cure and ACS, as well as professional societies and local healthcare institutions. The color pink is universally associated with breast cancer, and during these special awareness programs, there are constant reminders about the need for improved detection and treatment of the disease set against a background of pink.

Many breast cancer survivors have become activists and advocates for other women to prevent the disease and promote its early detection.

This awareness of breast cancer has dramatically changed the outlook and treatment for those diagnosed with breast cancer. In the past two decades, thousands of women have walked in awareness races, raised money for research and screening, participated in screening, and enrolled in clinical trials with the hope of improving the outcomes for those diagnosed with breast cancer.

Historical Perspectives

An examination of the history of breast cancer treatment enables women and healthcare providers to understand how much progress has been made, yet it also leaves questions about what yet needs to be done. As early as 400 BC, Hippocrates speculated on the systemic nature of the disease (Foster, 2003). Galen (AD 130–200) believed breast cancer to be a local/regional disease requiring complete excision for cure. The early Romans performed a type of mastectomy that included removal of the pectoralis muscle. Throughout the Middle Ages and Renaissance periods, crude types of mastectomies often were attempted to potentially eradicate disease. These early physicians initiated the debate about whether breast cancer is a systemic disease, local/regional disease, or both.

During the middle of the 18th century, William Hunter identified and described the importance of the lymphatic system in the spread of cancer (Foster, 2003). Surgical techniques greatly improved in the mid-19th century with the introduction of general anesthetics and more antiseptic techniques. In the late 19th century, Thomas Beatson of Scotland reported that oophorectomy resulted in the regression of advanced breast cancer. This early finding was just the beginning of hormonal manipulation as an effective adjuvant therapy in the treatment of breast cancer.

Although considered controversial in his time, William Halsted believed that breast cancer was a local/regional disease and is well known for promoting the Halsted radical mastectomy, which quickly became the standard of care for more than the first half of the 20th century. This radical surgical procedure often was combined with radiation therapy, which was also an emerging science at that time (Foster, 2003). Surgical treatment typically involved a "one-step procedure," in which a woman undergoing a biopsy with general anesthesia also would consent to an immediate mastectomy if the frozen section showed malignancy. It was not until the woman woke up that she would know the actual diagnosis and extent of surgery. Women typically were offered little choice in treatment.

The middle of the 20th century brought about a push toward clinical trials and decreasing the morbidity and mortality associated with breast cancer. These trials have had an enormous impact on breast cancer treatment and have led to the view that breast cancer is systemic and not just a local/regional disease. Because of these trials, lumpectomy followed by radiation therapy is now an appropriate local/regional control strategy for many women. The one-step biopsy procedure was gradually eliminated as biopsy techniques became more refined and women could make informed decisions about local/regional management. Adjuvant therapy trials have greatly changed systemic treatment for breast cancer. The National Surgical Adjuvant Breast and Bowel Project (NSABP) has enrolled more than 40,000 women in more than 30 trials (Foster, 2003).

In the 1970s, the concept of screening for early breast cancer gained more acceptance. Women were encouraged to practice breast self-examination. Mammography gradually became more readily available and more sensitive in detecting early malignancies. Screening continues to be refined with digital mammography, and breast magnetic resonance imaging is showing promise as a detection tool in some high-risk groups.

Prevention of breast cancer is not yet a reality, although it may eventually be one. The NSABP P-1 trial clearly demonstrated that tamoxifen may be beneficial in some high-risk women to reduce the risk of, delay the development of, or prevent breast cancer. Genetic testing is now readily available for two hereditary breast cancer susceptibility genes *(BRCA1/2)*. Women with a known mutation can be offered prophylactic surgeries to prevent the development of breast cancer.

Social movements, as well, have influenced the treatment of breast cancer. Prior to the 1970s, breast cancer was considered a stigma. It was not discussed. The diagnosis of breast cancer in several prominent women, including Shirley Temple Black, Betty Ford, Happy Rockefeller, and Betty Rollin, changed public opinion about the disease in a relatively short period of time. These women used their popularity to encourage other women to engage in early detection practices and to be open about their diagnosis. They increased public awareness

of the disease and, along with many other women, challenged the breast cancer practices of the time (including the Halsted radical mastectomy) and lobbied for increased accountability and accessibility in mammography (Kolker, 2004). These efforts ultimately led to significant federal funding for more research related to breast cancer.

The trend toward shorter hospitalization is another social movement that has dramatically affected breast cancer treatment. Twenty-five years ago, women would recover for 10 days to two weeks in the hospital. Today, for many women, same-day or one-night stays are now the norm after surgical management of the disease. These women still go home with physical limitations and emotional concerns but often with much less support from the healthcare team. This creates new challenges for patients and their families.

Consumerism also has affected breast cancer (Klawiter, 2004). Two decades ago, few resources were available to women other than the ACS and its "Reach to Recovery" program. Minimal printed resources existed, and the Internet had not been developed yet. Women faced the disease and its treatment, often with a limited understanding of the pathophysiology of the disease and its treatment. Today, society promotes the concept that women should be active partners in decisions regarding treatment. The National Cancer Institute and numerous other organizations encourage women to ask questions and provide educational resources in many formats.

Epidemiologic Perspectives

Some epidemiologic trends in breast cancer have occurred that merit notice. Breast cancer risk increases with age. During 1998–2002, 95% of the new cancers and 97% of breast cancer deaths occurred in women age 40 and older (ACS, 2005). During this same time period, the median age at diagnosis was 61.

Many women believe that breast cancer has become increasingly more common. Since 1975, three basic incidence trends have occurred (ACS, 2005). From 1975 to 1980, the incidence was relatively constant. Between 1980 and 1987, the incidence increased by 4% per year. This increased incidence is attributed to more widespread use of mammography and the detection of nonpalpable lesions. The most recent data available are for 1987–2002, in which the incidence rates have increased 0.3% per year. Epidemiologists speculate that the recent increase in incidence is related to changing reproductive patterns, including delayed childbearing and fewer pregnancies.

Despite the increasing incidence, mortality rates are decreasing. Between 1990 and 2002, the mortality rate decreased by 2.3% annually (ACS, 2005). Recent estimates suggest that at least 2.3 million women are alive with a diagnosis of breast cancer (ACS, 2005). Long-term survival rates continue to improve. Currently, of all the women diagnosed, 88% are alive 5 years after the diagnosis; 80% are alive 10 years after the diagnosis; 71% are alive after 15 years; and after 20 years, 63% are still alive (ACS, 2005).

Clinical Perspectives

Women understandably worry about their risk for developing breast cancer. Understanding this concept is a challenge both for women to comprehend and for healthcare professionals to communicate. Multiple means are available to express risk. Healthcare providers are encouraged to find a risk assessment that correctly conveys risk and is appropriate for the woman. This usually includes a combination of figures including relative, absolute, and, in some cases, attributable risk. The primary reason for conducting a risk assessment is to use it to guide decisions about screening.

The Human Genome Project has greatly changed risk assessment processes, especially in the area of breast cancer risk. Approximately 10% of all breast cancers likely have a hereditary component (Daly et al., 2006). The identification of women with hereditary risk is an ever-emerging role in oncology. Once identified through risk assessment, these women need comprehensive, balanced counseling so that they can make an informed decision about genetic testing. Genetic testing has major ramifications for both the individual tested and for other relatives. For those who test positive for a known mutation, difficult choices can arise regarding prevention, including the possibility of prophylactic surgery.

For all women, the risk assessment guides screening recommendations. Multiple screening recommendations are available from numerous organizations. These recommendations usually include some combination of breast self-examination, a professional clinical breast examination, and mammography. For those with significant risk, other modalities such as magnetic resonance imaging may be added, as well as more frequent screening. When making screening recommendations, healthcare providers need to inform women about why a particular guideline is being utilized, as well as the potential risks, benefits, and limitations associated with a particular screening modality.

Ideally, all breast cancer would be prevented; however, limited strategies currently exist that are routinely used in the prevention of breast cancer. All women should be counseled about the benefits of a low-fat diet, weight control, and regular exercise. The role of exogenous hormone use in the development of breast cancer is still poorly understood. Tamoxifen, however, has shown some promise for the prevention of breast cancer. Clearly, more chemoprevention trials are needed to identify more agents and offer women some choice for the prevention of breast cancer. For women with a hereditary predisposition for developing breast cancer, recommended prevention measures may include prophylactic mastectomy and oophorectomy, but both of these surgeries are not without significant physiologic and psychological consequences.

The diagnostic process for evaluating any breast abnormality can be terrorizing for women. On a positive note, biopsy techniques continue to become less invasive. For most, the workup will result in a benign finding. These women usually feel a great sense of relief and ideally a heightened awareness of the importance of the early detection of breast cancer. For those with a positive finding, they are suddenly thrown into an unfamiliar and potentially frightening arena of health care. Being sensitive to the needs of these women is critical to promote their overall adjustment to the diagnosis.

Treatment for breast cancer has changed greatly. Mastectomy is no longer the only choice for many women. The Halsted radical mastectomy is no longer the norm. For many women, breast-sparing procedures are more than adequate treatment. Lymph node sampling techniques have improved with the hope of reducing lymphedema. Women, however, must make decisions about which treatment(s) to undergo, and this decision-making process can be extremely stressful for some.

Breast restoration also has improved dramatically. Women have many options in breast and reconstructive surgery. Patients with breast cancer need much guidance, support, and education as they make choices about reconstructive surgery. Although often forgotten, prosthetics also are an appropriate and satisfactory choice for women. They should not be considered as a "second rate" choice or reserved simply for women who are not good surgical candidates. The choices in prosthetics are numerous. Similarly, bras, undergarments, and swimsuits no longer need to be ugly. Women need to be counseled and encouraged to learn about these different options.

The past decades have demonstrated great strides in understanding the pathology of breast cancer and how it influences treatment. Two decades ago, treatment was limited to a few chemotherapeutic agents and tamoxifen. Treatment now includes multiple chemotherapeutic agents, immunomodulating agents, radiation therapy, and hormonal manipulation. Each of these areas continues to expand, and many active research trials are currently available.

These advances in treatment, however, have not come without a price. The acute toxicities associated with surgery and adjuvant therapy can be significant. Many research efforts are being expended to determine how to more accurately assess, prevent, and manage these side effects. In addition to short-term side effects, many breast cancer survivors cope with long-term consequences. The pool of survivors is steadily increasing, and with longer survival rates, the possibility of long-term complications increases. Most notably, the past decade has seen a significant number of survivors coping with the consequences of early menopause, osteoporosis, and mental changes. Addressing the needs of this patient population through tertiary prevention practices is an ever-expanding role for nurses.

Breast cancer can be an overwhelming diagnosis for both patients and those close to them. Many women cope with the diagnosis and ultimately may have a renewed sense of purpose in life. For others, it can be devastating. The psychological ramifications of the diagnosis are significant. It forces women to confront mortality. The body image changes that result from surgery and related treatment serve as a constant reminder of the diagnosis. Role changes during treatment disrupt many family routines. Women worry about hereditary susceptibility and whether a child has inherited increased risk for developing the disease. The diagnosis is accompanied by many unknowns, including prognostic factors, treatment issues, and how family and friends will react to the diagnosis. These unknowns contribute to stress with the diagnosis. The psychological care of these women and their families requires ongoing intervention by healthcare providers. For those women for whom breast cancer cannot be cured and who will die from the disease, there is an ongoing need to recognize and implement palliative care interventions in a timely fashion.

Research in breast cancer and its treatment continues. Researchers are actively looking for ways to detect breast cancer as early as possible. Much effort is being made to find effective and tolerable prevention strategies. Genetic markers continue to be identified to better stratify risk. Management of the long-term complications of surgery and treatment continues to provide challenges to healthcare providers. Women need to continue to be offered clinical trials to build an evidence-based practice for the management of breast cancer.

Conclusion

This book seeks to address issues related to cancer control, breast cancer treatment, psychosocial concerns, and management of complications related to cancer and its treatment in depth. Many issues in breast cancer are controversial. Patients and healthcare providers need to consider all issues, and then each woman needs to make choices that are consistent with her value system and place in life. In some cases, no single correct answer exists. New questions and challenges will continue to arise.

Many resources are available to healthcare providers who care for women with breast cancer. A more comprehensive list is provided in Appendix 1. Healthcare providers also need to continually be aware of the recommendations and position statements of respected professional organizations. The Oncology Nursing Society has published several position statements on topics that are especially relevant for the care of women with breast cancer. These include breast cancer screening, cancer predisposition genetic testing and risk assessment counseling, rehabilitation of people with cancer, and prevention and early detection of cancer in the United States (see Appendices 2, 3, 4, and 5).

For many diagnosed with breast cancer, nurses truly will make an enormous difference in how they cope with treatment and its associated complications. Each phase of the breast cancer trajectory is accompanied by different needs and concerns. Nurses are challenged to consider the past history of breast cancer treatment and to provide information and care in a way that promotes health, hope, and well-being for the women and families affected by the diagnosis of breast cancer.

References

American Cancer Society. (2005). *Breast cancer facts and figures, 2005–2006.* Atlanta, GA: Author.

American Cancer Society. (2007). *Cancer facts and figures, 2007.* Atlanta, GA: Author.

Daly, M.B., Axilbund, J.E., Bryant, E., Buys, S., Eng, C., Friedman, S., et al. (2006). Genetic/familial high-risk assessment: Breast and ovarian. *Journal of the National Comprehensive Cancer Network, 4,* 156–176.

Foster, R.S., Jr. (2003). Breast cancer detection and treatment. A personal and historical perspective. *Archives of Surgery, 138,* 397–408.

Klawiter, M. (2004). Breast cancer in two regimes: The impact of social movements on illness experience. *Sociology of Health and Illness, 26,* 845–874.

Kolker, E.S. (2004). Framing as a cultural resource in health social movements: Funding activism and the breast cancer movement in the U.S. 1990–1993. *Sociology of Health and Illness, 26,* 820–844.

CHAPTER 2

Risk Factors

Suzanne M. Mahon, RN, DNSc, AOCN®, APNG

Introduction

A risk factor is a trait or characteristic that is associated with a statistically significant increased likelihood of developing a disease. In the case of breast cancer, the presence of a risk factor does not absolutely mean that a woman will develop breast cancer, nor does the absence of risk factors make her immune to developing the disease.

Many women are very worried about developing breast cancer. This stems from extensive media coverage of the topic that is often confusing and conflicting. Most women know someone who has been affected by the diagnosis of breast cancer. This pervasive worry is compounded by the fact that the best way to assess and manage breast cancer risk is not always completely clear. Women who receive breast cancer screening and other health care would like to better understand their risk for developing breast cancer and what specifically can be done to reduce their risk and anxiety about the disease. Breast cancer risk assessment is the critical initial step in helping people to better comprehend the ramifications of the disease and to take appropriate steps to prevent and/or detect it early, when it is most treatable.

Basic elements of a breast cancer risk assessment generally include a review of medical history, a history of exposures to carcinogens in daily living, and a detailed family history. Once all information is gathered, it must be interpreted for the patient in reasonable terms. This is paramount in communicating breast cancer risk. Risk assessment guides not only screening decisions but also decisions about treatment. Genetic testing (a tool for breast cancer risk assessment) affects and guides treatment decisions. Decisions based on genetic testing are often significant and can have many ramifications, such as prophylactic surgery. This underscores the importance of constructing an accurate risk assessment, so that genetic testing and prophylactic measures can be implemented appropriately in individuals who stand to gain the most benefit.

Because risk communication alters screening and treatment decisions, nurses need to understand the known and suspected risk factors for breast cancer and their physiologic basis. Genetic predisposition testing for breast cancer susceptibility genes is readily available on a commercial basis, and people need sufficient, accurate information to make appropriate choices about testing. To provide effective education and support for women concerned about breast cancer risk and genetic testing, nurses must use clear communication strategies regarding cancer risk. This chapter will provide a discussion of conceptual issues in risk assessment, a review of risk factors associated with the development of breast cancer, considerations in genetic testing for breast cancer susceptibility genes, and issues in breast cancer risk communication.

Types of Risk Utilized in Breast Cancer Risk Counseling

Absolute Risk

Absolute risk is a measure of the occurrence of cancer, by either incidence (new cases) or mortality (deaths), in an identified population. Absolute risk is helpful when patients need to understand what the chances are for all individuals in a population of developing a particular disease. Absolute risk can be expressed either as the number of cases for a specified denominator (for example, 131 cases of breast cancer per 100,000 women annually) or as a cumulative risk up to a specified age (for example, one in eight women will develop breast cancer if they live to age 85) (American Cancer Society [ACS], 2007). Another way to express absolute risk is to discuss the average risk of developing breast cancer at a certain age. For example, a woman's risk of developing breast cancer may be 2% at age 50, but at age 85, it might be 13%. Risk estimates will be much different for a 50-year-old woman than for an 85-year-old woman, as approximately 50% of breast cancer cases occur after age 65 (ACS) (see Table 2-1).

Women need to understand that certain assumptions are made to reach an absolute risk figure for breast cancer. For

Table 2-1. Absolute Risk of Developing Breast Cancer Over Time*	
Age	**Risk**
0–39 years	0.48% (1 in 210 women)
40–59 years	3.98% (1 in 25)
60–69 years	3.65% (1 in 27)
70 or more years	6.84% (1 in 15)
*Lifetime risk is 12.67% (one in eight women). *Note.* Based on information from American Cancer Society, 2007.	

example, the one-in-eight figure describes the "average" risk of developing breast cancer in Caucasian American women, and its calculation considers other causes of death over the life span. This figure will overestimate breast cancer risk for some people with no risk factors and will greatly underestimate the risk for people with several risk factors, such as a genetic mutation. What this statistic actually means is that the average woman's breast cancer risk is 0.48% until age 40, 4.11% for ages 40–60, 3.82% for ages 60–69, and 4.81% for ages 70 and older. The 13.22% or one-in-eight risk figure is obtained by adding the risk in each age category (0.48% + 4.11% + 3.82% + 4.81% = 13.22%). When a woman who has an average risk reaches age 40 without a diagnosis of breast cancer, she has passed through 0.48% of her risk, so her lifetime risk is 13.22% minus 0.48%, which equals 12.74%. When she reaches age 70 without a diagnosis of breast cancer, her risk is 13.22% – 0.48% – 4.11% – 3.82% = 4.81%. Time always must be considered for the risk figure to be meaningful.

Relative Risk

The term *relative risk* refers to a comparison of the incidence or deaths among those with a particular risk factor compared to those without the risk factor. By using relative risk factors, patients can determine their risk factors and thus better understand their chances of developing a specific cancer as compared to people without such risk factors. If the risk for a woman with no known risk factors is 1.0, one can evaluate the risk of those with risk factors in relation to this figure (see Table 2-2).

The use of relative risk factors can be confusing to some patients. When providing information about relative risk, it is important to specify exactly what comparison is being made. Often, percentages are confusing when used with relative risk. If a news report states that taking a particular hormone therapy after menopause causes a 30%–50% increase in breast cancer risk, in absolute numeric terms this means that 0.6 more cases of breast cancer will occur per 100 women ages 50–70. The same concept applies if a person has a 1% chance of develop-

ing cancer. This means that the risk has increased from 1 in 10,000 to 1.3 in 10,000 (Rothman & Kiviniemi, 1999).

Attributable Risk

Attributable risk is the amount of disease within the population that could be prevented by alteration or elimination of a risk factor. Attributable risk has enormous implications for public health policy. A risk factor could convey a very large relative risk but be restricted to a few individuals; so, changing it would benefit only a small group. Conversely, some risk factors amenable to change could potentially decrease the morbidity and mortality associated with malignancy in a significant number of people. Little is known about attributable risk in breast cancer, and most gains at this point are probably small. For example, a package insert might report a relative risk of 2.35 for developing breast cancer in women younger than age 35 whose first exposure to an oral contraceptive (OC) drug was within the previous four years. Because the annual incidence rate (absolute risk) for women ages 30–34 is 26.7 per 100,000, a relative risk of 2.35 increases the possible risk from 26.7 to 62.75 cases per 100,000 women. The attributable risk of breast cancer is calculated to be an additional 3.38 per 10,000 women per year. This increase in the number of cases possibly is associated with the use of a pharmacologic agent. Public health policy related to the use of this agent will need to incorporate a harm-versus-benefit analysis to determine whether the recommendation for the agent should be altered to decrease breast cancer risk.

Risk Factors for Breast Cancer

When nurses discuss risk factors for breast cancer with patients, they need to carefully articulate the type of risk (absolute, relative, or attributable) and the physiologic basis of the risk factor, if known. Much research has been conducted to better understand risk factors for the development of breast cancer. Known risk factors for developing breast cancer are associated with aging, reproductive history, exogenous hormone exposure, family history, and other environmental exposures. Much remains unknown about the influence and interaction of these risk factors, and at present, they provide only a modest explanation at best for the risk of developing breast cancer. Other factors that probably have significantly contributed to the increasing incidence of breast cancer in the past 30 years include better nutrition leading to an earlier menarche, delayed or no childbearing related to career and societal expectations, and increased exogenous hormone use, including OCs and hormone replacement therapy (HRT). Women would like to have a simple explanation as to why they may be at risk for breast cancer, but the interaction of risk factors makes this a nearly impossible challenge (Ganz, 2002). Clearly, some risk factors are under the control of individuals, and others are not.

Table 2-2. Relative Risk Factors for Developing Breast Cancer		
Risk Factor	**Comparison Category**	**Relative Risk**
Early menarche (before age 12)	Menarche after age 15	1.3
Late menopause (after age 55)	Menopause age 45 or younger	1.2–1.5
First live birth between ages 25–29	First live birth before age 25	1.5
First live birth after age 30	First live birth before age 25	1.9
First live birth after age 35	First live birth before age 25	2.0–3.0
Nulliparous	First live birth before age 25	3.0
Biopsy-proven proliferative disease	No proliferative disease	1.9
Biopsy-proven proliferative disease with atypical hyperplasia	No proliferative disease	4.4–5.3
Lobular carcinoma in situ	No proliferative disease	6.9–16.4
Alcohol intake (two or more drinks per day)	No alcohol intake	1.2
Obesity/increased body mass (80th percentile or higher at age 55)	Body mass 20th percentile or less	1.2
First-degree relative with postmenopausal breast cancer	No first-degree relative with breast cancer	1.8
First-degree relative with premenopausal breast cancer	No first-degree relative with breast cancer	3.3
Two first-degree relatives with postmenopausal breast cancer	No first-degree relative with breast cancer	3.6
Two first-degree relatives with premenopausal breast cancer	No first-degree relative with breast cancer	7.1
Past history of invasive breast cancer	No past history of invasive breast cancer	6.8
Radiation exposure for Hodgkin disease	No exposure	5.2
Current hormone replacement therapy user with estrogen and progesterone for at least five years	No history of use	1.3–1.8
Age older than 55 years	Age younger than 45 years	1.2–1.5

Note. Based on information from Bilimoria & Morrow, 1995; Lee et al., 2003; Singletary, 2003.

The risk factor assessment for breast cancer is based on past medical history, lifestyle behaviors, and family history.

Age

One of the most consistently documented uncontrollable risk factors for the development of breast cancer is increasing age. Table 2-1 illustrates how at different ages women have different statistical risks for developing breast cancer. One way to consider this risk is that if all women younger than 65 years of age are compared with women ages 65 and older, the relative risk of breast cancer associated with increased age is 5.8 (Singletary, 2003).

Reproductive Factors

A woman's hormone levels normally change throughout her life for a variety of reasons. These hormonal fluctuations can lead to changes in the breast tissue. Hormonal changes occur during puberty, pregnancy, and menopause. Multiple studies have linked the age at menarche, menopause, and first live birth to breast cancer risk. Collectively, the patterns of risk associated with reproductive history suggest that prolonged exposure to ovarian hormones increases breast cancer occurrence. Although results are mixed, research suggests that the number of menstrual cycles during a lifetime may have a greater impact on risk than the number of cycles until the first full-term pregnancy (Chavez-MacGregor et al., 2005). Support for this theory stems from the observation that women who have had both ovaries removed before the age of 40 show a 45% reduction in breast cancer risk compared with women who undergo a natural menopause between ages 50–54 (Singletary, 2003). Thus, women who experience menarche before age 12 or menopause after age 50 are considered at somewhat higher risk because of the total increased number of ovulatory cycles in their lifetime.

Specific pathways involved in estrogen metabolism that may play a role in the etiology of breast cancer are not as well understood. It has been hypothesized that breast tissue damage or aging starts at a constant rate at menarche and continues at that rate until the time of first pregnancy, at which point the rate of tissue aging decreases. This continues until menopause, when there is an additional decrease, and after menopause, when there is a more constant but decreased rate (Colditz, 2005). Researchers speculate that if the first full-term pregnancy is delayed, the proliferation due to pregnancy hormones would be acting on a more damaged or aged set of DNA and would carry a greater adverse effect. Furthermore, it has been noted that when the interval between births is shortened, there is a lower rate of tissue aging and incidence of breast cancer. As a society, the interval has been greatly lengthened between menarche and the first full-term pregnancy because of increasing education and more effective contraception.

After a transient increase in risk after childbirth, a long-term reduction occurs in breast cancer risk (Collaborative Group on Hormonal Factors in Breast Cancer, 2002). The same is true of miscarriage (Brewster, Stockton, Dobbie, Bull, & Beral, 2005; National Cancer Institute [NCI], 2005). The degree of risk reduction appears to be related to age. Increasing parity is associated with a long-term reduction in breast cancer risk, presumably because of the interruption of estrogen cycling (NCI). In addition, breast-feeding is associated with a decreased risk of breast cancer (Collaborative Group on Hormonal Factors in Breast Cancer; Furberg, Newman, Moorman, & Millikan, 1999). Reproductive risk factors also may interact with other predisposing genotypes, placing some women at high risk for developing breast cancer.

Although modulation of reproductive risk factors or hormonal interventions that simulate the preventive effects of early pregnancy or early menopause are theoretically possible, these types of interventions may not be effective for all women, including those with a family history of breast cancer (Colditz, 2005). Chemoprevention is an example of this expanding area of research to modulate risk factors in the development of breast cancer.

History of Benign Breast Disease

A history of benign breast disease often is reported to be a risk factor for developing breast cancer. The key to understanding the usefulness of this risk factor is to be very careful to review the findings of all pathology reports. Defining this risk is becoming increasingly important as more women undergo breast biopsies for asymptomatic abnormalities found on mammography and, more recently, breast magnetic resonance imaging, which creates a larger pool of "higher risk" women. This risk factor can be stratified only when fibrocystic or benign breast disease is quantified according to a histology/pathology report. Nonproliferative lesions (which account for more than 70% of all breast biopsies [Colditz, 2005]) include

adenosis, fibrosis, cysts, mastitis, duct ectasia, fibroadenomas, and mild hyperplasia and confer no added risk for developing breast cancer. Of concern are pathology reports that suggest the presence of atypical hyperplasia or lobular carcinoma, although an accurate risk figure associated with this finding is difficult to quantify.

Oral Contraceptive Use

The exact risk of breast cancer conferred by the use of OCs is controversial. The composition of OCs has changed greatly over time. Early formulations of OCs used in the 1960s and 1970s contained larger amounts of estrogen and progestin than current formulations. Large randomized controlled trials are not readily available and present many methodologic and ethical concerns that make them very challenging to conduct. Interpretation of these studies is further confused by the different end points. Different risks of specific histologic types may exist based on the type and duration of OC used (Newcomer, Newcomb, Trentham-Dietz, Longnecker, & Greenberg, 2003).

Marchbanks et al. (2002) reported one of the largest case-control studies among former and current users of OCs. These researchers interviewed 4,575 women with breast cancer and 4,682 controls. They concluded that among women ages 35–64, former OC use was not associated with a significantly increased risk of developing breast cancer. OCs have been associated with a small increased risk of breast cancer in current users that gradually diminishes over time.

Hormone Replacement Therapy

Like OC use, HRT is associated with a slightly increased risk for developing breast cancer, but the amount of risk is not clear. HRT has been readily available since the 1970s, but it was not until the later 1990s that reports began to link HRT use with the development of breast cancer (Singletary, 2003).

Evidence supporting an association between the use of exogenous hormones after menopause and breast cancer is more consistent than that for OC use. The landmark Women's Health Initiative (WHI) study has suggested that HRT may not be as safe or as effective as originally thought (WHI Steering Committee, 2004). Combination HRT using an estrogen and progestin is associated with an increased risk of developing breast cancer. The exact risk is unclear because of the multiple forms of HRT available and the varying number of years of use, but it is thought to be approximately a 24% increase overall. The evidence is mixed concerning the association between estrogen-only therapy and breast cancer.

Alcohol Consumption

Clear, documented evidence shows that alcohol consumption of more than two drinks per day increases the risk of developing breast cancer. The proposed mechanisms for this phenomenon are that alcohol stimulates the metabolism of carcinogens, such as acetaldehyde, and more global mechanisms, such as decreased DNA repair efficiency or poor nutritional intake of protective nutrients (Singletary, 2003).

Individual data from 53 case-control and cohort studies were included in a British meta-analysis (Hamajima et al., 2002). Results showed that the relative risk of breast cancer increased by approximately 7% for each 10 g (one drink) of alcohol per day. The same result was obtained even after additional stratification for race, education, family history, age at menarche, height, weight, breast-feeding history, OC use, HRT use, and type of and age at menopause.

Increased Body Mass

Increased body mass may be a more important risk factor in postmenopausal women than in premenopausal women. Adipose tissue is an important source of extragonadal estrogens in postmenopausal women. The more tissue that is available, the higher the circulating levels of these estrogens, theoretically (Singletary, 2003). Obesity is associated with increased breast cancer risk, especially among postmenopausal women. The WHI Observational Study looked at 85,917 women ages 50–79 and collected information on weight history as well as known risk factors for breast cancer (Morimoto et al., 2002). Increased breast cancer risk was associated with weight at entry, body mass index (BMI) at entry, BMI at age 50, maximum BMI, adult and postmenopausal weight change, and waist and hip circumferences. Weight was the strongest predictor, with a relative risk of 2.85.

Additionally, women who have lower body mass may exercise more. Exercise can decrease the number of ovulatory cycles. This may offer a small amount of protection against breast cancer in women who are physically active on a regular basis (Singletary, 2003).

Ionizing Radiation

Exposure of the breast to ionizing radiation is associated with an increased risk of developing breast cancer, especially when the exposure occurs at a young age. The evidence of this emerged from cohort and case-control studies. This finding supports the avoidance of unnecessary breast irradiation. Women treated for Hodgkin lymphoma before age 16 may have a subsequent risk as high as 35% of developing breast cancer by age 40, with higher doses of radiation (median dose is 40 gray [Gy] in breast cancer cases) and treatment between 10–16 years of age corresponding with higher risk (Travis et al., 2003). When radiation therapy was administered after age 16 but before age 30, the risk of developing breast cancer also increased, but to a lesser degree. Unlike the risk for secondary leukemia, the risk of treatment-related breast cancer did not abate with duration

of follow-up, and the increased risk persisted for more than 25 years after treatment.

In theory, patients with breast cancer who were treated with lumpectomy and radiation therapy (L-RT) may be at increased risk for second breast or other malignancies, compared with those treated by mastectomy. Outcomes of 1,029 patients treated with L-RT were compared with 1,387 patients treated with mastectomy. After a median follow-up of 15 years, results showed no difference in the risk of second malignancies (Fisher, Anderson, et al., 2002). Another study of 701 women randomized to radical mastectomy or L-RT demonstrated the rate of contralateral breast carcinomas per 100 woman-years to be 10.2 versus 8.7, respectively (Veronesi et al., 2002).

Abortion

The possibility of an association between induced abortion and subsequent breast cancer development has been suggested, although the exact risk is not clear, and this risk factor is controversial. Initial research was based on studies using recalled information in populations where induced abortion had a negative social or religious stigma (Singletary, 2003). Trials done in social environments where abortion is accepted have not shown an increased risk (Mahue-Giangreco, Ursin, Sullivan-Halley, & Bernstein, 2003; Singletary).

Diet and Vitamins

A low-fat diet might influence breast cancer risk. Epidemiologic studies show a positive correlation between international age-adjusted breast cancer mortality rates and the estimated per capita consumption of dietary fat (Smith-Warner et al., 2001). When case-control studies have been used to evaluate the hypothesis that dietary fat is related to breast cancer risk, the results have been mixed.

Fruit and vegetable consumption (or specific fruits or vegetables) has been thought to be associated with reduced breast cancer risk. A pooled analysis of adult dietary data from eight cohort studies, which included 351,823 women in whom 7,377 incident cases of breast cancer occurred, provided little support for an association (Smith-Warner et al., 2001). When examining the dietary data treated as continuous variables (based on grams of intake/day), no association was present. These studies suggest that if there is any decreased risk of breast cancer associated with consumption of fruits and vegetables, the association is probably weak.

Micronutrient intake also may play a small role in the development of breast cancer. Case-control studies show an inverse association between dietary beta-carotene intake and breast cancer risk (Zhang, Hunter, Forman, et al., 1999). High intake of foods containing folate, beta-carotene, and vitamins A and C may reverse the increased risk associated with alcohol use (Zhang, Hunter, Hankinson, et al., 1999). In the Women's Health Study, in which 39,876 women were assigned to take beta-carotene or placebo, cancer incidence was unaffected at two years. Similarly, in this same study, no overall effect on cancer was seen in women taking 600 IU of vitamin E every other day (Zhang et al., 1999).

Family History of Cancer

Assessment of risk for breast cancer would be incomplete without an accurate assessment of hereditary risk. This may be the most quantifiable of all the risk factors as well as the most clinically significant. Assessment of hereditary risk for breast cancer is confusing to many patients. It often is incorrectly assumed that any family history of cancer automatically infers a higher risk of developing the disease. In a subgroup of families, however, this is indeed the case, but for many women, the presence of one or two relatives with breast cancer does not contribute to a substantially increased risk. Breast cancer is a common malignancy in women; consequently, it is plausible that a woman may have one or two relatives with the diagnosis, especially if the age at onset was older. Assessment of the family history is important primarily to determine who may have a genetic predisposition for developing breast and/or other cancers. These family members should be offered information on the risks and benefits associated with genetic testing.

Traditionally, risk has been assessed for an individual. Because families share a pool of genes, they also share similar risks for inheriting a predisposition to a particular cancer. Genetic risk assessment, therefore, must include not only individuals but also entire families. Genetic testing is one of the tools used in the cancer risk assessment process to accurately quantify risk.

Approximately 10% of all cases of breast cancer are related to a hereditary predisposition. This predisposition usually results from the inheritance of a single germ-line mutation, which is usually autosomal dominant. Most commonly this is a mutation in *BRCA1* or *BRCA2*, for which commercial testing is available. Other genetic syndromes associated with a family history of breast cancer are shown in Table 2-3. Given the high incidence of breast cancer, even a seemingly small incidence of 10% potentially translates into a large number of affected patients.

The prevalence of deleterious *BRCA1* mutations is estimated to be 1 in 800 in the general population. Several mutations in *BRCA1* and *BRCA2* have been observed to occur with a higher frequency among individuals of Ashkenazi Jewish descent. These mutations include 185delAG and 5382insC for *BRCA1* and 6174delT for *BRCA2* (Frank et al., 1998).

BRCA1 and *BRCA2* are tumor suppressor genes. These genes are normally present in every human and function to suppress tumor cell growth. The presence of a germ-line mutation in either *BRCA1* or *BRCA2* renders an individual significantly more likely than others in the general population to develop breast and/or ovarian cancer. These are autosomal dominant genes, so each first-degree relative has a statistical

Table 2-3. Common Hereditary Breast Cancer Syndromes		
Syndrome/ Incidence	Gene	Common Features
Breast-ovarian cancer syndrome 1 in 800–2,500	*BRCA1* at 17q21 *BRCA2* at 13q21 Autosomal dominant 85% penetrant	• Premenopausal breast cancer • Multiple generations with multiple relatives • Family history of ovarian cancer
Li-Fraumeni syndrome Very rare	*TP53* at 17p13.1 Autosomal dominant 90% penetrant	• Premenopausal breast cancer • Uterine sarcomas • Childhood sarcoma, brain tumor, leukemia, and adrenocortical carcinoma
Cowden syndrome 1 in 200,000– 250,000 in Dutch population	*PTEN* at 10q23 Autosomal dominant 50% penetrant	• Excess of breast, gastrointestinal, and thyroid disease, both benign and malignant • Skin manifestations including multiple trichilemmomas, oral fibromas, and acral, palmar, and plantar keratoses
Ataxia telangiectasia 1 in 30,000– 100,000	*ATM* at 11q22.3 Autosomal recessive Almost 100% penetrant	• Characterized by neurologic deterioration, telangiectasias, immunodeficiency states, and hypersensitivity to ionizing radiation • Increased risk of hematologic and breast cancers
Peutz-Jeghers syndrome 1 in 120,000	*STK11* at 19p13.3 Autosomal dominant 50% penetrant	• Characterized by melanocytic macules on the lips, perioral, and buccal regions • Multiple gastrointestinal polyps • Multiple cases of breast, colon, pancreatic, stomach, and ovarian cancers

Note. Based on information from Schneider, 2002.

50% chance of inheriting the mutation and the associated cancer risk.

Current estimates suggest that *BRCA1* and *BRCA2* mutation carriers have up to an 82% lifetime risk of developing at least one breast cancer and approximately a 30%–50% risk of developing ovarian cancer (Frank et al., 2002; King, Marks, Mandell, & New York Breast Cancer Study, 2003). Approximately half of the women with a *BRCA1* or *BRCA2* mutation develop breast cancer by age 50.

Certain features of a family history should raise suspicion that a hereditary breast cancer syndrome may be present (see Figure 2-1). It is usually best to begin a hereditary assessment by constructing a family tree or pedigree as shown in Figure 2-2. A pedigree should include the ages and causes of death for three generations. Paternal and maternal sides should both be assessed and recorded, as most hereditary susceptibility genes are located on autosomes and can be passed with equal frequency from either side. For family members diagnosed with cancer, the pedigree also should include the type of primary cancer(s) and age(s) at diagnosis. In many cases, patients may be unsure of the accuracy of the information, and ideally, they should use pathology reports, medical records, and/or death certificates to confirm information about cancers. Once such records are collected, the family history often appears very different, and this ultimately may change recommendations regarding testing. For example, when considering testing for *BRCA1* and *BRCA2* in a family, a reported case of ovarian cancer that is later confirmed by report to be cervical cancer might greatly alter the risk assessment. Family members

can find this process extremely stressful. An accurate family history also can be challenging to collect if records are lost or if there is a small family size, underlying emotional or psychiatric problems, or cultural or family taboos regarding discussing cancer (Sadler, Wasserman, Fullerton, & Romero, 2004). Nurses need to educate patients on the importance of this activity and encourage them to collect the data. Figure 2-3 describes limitations of pedigree assessment.

Ethnic background also is a consideration when deciding whether testing may be appropriate, and this information may alter testing strategies. More than 2% of Ashkenazi Jews are estimated to carry *BRCA1* and *BRCA2* mutations associated with increased risk for breast, ovarian, and prostate cancers (Struewing et al., 1997). This results from a phenomenon referred to as a *founder effect,* when a population has descended from a relatively small number of people without other groups.

Interpreting family trees is further complicated by the concept of penetrance. Not everyone with a mutation will go on to develop the cancer(s). Mutations in *BRCA1* and *BRCA2* are about 85% penetrant, meaning that approximately 85% of the women with the mutation will go on to develop breast cancer by age 70 (Lynch, Snyder, Lynch, Riley, & Rubinstein, 2003). Sometimes a family will have members who have the mutation but for whatever reason have not gone on to develop the cancer. This makes evaluation of family histories challenging.

Figure 2-1. Key Indicators of Hereditary Breast-Ovarian Cancer

- Several relatives with breast and/or ovarian cancer. In general, the pedigree will show two or more first-degree relatives who have developed the same or related cancers.
- Cancers are diagnosed at an age that is younger than seen in the general population. Often this is 10–15 years earlier than if it were a sporadic cancer. This is especially true with breast cancer before the age of 40 and ovarian cancer before the age of 60.
- A pattern of autosomal dominant transmission is evident. Usually the cancer is seen in more than one generation, and there is evidence of vertical transmission. First-degree relatives have a 50% statistical chance of developing the cancer.
- Unique tumor site combinations may be present. Individuals with a mutation in one of the *BRCA* genes may have a history of breast and ovarian cancers.
- An excess of multifocal or bilateral cancers may exist. This can include more than one cancer in the same organ or cancers that occur in both paired organs, for example, bilateral breast cancer.
- There can be an excess of multiple primary tumors. After successful treatment of one cancer, individuals from these families might go on to develop a completely new cancer, such as ovarian cancer after breast cancer.
- The family is of an Ashkenazi Jewish background.
- A history of male breast cancer exists in the family.
- The lifestyle history excludes a history of environmental risk factors.
- There is a confirmed *BRCA1/2* or other known mutation associated with breast cancer.

Figure 2-2. Three-Generation Pedigree of a Family at Risk for Developing Breast and/or Ovarian Cancer

This is a typical pedigree constructed with the purpose of visually portraying hereditary risk of developing breast and/or ovarian cancer. The arrow indicates the proband or the member initiating inquiry about risk. Circles represent women, and squares represent men. Three generations are recorded. Current age or age at death is listed. A slash indicates a deceased family member. Cancer diagnoses and age at diagnosis are listed. This pedigree also illustrates how a male can pass the mutation on to a female because the mutation is on an autosome, not a sex chromosome.

BRCA1-2 Hereditary Breast Cancer

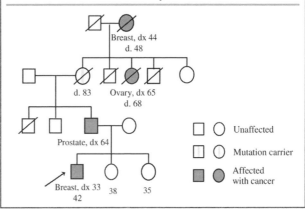

Figure 2-3. Limitations of Pedigree Assessment

- Most hereditary cancer syndromes have incomplete penetrance. In most families, there are carriers of the mutation who have lived to older ages without development of cancer.
- Family histories often are incomplete or inaccurate. Families may have inaccurate information, or family dynamics may lead to incomplete information because family members are unable or unwilling to communicate with each other.
- Sometimes family members who have the mutation may have died early from other causes such as accidents, infections, or other unexpected deaths.
- There may be false paternity. This creates challenges when counseling family members about the pedigree. The same conflicts arise if an individual learns he or she is adopted. Adoptees may have difficulty obtaining family records.
- There may be a phenocopy in the family. This means that a person develops a sporadic cancer that is the same as the cancer for which the family has hereditary risk. For example, two sisters are diagnosed with breast cancer in their mid-40s. One tests positive for a mutation, and one does not. The sister that tests negative is a phenocopy, meaning that on paper assessment, she appears to have genetic risk because she has early-onset breast cancer, but genetically, she did not inherit the mutation; rather, she developed a sporadic cancer.
- Medical records are sometimes destroyed or impossible to obtain, so an accurate pedigree cannot be constructed.
- The family may be very small or have only a small number of female relatives in the case of assessing breast/ovarian cancer risk. A statistical 50% chance of developing hereditary cancers may not be evident.
- Sometimes women who are mutation carriers may have already had prophylactic surgery, especially an oophorectomy, which might mask their risk or may have prevented them from developing the cancer.

Note. Based on information from Lynch et al., 2003.

The commercial availability of genetic testing for the cancer susceptibility genes associated with these hereditary breast-ovarian cancer syndromes has greatly changed oncology risk assessment practices. Cancer susceptibility genetic testing has the potential to identify whether a person is at increased risk for a particular cancer or cancers associated with a hereditary breast-ovarian cancer syndrome. These tests, however, cannot predict when, where, or if the individual will be diagnosed with the cancer. One of the challenges in the communication of genetic risk information and genetic test results is that probabilities and uncertainties surround genetic information. Benefits of cancer risk assessment are shown in Figure 2-4.

Genetic tests are relatively simple to order. The clinical challenge is to provide patients and their families with enough information regarding genetic testing so that they can make an informed decision that is best for their individual situation and consistent with their values. Whether a patient might benefit from predisposition genetic testing will depend on the patient's degree of genetic risk, whether testing is likely to address the patient's needs, the individual's motivation to actively engage in prevention strategies, and the availability of an appropriate cancer predisposition test. Because of the high cost of some genetic tests (approximately $3,200 for full sequencing of *BRCA1/2*), reimbursement factors may need to be considered. Most insurers cover some or all of the cost of genetic testing in patients who meet eligibility criteria set by the insurer. There may be additional costs for counseling and education. The final testing decision, however, will depend upon patients' understanding of the potential risks and benefits and whether they want to proceed.

Deciding who is the most appropriate candidate for cancer predisposition testing requires clinical judgment because of the complexity of the issues involved. Ideally, an affected family member will be the first one to be tested. In the case of testing for *BRCA1/2,* a woman who has been diagnosed with breast (particularly premenopausal) or ovarian cancer usually will be the most informative for the rest of the family. If an affected relative has been tested and found to carry a deleterious mutation known to be associated with increased cancer risk, then at-risk unaffected family members are likely to benefit from single-site testing for the same mutation (which is significantly less expensive, usually costing $375–$400).

Figure 2-4. Benefits of Breast Cancer Risk Assessments

- Provide women with informed consent so they can choose appropriate screening recommendations.
- Develop a plan for cancer screening and prevention that is consistent with the values and needs of the woman at risk.
- Provide an educational opportunity to instruct women on basic information about breast cancer, including incidence, mortality, survival trends, and signs and symptoms that merit immediate evaluation.
- Detect cancers at an early stage, when treatment is most likely to be effective and less drastic.
- Identify psychosocial concerns related to cancer risk, and provide appropriate support and encouragement.
- Identify families who might be at risk for a hereditary predisposition. If a mutation is identified in a family, predictive testing can be offered to other at-risk members. For those who test positive, a detailed and aggressive plan for cancer prevention and detection needs to be developed. For those who test negative for a known mutation in the family, recommendations for cancer screening and prevention should reflect those used in the general population. This strategy allows financial healthcare resources to be spent in a sound way.

Note. Based on information from Lynch et al., 2003; Mahon, 2003.

The Oncology Nursing Society (ONS, 2004) has issued a position statement outlining considerations for genetic testing. This statement emphasizes that risk assessment and genetic testing are components of comprehensive cancer care and that cancer predisposition genetic testing requires informed consent. Qualified healthcare professionals should provide pre- and post-test counseling and education.

When deciding whether to pursue cancer predisposition genetic testing, each patient and family member must weigh the options, risks, and benefits in light of one's own unique situation. The decision is a very personal one, and for each family member the issues will be different. Just because a person has a personal or family history putting him or her at increased risk for carrying a genetic mutation does not mean that the individual will want to know his or her genetic status. For other people, the uncertainty may be causing them great anxiety or interfering with their ability to make informed choices about their health. The physical risks of having a blood sample drawn are minimal. The real risks are associated with the psychological and psychosocial impact of knowing one's genetic status.

Pretest counseling may identify potential psychological problems. Patients found to carry a cancer susceptibility mutation may experience anxiety, depression, anger, and feelings of vulnerability or guilt about possibly having passed the mutation to children. Those found not to carry a mutation might experience guilt known as survivor's guilt, especially if close family members are found to carry the mutation. Psychological issues to be considered also include fear of cancer or medical procedures, past negative experiences with cancer, unresolved feelings of loss and sorrow, feelings of guilt about passing on a mutation to children, anxiety about learning test results, and concern about the effect of results on other family members. Some families may need information on how to access additional support services such as counseling, social work, or support groups.

The informed consent process for predisposition genetic testing must include both educational and decision-making components. Components of informed consent for genetic testing include risks, benefits, cost, accuracy, and purpose of the specific genetic test being ordered; alternatives to genetic testing; implications of a positive, negative, or uncertain test result; how results will be communicated; psychosocial implications; confidentiality issues; and options for medical surveillance and risk reduction for both positive and negative results.

Results of cancer predisposition genetic tests generally fall into several categories, including positive, negative, and indeterminate. It is critical that individuals understand the issues associated with predisposition genetic testing along with all the potential testing outcomes prior to initiating the testing process.

Positive Test Result

A positive result for a *BRCA1* or *BRCA2* mutation is associated with an increased risk for developing both breast and ovarian cancers. If the patient has already been diagnosed with cancer, a positive test result can have implications for the individual's risk of developing a second primary cancer or a cancer recurrence associated with that mutation.

Negative Test Result

A negative test result can occur in two situations. The first is where a known mutation exists in the family and the patient has been tested specifically for that same mutation. The second situation is when no known mutation exists in the family and the patient is tested for one or more mutations associated with increased cancer risk.

Ideally, a person who has been diagnosed with cancer is tested first. If a mutation is identified, subsequent family members can be tested for the same mutation. When a known mutation is identified in the family and an unaffected (no cancer diagnosis) person tests negative, his or her risk of developing cancer approaches the risk of the general population. The patient's cancer risk still may be increased, however, because of nonhereditary cancer risk factors related to lifestyle, diet, environment, or carcinogen exposure.

In a patient without a cancer diagnosis with no known mutation in the family, several possible interpretations of a negative test result exist. The first possibility is that the cancer in the family is caused by a known mutation for which the patient was tested and did not inherit (true negative result). A second possibility is that the cancer in the family is due to a different gene mutation for which the patient was not tested. A third possibility is that the cancer in the family is caused by environmental or other nonhereditary risk factors. Because it is not possible to know which outcome is true for the patient, it is recommended to first test a blood relative who has been diagnosed with cancer for a mutation known to be associated with that type of cancer. The rationale is that if there is a mutation in the family, it will most likely be found in a family member already diagnosed with cancer. If a mutation is found in an affected family member, then the unaffected family members can be tested for that specific mutation. If a mutation is not found, the family still may be at risk and may want to consider more aggressive screening measures and participation in a research study.

Variation of Uncertain Significance

A variation of uncertain significance is when the genetic test indicates that a change in the gene was found, but the cancer risk associated with that change is not yet known. This can occur when a new mutation or variant is found or if the variant is uncommon and not enough information is available to determine whether the variant is a deleterious mutation (associated with an increased cancer risk) or a harmless variant. Some genes, such as *BRCA1* and *BRCA2,* are very large genes with hundreds of known deleterious mutations. Not all gene changes or variants are deleterious, however, and it is possible for a gene change to be present that does not interfere with protein function and, therefore, does not increase cancer risk.

Patients with this result will need to be informed that the significance of the mutation found is not yet known. These patients may experience disappointment, anxiety, anger, or depression because the test result did not provide the information they expected. They also may feel confused and uncertain about how to make healthcare decisions regarding cancer surveillance. Until a number of families with the same mutation have been studied, it is impossible to know if an increased cancer risk may be associated with the mutation found. This can be a difficult situation for some patients because of the uncertainty. It may be helpful to test more family members to find out whether the mutation is found only in the affected individuals, but this may not necessarily give concrete answers. Another option is to encourage patients to become part of a research study or confidential registry for people who carry genetic variants in hopes that more information about the particular variant will be known as more people are tested. These patients need to be informed that, as more information about specific variants becomes available, it may be possible to determine whether the particular variant for which they tested positive is deleterious or not. Decisions about cancer surveillance, early detection, and risk reduction are based on patients' personal and family history of cancer and nonhereditary cancer risk factors.

Confidentiality of Genetic Information

Given the sensitivity of genetic information, patients need to know that their genetic information will not be released to any third party without their specific written informed consent. When a healthcare provider refers patients to a cancer genetics program for predisposition genetic testing, patients must sign a written consent form before cancer genetic counseling and predisposition testing information can be released to their healthcare provider. If patients have a positive genetic test result and choose not to release their cancer predisposition test results to their healthcare provider, it may be difficult for the healthcare provider to order appropriate cancer screening tests, offer chemoprevention or prophylactic surgery, and provide appropriate clinical examinations.

The genetic counseling process often involves obtaining medical records on the patient from one or more sources, as well as medical records on one or more family members. The presence of these records in the patient's medical chart creates an additional responsibility in relation to maintaining the confidentiality of information about the patient as well as other family members. When a patient's medical record contains secondary records (i.e., medical records on a family member or patient records from another institution), these records should not be released to a third party, even with written informed consent from the patient. The third party needs to go to the original source to obtain those records. This is especially important now that the Health Insurance Portability and Accountability Act privacy rules have been enacted.

Confidentiality is necessary to protect patients from genetic discrimination. Genetic discrimination occurs when individuals experience workplace or insurance discrimination based on information about their genetic makeup. Patients found to have a positive genetic test are at risk for genetic discrimination based solely on their genetic makeup. Individuals who are asymptomatic but have a positive predisposition genetic test are at the greatest risk for genetic discrimination. Patients should be informed of the risks of discussing their genetic history in the workplace. They also may want to consider purchasing additional life insurance before testing to prevent higher premiums resulting because of a known genetic predisposition.

Challenges in Risk Communication

After completion of the breast cancer risk assessment, the next challenge for healthcare providers is to communicate the risk assessment to women who may be anxious or concerned about their risk for developing breast cancer. This anxiety often affects patients' ability to completely grasp and comprehend the meaning of the assessment and their actual risk. Nurses providing breast cancer risk assessment services need to interpret the assessment so that women can make informed and appropriate choices for prevention and early detection. Central to this communication is selecting an appropriate risk-prediction model.

Selecting a Prediction Model

Several factors influence the selection of a risk-prediction model. Different methods may be appropriate in different settings (Armstrong, Eisen, & Weber, 2000). Simply considering the patient's age may be sufficient for a woman 40–49 years of age to decide about using the screening tool of mammography. Conversely, simply using the patient's age to determine whether tamoxifen may be effective in reducing breast cancer risk in a 45-year-old woman is probably inappropriate, because chemoprevention is best used in those with a moderate to high risk of developing a breast cancer. Furthermore, decisions about whether to undergo a prophylactic surgical procedure are best made after genetic testing. Prophylactic surgery involves too many physical and psychological risks to be used with those of average or moderate risk for developing cancer (Vogel, 2000). It is reserved only for those with a high risk that is probably best identified through genetic testing. Clearly, clinicians need to consider which risk-prediction model they should use and whether it is appropriate to provide guidance for selecting a screening or prevention measure or offering genetic testing.

In general, models for prediction of breast cancer risk focus on two separate types of risk. The first type of risk information generally offered to patients describes their chance of developing breast cancer. Often this information is presented as an estimated chance of developing breast cancer both in the next five years and over their lifetime. Stopfer (2000) emphasizes that patients must be informed of the imprecision of these cancer risk assessment models because risk models may not always be able to capture all salient features of family history or incorporate a significant risk factor. Furthermore, the significance and interaction of all risk factors in the subsequent development of cancer is not known. The Gail and Claus models typically are used to describe an individual woman's risk of developing breast cancer (see Table 2-4).

The second type of risk information usually is given to those with a family history that suggests hereditary suscepti-

bility and is an estimate of the chance that an individual carries a mutation in a particular cancer susceptibility gene (see Table 2-4). Sometimes this is referred to as the *prior probability* of carrying a gene mutation (Stopfer, 2000). Calculating and interpreting this risk figure is important for those who desire genetic testing. Generally, offering genetic testing is appropriate if at least a 10% prior probability exists for detecting a mutation in a cancer susceptibility gene and the presence of such a mutation ultimately will have an impact on prevention and treatment decisions.

Selection of a proper model is further complicated by genetic heterogeneity (see Table 2-3). Both *BRCA1* and *BRCA2* mutations are associated with hereditary breast and ovarian cancer. Hereditary breast cancer also may be the primary

Table 2-4. Risk Models for Hereditary Breast and Ovarian Cancer

Model	Reference	Indications	Strengths	Limitations
Gail model	Gail et al., 1989	• Estimates breast cancer risk • Most effectively used in women with a limited to moderate family history of breast cancer • Often used to determine whether the patient should be enrolled in a chemoprevention trial or treatment	• Readily available to use on computers and handheld devices • Inexpensive and simple to use • Considers previous biopsies • Considers previous pregnancies	• Does not consider personal or family history of ovarian cancer • Does not consider the age at which other relatives were diagnosed (the model does not take into account the impact of early-onset breast cancer in the family) • Does not consider paternal side of family with a diagnosis of breast and/or ovarian cancer • Does not consider second-degree relatives with a diagnosis of breast and/or ovarian cancer • Has not been used extensively with many ethnic minorities and may have limited usefulness
Claus model	Claus et al., 1994, 1996	• Provides age-specific estimates for the risk of developing breast cancer • Most effectively used in women with a significant family history of breast cancer	• Considers the age at diagnosis of breast cancer • Considers both maternal and paternal family history • Calculates risk in 10-year increments, which is helpful to younger women or when trying to keep risk in perspective	• Does not consider ethnicity • Does not consider ovarian cancer history • Might significantly underestimate risk in people with a *BRCA1/2* mutation
Couch model	Couch et al., 1997	• Estimates the chance of carrying a *BRCA1* mutation • Most effectively used in women with a family history of multiple cases of breast cancer, especially early-onset breast cancer	• Considers the average age of onset of breast cancer in the family • Takes ethnicity factors into consideration	• Predicts *BRCA1* mutations only • Reported to be less sensitive in small families

(Continued on next page)

Table 2-4. Risk Models for Hereditary Breast and Ovarian Cancer *(Continued)*				
Model	**Reference**	**Indications**	**Strengths**	**Limitations**
Shattuck-Eidens model	Shattuck-Eidens et al., 1997	• Estimates the chance of carrying a *BRCA1* mutation • Most effectively used in women with a family history of multiple cases of breast cancer, especially early-onset breast cancer	• Considers the age of onset of breast cancer in family • Considers both first- and second-degree relatives • Considers breast and ovarian cancer history • Considers the significance of Ashkenazi Jewish background	• Predicts *BRCA1* mutations only • Limited data in ethnic minority groups
Berry model (Duke model, BRCAPRO model)	Berry et al., 1997, 2002	• Calculates the chance of having a *BRCA1* or *BRCA2* mutation	• Considers the age of onset of breast cancer in family • Considers both first- and second-degree relatives • Considers breast and ovarian cancer history	• Readily available in the BRCAPRO computer program • Limited data in some minority groups
Frank model (Myriad II model)	Frank et al., 1998	• Calculates the chance of having a *BRCA1* or *BRCA2* mutation • Most effectively used in women with breast cancer diagnosed before the age of 50	• Considers the age of onset of breast cancer in family • Considers both first- and second-degree relatives • Considers breast and ovarian cancer history	• Most useful in premenopausal women • Less useful in small families • Limited data available in some minority groups • Readily available in the BRCAPRO computer program

manifestation of Cowden disease or Li-Fraumeni syndrome because of mutations in the *PTEN* gene or the *TP53* gene. Knowledge about differentiating clinical features is important for identifying the correct syndrome and highlights the need for both physical examination and a thorough family history prior to interpreting the risk assessment and possibly selecting a genetic test to order (Weitzel, 1999).

As Stopfer (2000) noted, these models sometimes can produce inconsistent risk assessments for the same individual. This is seen in Table 2-5, in which the same woman has a 29%–48% likelihood of carrying a mutation depending on the model used. Each model is based on unique combinations of information. This can be a source of confusion for both patients and health professionals. Those using risk-assessment models need to explain to patients why they are using a particular risk assessment and what it means. They also should distinguish between risk models that calculate a patient's chances for developing a particular cancer(s) and those that assess one's risk of carrying a specific mutation. Because multiple models are used, families often receive conflicting information, which can lead to increased stress and confusion. Some recommend using one model consistently and explaining its inherent strengths and weaknesses; others recommend using multiple models to give a range of risk (Rosser, Hurst, & Chapman, 1996).

Communication of cancer risk also is challenging because it includes both a quantitative and qualitative component (Fischhoff, 1999). The quantitative component usually is more straightforward. It typically involves risk figures such as abso-

lute or relative risk or the probability of having a mutation in a cancer susceptibility gene. Numeric data can be presented to patients and families. Some individuals have a greater capacity than others to comprehend the meaning of numeric data. Fischhoff stated that qualitative information should follow the presentation of quantitative data. This includes a discussion of what the quantitative data specifically means for the patient. Many experts in risk communication believe that all discussions of risk should include both a qualitative and quantitative component (Rothman & Kiviniemi, 1999).

Risk factors do not necessarily increase in a simple mathematical fashion. For example, if one risk factor gives a woman a 14% risk of developing breast cancer and another gives the woman a 16% risk, the two numbers cannot be assumed to mean the woman now has a 30% chance of developing breast cancer. The interaction of risk factors is complicated. Breast cancer is a multifactorial disease that has many causes that interact in ways that are not fully understood. Furthermore, some researchers have estimated that 70% of breast cancers occur in women without any of the classic risk factors for it (Madigan, Ziegler, Benichou, Byrne, & Hoover, 1995). Healthcare professionals must be aware of the strengths and limitations of risk factors and communicate all of these considerations to patients.

Consideration also must be given to an individual's ability to understand risk assessment. Some groups of patients may be more likely to seek information about cancer risk assessment. This may be related to a variety of factors, including educational level and the ability to understand complex technical

Table 2-5. Variations in Risk of Carrying a *BRCA* Mutation Using Different Models for the Same Woman of Ashkenazi Jewish Background	
Model	**Predicted Risk**
Couch	0.286
Shattuck-Eidens	0.396
Berry	0.479
Frank	0.306

Note. Pedigree includes 14 family members (3 with premenopausal breast cancer, 1 with ovarian cancer, and 1 with both breast and ovarian cancers).

concepts. Communication of risk information should be given according to how much the patient or family wishes to know (Hopwood, 2005). Timing also may be important. Messages suggesting increased susceptibility to breast cancer may be less effective if delivered too soon after the breast cancer diagnosis of a close relative, but they might be appropriate several months after the diagnosis (Rimer, Schildkraut, Lerman, Lin, & Audrain, 1996).

Many factors influence the perception of risk. All individuals have their own perception of risk, and it often is difficult to determine which risks they deem acceptable and which risks are not acceptable. For some, personal beliefs and perceptions of risk are so strong that they prevent many individuals from going on to adopt healthy behaviors (Rodgers, 1999).

Many women with a family history of breast cancer incorrectly assume that it is not an issue of whether they will be diagnosed with breast cancer, but when they will be diagnosed. Kelly (2000) stated that as women approach the age at which their mothers were diagnosed with breast cancer, their anxiety often increases. As they pass that age, they may begin to feel their risk is sufficiently different and believe they might not get breast cancer after all. Unfortunately, some may become overconfident and then fail to get adequate screening. Critical to the process of cancer risk assessment is determining a person's beliefs about cancer. All people have beliefs about cancer. Some fit with current scientific findings, and others do not. Health professionals must have an understanding of these beliefs because they will influence what information is understood and how it is interpreted in the risk assessment.

A great deal of information can be obtained by listening carefully to people describe their past experiences with cancer. Individuals may realize intellectually that improved treatments are now available but continue to remember, and dread, the disease as experienced by a friend or relative. For example, a woman whose mother was treated with a Halsted radical mastectomy may fear the same treatment for herself and consequently ignore a breast lump, despite the availability of more cosmetically acceptable forms of treatment. Such fears need to be assessed in order to correct misconceptions.

In addition to understanding patients' perceptions of the disease, it is important to determine their assessment of their own personal risk for a particular cancer. This information can elucidate the patient's level of concern related to developing cancer. In some cases, an individual may have an actual numeric risk in mind. It is also important to understand whether the patient is considering absolute or relative risk. In some cases, people tend to underestimate their risk, which is termed *optimistic bias*. In cancer risk assessment, the opposite phenomenon also occurs, which is known as *pessimistic bias*. Those with pessimistic bias often will suffer unnecessary anxiety and concern. These biases may occur because people have inaccurate information or are unable to comprehend complex technical information, or the preconceptions may reflect a psychologically protective coping mechanism.

The Challenge of Uncertainty

Uncertainty exists regarding recommended prevention and detection strategies. This may be the most serious limitation of risk assessment and genetic testing (Kash et al., 2000). No screening strategy is completely effective in detecting cancer early. The sensitivity and specificity of screening tests are widely variable. Furthermore, many of the prophylactic measures, and sometimes the chemoprevention recommendations, are not based on firm, scientific knowledge. Often the data are extrapolated from other studies and information. This means that the certainty with which recommendations can be made often is limited at best.

Testing for genetic predisposition provides information about risk, but much uncertainty still exists for most patients (Bottorff, Ratner, Johnson, Lovato, & Joab, 1998). For those who test negative, the risk is not completely eliminated. These people still carry the same probability or risk of developing a sporadic cancer as those in the general population. For those who undergo testing that shows they have a change of indeterminate significance, the uncertainty is very large. These individuals have not gained any new or helpful information from the genetic testing process.

Variable penetrance is another feature of uncertainty that must be addressed in cancer genetics counseling (Cornelisse & Devilee, 1997). Penetrance can change with age and specific mutation and may vary considerably among different families. Additional genetic factors likely are associated with different mutations that modify the risks of gene carriers. To date, these additional factors are largely unknown. Thus, patients who test positive trade the uncertainty of not knowing if they really are at significant risk for developing a malignancy for the uncertainty of when (if at all, in some cases) and what type of cancer will develop.

Techniques for Communicating Breast Cancer Risk Assessments

Those who communicate cancer risk assessments to patients must be aware of the patients' perceptions of risk and remind them of the fundamental purposes for conducting a risk assessment, which include determining appropriate cancer prevention strategies when known and developing a reasonable schedule for cancer screening. Communication of the risk information should begin by reminding patients of the strengths and limitations as well as the purpose of a cancer risk assessment. In most cases, the next step is to provide basic information about the cancer for which the person is at risk (e.g., number of people affected annually, average age at diagnosis, clinical presentation). A review of basic anatomy and physiology using diagrams and models may be indicated to provide necessary background information. Information about the general population can serve as a baseline against which individuals can measure the magnitude of their increased risk. Adequate opportunity for patients to ask questions and express concerns must be provided to make the cancer risk assessment process effective and the interview truly informative. Depending on the magnitude of the risk and the ability and desire of the patient to understand the content, the discussion can be expanded to include a more detailed conversation about absolute or relative risk (perhaps including information such as that found in Tables 2-1 and 2-2). Care should be given to distinguish between absolute and relative risk and to reinforce the fact that risk factors do not combine in a simple mathematical fashion.

After the data for risk assessment are collected, one must choose the best method to communicate the assessment. Risk can be presented as a numeric risk, a statistical comparison to an average or anchor risk, given as a risk category (low, average, or high), expressed in qualitative terms (e.g., telling a patient she is more likely to develop this disease than a person who does not smoke), or using graphical or pictorial presentations. The numeric results of a quantitative risk assessment can appear to be highly scientific (such as an absolute or relative risk figure) and difficult for many patients to understand. Conversely, using verbal terms such as high or low risk can be equally confusing. A high risk to one woman might mean a 100% chance of developing breast cancer, whereas for another, it may mean a 25% chance.

The manner in which the information is communicated (sometimes referred to as *framing*) is also important (Salovey, Schneider, & Apanovitch, 1999). If material is presented in a negative fashion, patients may assume the risk is more than it actually is. If the discussion is too positive, patients may underestimate or minimize the magnitude of risk. Framing also occurs with statistics. If an individual is told that he has a chance of a particular occurrence of 1.3 in 10,000 compared to the general population's chance of 1 in 10,000, it is not particularly impressive to most individuals. If the same risk

is communicated using the format that the individual has a 30% greater risk than the general population, the situation is likely to be seen as "riskier," even though the two situations are equivalent (Bottorff et al., 1998). Clearly, this is the most challenging aspect of cancer risk assessment communication. The goal is to not frighten a patient unnecessarily; however, if the risk is minimized too much, the patient may not see the value in recommended cancer prevention and screening activities. Information about lifestyle factors amenable to change (attributable risk) should be discussed. For example, women with a strong family history of breast cancer may need to weigh the benefits and risks of taking OCs or HRT. A discussion of these risks is critical so that the patient can make an informed decision about what may be the best action in her individual situation.

Patients also should receive information about the strengths and limitations of screening tools, including information about the recommended time interval for using each tool. For most patients, the standard recommendations endorsed by an organization such as ACS (2007) will be appropriate (see Figure 2-5). People with significantly higher risk may need more aggressive screening and should understand the rationale, strengths, and limitations of such a schedule, as well as the strengths and limitations associated with chemoprevention agents and prophylactic surgery. Signs and symptoms that require immediate attention also should be discussed.

Figure 2-5. American Cancer Society Recommendations* for the Early Detection of Breast Cancer

- Yearly mammography beginning at age 40 is recommended. The age at which to stop mammography should be individualized based on the potential risks and benefits of screening in light of the overall health of the woman.
- A clinical breast examination is recommended about every three years for women in their 20s and 30s and annually for women age 40 and older.
- Breast self-examination is an option for women to consider on a monthly basis beginning in their 20s.

*These recommendations are for asymptomatic women without significant risk or hereditary risk for developing breast cancer.

Note. Based on information from American Cancer Society, 2007.

Role of Visual Aids in the Communication of Risk Data

Graphics can be a very effective means to communicate risk. They can be especially effective in communicating numeric risk (Lipkus & Hollands, 1999). Graphics often can reveal data patterns that may otherwise go undetected. Graphs also hold people's attention for longer periods of time, which might increase the understanding of data. To be useful, graphs must communicate the magnitude of risk, relative risk, cumulative risk, uncertainty, and interactions among risk factors. Despite the popularity of using graphics, little research exists on the impact of graphics in communicating risk data. In many cases, a combination of different formats is used to present risk, including numeric, visual, and explanatory (Press, Fishman, & Koenig, 2000). Graphs should decrease the number of mathematical computations that the user must make.

Often, a risk ladder is used to describe and display a range of risk magnitudes by showing increasing risks portrayed higher up on the ladder (see Table 2-6). Perceptions of risk are influenced by the location on the ladder. The ladder helps people to anchor their risk to upper and lower reference points.

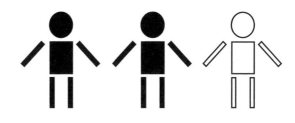

Figure 2-6. Stick Figures to Communicate Risk

One in three Americans will develop cancer over the course of a lifetime. The white figure represents the one American who will develop cancer.

Table 2-6. Risk Ladder for Having a *BRCA* Mutation Based on Family History in a 48-Year-Old Woman With a Personal History of Breast Cancer Diagnosed at Age 45	
Risk Variable	**Percentage**
Breast cancer and ovarian cancer in one relative younger than age 50	40.7%
Breast cancer in more than one relative younger than age 50	30.7%
Ovarian cancer in more than one relative	27.3%
Ovarian cancer in one relative	17.6%
Breast cancer in one relative younger than age 50	16.3%
No family history	6.9%

This figure demonstrates lower and upper percentages of risk based on family history. Women can use this graphic to visually anchor where their personal risk falls.

Note. Based on information from Myriad Genetic Laboratories, Inc., 2005.

Figure 2-7. Using Line Graphs in Cancer Risk Communication

Line graphs often are useful to illustrate trends over time, such as mammography use.

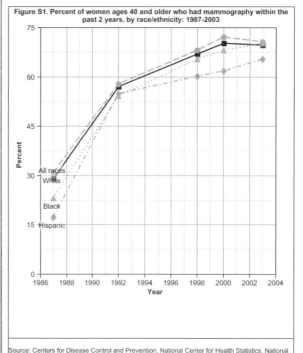

Note. From *Cancer Trends Progress Report—2005 Update,* by the National Cancer Institute, National Institutes of Health, Department of Health and Human Services, 2005, Bethesda, MD: Author. Retrieved May 11, 2006, from http://progressreport .cancer.gov

In addition, stick figures frequently are used to communicate relative risk. They also are used to illustrate how many people out of a certain number may go on to develop a particular disease (see Figure 2-6). When a small number of figures are used, patients often perceive the risk to be higher (Lipkus & Hollands, 1999). If the number of figures is increased, the impact may not be as strong.

Line graphs are effective for communicating trends and changes in data (see Figure 2-7). They are commonly used to show changes in incidence or mortality over time. Pie charts are commonly used to effectively communicate information about proportions (see Figure 2-8). Most individuals are able to understand line graphs and pie charts. Pie charts may be combined to explain subcategories of data.

Histograms or bar graphs also are commonly used (see Figure 2-9). Most individuals have some understanding of

how to read a simple histogram. Lipkus and Hollands (1999) stated that histograms often will convey the magnitude of the risk more clearly than just using numbers.

Figure 2-8. Using Pie Charts to Communicate Risk Data

This pie chart demonstrates a useful way to communicate proportions of the population affected by hereditary predisposition to developing breast cancer. The inset chart represents the proportions represented by specific mutations.

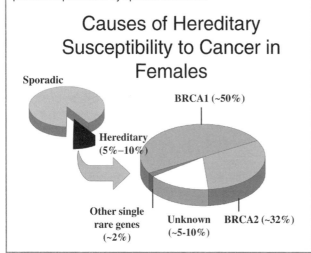

Causes of Hereditary Susceptibility to Cancer in Females

Sporadic

Hereditary (5%–10%)

BRCA1 (~50%)

Other single rare genes (~2%)

Unknown (~5-10%)

BRCA2 (~32%)

Note. Based on information from Frank et al., 2002.

Figure 2-9. Using a Bar Chart to Communicate Breast Cancer Risk

This bar chart is a convenient way to compare the incidence of breast cancer in women with and without a *BRCA1/2* mutation.

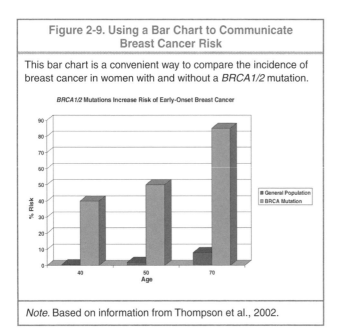

BRCA1/2 Mutations Increase Risk of Early-Onset Breast Cancer

■ General Population
■ BRCA Mutation

% Risk

Age

Note. Based on information from Thompson et al., 2002.

Ethical Concerns

A number of ethical concerns and principles should be considered in communicating a risk assessment. Healthcare professionals communicating risk assessments have an obligation to honestly disclose any biases or concerns related to the risk assessment.

One concept involved in cancer risk assessment is *autonomy,* which implies that each individual has the right to choose his or her own course. In relation to cancer screening, patients need information to make appropriate choices about lifestyle habits and screening behaviors, and these decisions can be made only after receiving a realistic and accurate assessment of risk.

The concept of *beneficence* applies to the obligation to inform individuals of a real health risk. The principle of *nonmaleficence* applies to the obligation to not hide, cover up, or otherwise fail to communicate risk information. In the case of cancer risk assessment, information should not be over-interpreted to create a climate of fear or anxiety regarding nonexistent risks. Patients must accurately understand their risk for developing a particular cancer, the potential consequences of not changing a particular behavior or having a particular screening test done, and the strengths and limitations of screening tests. Beneficence also applies to families with a known predisposition mutation and the manner in which other potentially at-risk members are informed of their risk.

Those who communicate a risk assessment also have an obligation to convey as clearly as possible any biases or assumptions that have been made in constructing the risk assessment. For example, a risk assessment may be less accurate if a woman reports that a first-degree relative had breast surgery and it is assumed it was for malignancy when, in reality, it was for a benign cyst. The person conveying the risk information is obligated to explain that the risk would be higher if the surgery was for a malignancy, but if the surgery was for a cyst, it means little in terms of the patient's risk of eventually developing breast cancer. One of the most challenging points can be deciding when a risk is significant and therefore should be communicated.

Accurate assessment is very important when explaining risk issues to a family with an apparent genetic predisposition to cancer. These family members need to understand why their risk is elevated, what preventive means are available, the strengths and limitations of available standard screening tests, and what is involved in genetic testing. To make an informed decision about genetic testing for breast cancer susceptibility, a number of points must be communicated to and comprehended by potential patients. Each family member is autonomous and has the right to make an individual decision regarding genetic testing. Healthcare professionals who obtain a family history suggestive of a genetic susceptibility to developing cancer have an obligation to inform the individual and, if possible, other family members.

Psychological Concerns

Clearly, the overall impact of risk assessment on quality of life is poorly understood. Similarly, it is not clear why two women with similar risk factors for developing breast cancer who receive risk factor information in a similar format can respond so differently to the information.

Performing risk assessment and giving patients information about risk factors do not affect their risk of developing cancer. However, such information about risk may influence patients' choices regarding screening and may change the way in which some people think about themselves and their lives. A risk factor assessment can potentially improve patients' health care and ultimately their quality of life if it results in regular screenings and possibly the early detection of a malignancy or if a woman with a known *BRCA* mutation elects for a prophylactic mastectomy and oophorectomy. Conversely, if a person is distressed or upset by the information conveyed in a risk assessment, the individual may ignore recommendations for screening or may experience psychological harm and possibly increased morbidity if a malignancy is not detected early.

The psychosocial impact of risk factor communication has not received much attention (Lerman et al., 1995). Some degree of concern or anxiety about breast cancer might heighten a woman's vigilance and motivation to seek reassurance through repetitive breast screenings. Conversely, such notification may result in anxiety and cancer worries with a reduction in breast self-examination and regularly scheduled clinical breast examinations as well as reductions in the frequency of regular mammography. Of concern would be the potential for inappropriate decisions about the use of prophylactic mastectomy in women who overestimate their risk of breast cancer (Bilimoria & Morrow, 1995).

Long-term follow-up is essential after a patient's cancer risk is communicated and genetic testing is completed or declined. Early studies suggest that depression might occur 6–12 months after genetic risk counseling and testing is completed (Hopwood, 2005). As more people receive cancer risk genetics counseling, assurance needs to be made that long-term follow-up includes assessment for depression and other negative sequelae associated with accepting or declining the testing process.

Those who counsel about genetic testing and risk must be aware of underlying beliefs and psychological distress and how these motivate testing decisions. Several unique considerations exist in cancer genetics risk counseling. Unlike acquired cancer risk factors, such as a poor diet, lack of physical activity, or smoking, patients cannot alter their genetic risk for developing cancer. This can lead to a sense of fatalism (Croyle & Lerman, 1999). The risk assessments completed in a cancer genetics counseling session have implications for the entire family, not just one individual. Helping families to find the best way to share this information with other members is very challenging. Test findings can permanently alter relationships within families. Family communication can be distressing, and responses to testing information will vary. Not knowing what to say and upsetting relatives may be significant barriers to disclosure (Hopwood, 2005).

How long a person can retain information after counseling about cancer risk factors is unclear. Information about risk and recommended screening can be reinforced by sending patients a post-visit letter that summarizes the discussion of risk and recommendations for screening or other follow-up. Consideration must be given to how individuals will be retained in cancer screening programs and genetic counseling programs so that risk assessments can be updated, recommendations for screening can be modified if needed, and regular routine screening can be completed (see Figure 2-10).

Figure 2-10. Summary of Breast Cancer Risk Communication Considerations

Gather Information for the Risk Assessment
- Gather family history. This should include at least three generations, age at onset of cancer, and diagnoses.
- Confirm family history with pathology reports when possible.
- Assess reproductive history (age at menarche, age at first pregnancy, oral contraceptive use, hormone replacement therapy use, number of pregnancies, and age at menopause).
- Assess past history of breast biopsies (confirm with pathology report).
- Assess social risk factors (alcohol use, exercise patterns, dietary patterns).
- Assess what the patient's perceived risk of cancer is and how the perception was formed.

Construct the Risk Assessment
- Select a model to predict risk for the individual patient.
- When appropriate, select a model to predict patient's risk of carrying a mutation.

Communicate the Risk Assessment
- Include patient's absolute risk of developing breast cancer.
- Discuss the relative risk of developing breast cancer.
- Communicate the risk of carrying a mutation in families with a hereditary predisposition.
- Use graphics and written materials when possible.

Communicate Information About Cancer Prevention and Early Detection
- Discuss recommended strategies for cancer prevention, including strengths and limitations.
- Discuss recommended strategies for cancer detection, including strengths and limitations.
- Discuss signs and symptoms of malignancy that warrant immediate evaluation.
- Discuss prognosis of cancer when prevention and early detection strategies are implemented.
- Follow the office visit with a written letter summarizing the recommendations made in the office.

Address Psychosocial Concerns
- Provide an opportunity for the patient to describe any fears and concerns.
- Assess for depression, anxiety, or other signs that might suggest difficulty adjusting to the information. Refer the patient for further services when indicated.
- Provide guidance on discussing the risk assessment with family members, especially in the case of hereditary predisposition.

Long-Term Follow-Up
- Assess whether the patient is engaging in the recommended prevention and early detection strategies.
- Update family history and risk assessment. Revise recommendations as indicated.
- Assist patients with a hereditary risk in contacting and informing other family members who also may have hereditary risk.

Nursing Implications

Educational Issues

Risk assessment is the responsibility of many different healthcare professionals, including physicians, nurses, psychologists, and genetic counselors. Lerman et al. (1996) noted that formal and clinical education regarding risk assessment is limited in many professions. Education of healthcare professionals regarding the techniques and tasks of risk assessment is important because clinically, healthcare professionals make most of the recommendations for screening. Weitzel (1999) emphasized that many oncology professionals have learned about genetics through self-study and clinical practice. Although these professionals may understand oncology well, they may be less familiar with the principles of genetics. Knowledge of statistics also is critical.

Specific content regarding cancer risk assessment that should be incorporated into a curriculum includes basic epidemiologic concepts, specific types of risk (absolute and relative), risk factors for specific cancers and etiologic factors if known, basic statistics, information about cancer prevention and early detection measures, and counseling techniques.

Administrative Issues

Administrators who want to implement cancer risk assessments into a cancer screening program or other oncology programs need to consider a number of issues. First, they must look at the rationale for implementing such a program. If the institution is unable to provide the screening that will be recommended following a risk factor assessment (e.g., genetic testing), what arrangements will be made for patients who desire such services? Administrators cannot overlook the need to hire nursing or other personnel who have the expertise and skills needed to provide this essential and comprehensive service.

Clinical Considerations

At the clinical level, the delivery of cancer risk information takes time, and how people who provide such information should be reimbursed for their risk assessment and counseling services is unclear. Such charges may be bundled with other service charges such as mammography. Without adequate reimbursement, however, it may be more likely that risk assessment services will not be given adequate attention or will be provided by people with insufficient background and expertise.

When providing genetic services, many providers use a standard protocol that calls for individuals or families to be seen for two visits, each lasting about one to two hours, prior to testing and at least one appointment for results disclosure and discussion of recommendations. In the setting of genetic risk,

the use of multidisciplinary teams and multiple interactions is emphasized. The underlying concern is that individuals may be overwhelmed by all the information provided in a single one-hour visit. Such attention usually is not given to people with an average risk for developing malignancy.

Risk factor profiles should be reviewed at least annually. Patients should be questioned about any change in their family history since the last assessment, development of any new health problems that may be associated with increased risk, and whether they have started new medications that may change the risk profile (e.g., initiating HRT). If significant changes have occurred, screening recommendations may need to be modified. If no significant changes have occurred, an annual review of the risk factor assessment offers an excellent opportunity to reinforce information on cancer prevention and early detection. It also communicates an ongoing concern for the patient as a dynamic individual and identifies the nurse as a resource for further information should a problem develop.

The cancer risk assessment provides the foundation for the educational process related to cancer prevention and early detection. Oncology nurses have the opportunity to teach individuals about the epidemiology, risk factors, and signs and symptoms associated with various cancers. This provides the framework that individuals need to understand the importance of and rationale for primary and secondary cancer prevention strategies as well as information about signs and symptoms that merit further evaluation.

Staff nurses can serve as case finders to identify individuals at increased risk for developing cancer who will benefit from a more detailed risk assessment and possibly cancer genetics counseling. Staff nurses who work directly with patients and get to know their families are in the best position to initiate referrals as case finders and initiate the cancer risk assessment process. To be an effective case finder, nurses must understand basic cancer incidence, epidemiology, and the importance of an accurate family history.

Nurses with advanced practice degrees can perform more in-depth risk assessments, recommend cancer screening procedures, explain the risks and benefits of a particular screening examination, and, in many cases, actually perform the screening examination. For those who provide cancer genetics counseling, additional training in genetics and counseling is recommended. Currently, the means to obtain this additional training is variable. The International Society of Nurses in Genetics (www.isong.org) offers a process in which nurses can earn a credential by submitting a detailed portfolio that demonstrates their expertise.

As more and more nurses become involved in cancer risk assessment and genetic risk assessment, the need for nurses who have the background and expertise to provide this counseling will increase (Calzone, Stopfer, Blackwood, & Weber, 1997). Both undergraduate- and graduate-level nursing programs need to include content on genetics education. At present, there is limited recognition that genetics and risk assessment are relevant to nurses and that content must be included in educational curricula. Continuing education programs may help to bridge the gap in this knowledge for practicing nurses.

New risk factors seem to emerge every day. An important educational role for nurses is to help patients to understand which risks they should take seriously. Most people accept a wide variety of risks (e.g., driving faster than the posted speed limit, crossing a busy parking lot, riding a bike, flying across the country in an airplane) on a daily basis with little thought. For some reason, small news segments about cancer risk seem to conjure up more fear. Nurses must be aware of public news reports and go to primary sources when new risk factors are presented so that they can interpret this information accurately for patients. Nurses also need to communicate concepts related to breast and other cancer risks carefully when providing information to the media. This may include providing the media with primary sources and reports and more integrated state-of-the-art information. ACS and other resources should be consulted prior to speaking with the media to ensure that accurate statistics and figures are provided.

Each year ACS publishes *Cancer Facts and Figures* (ACS, 2007). This is a helpful reference that nurses can use to quickly gather incidence data about estimated cancer cases. The resource presents information in several different formats, including the projected number of new cases of specific cancers (incidence) and estimated mortality rates. The incidence rates also are given by state. Oncology nurses can obtain this publication free of charge from their local ACS office or through the ACS Web site (www.cancer.org) and may find it helpful to review to better understand the incidence of specific cancers in the geographical area of the country in which they practice. The publication also offers detailed information about primary and secondary cancer prevention of the major tumors as well as projected survival data by stage. Once they are familiar with the format of the publication, oncology nurses will find this to be an invaluable resource. Another source of commonly cited data is the Surveillance, Epidemiology, and End Results (SEER) Program. This information is available at the NCI Web site (http://seer.cancer.gov).

Research

Future research should evaluate the process of risk notification; the impact on knowledge, attitudes, emotions, and practices; and outcomes related to health and disease status. This research should include controlled clinical trials to evaluate different counseling protocols and provide information on the impact and effectiveness of cancer risk assessment and counseling. More research is needed to better understand how patients make decisions about genetic testing and how to facilitate positive outcomes.

Clearly, more information is needed on the roles of cognition, the affective state of the individual, developmental differences, personal values, and how these individual qualities affect cancer risk communication (Maibach, 1999). More research also is needed on the best people (including an interdisciplinary approach) to communicate cancer and genetic risks (Arkin, 1999). The effect of cancer risk assessment on cancer screening behaviors merits more attention.

Conclusion

Oncology nurses need to consider risk factor assessment as a wonderful opportunity for patient education not only on cancer risk factors but also on cancer prevention and early detection activities. Cancer risk assessment can be a technical process requiring expertise. Oncology nurses have an ethical responsibility to communicate risk information in understandable terms and as accurately as possible. Risk assessment is more than collecting assessment data from patients. A critical component of the process is communicating the information to patients in a meaningful way.

Breast cancer risk communication is a continuous process. The risk assessment is a large component of this process. It demands communication with women so that they are informed about the best possible choices regarding cancer prevention and early detection activities. Patients will continue to ask when more will be known about particular cancer risks related to breast cancer and when there will be improvements in treatment. Developments in genetics will undoubtedly change risk assessments for some patients.

Like many cancers, breast cancer is a multifactorial disease. Causes and risk factors come from both endogenous and exogenous sources that interact in ways that are not completely understood. Much of the data about risk factors is seen at the theoretical level. Many risk factors for cancer, including breast cancer, are not within the control of the individual. Helping patients to understand these risks, live with these risks, and make good choices about breast cancer prevention and early detection strategies are important oncology nursing responsibilities.

References

American Cancer Society. (2007). *Cancer facts and figures, 2007.* Atlanta, GA: Author.

Arkin, E.B. (1999). Cancer risk communication—what we know. *Journal of the National Cancer Institute Monographs, 25,* 182–185.

Armstrong, K., Eisen, A., & Weber, B. (2000). Assessing the risk of breast cancer. *New England Journal of Medicine, 342,* 564–571.

Berry, D.A., Iversen, E.S., Jr., Gudbjartsson, D.F., Hiller, E.H., Garber, J.E., Peshkin, B.N., et al. (2002). BRCAPRO validation, sensitivity of genetic testing of BRCA1/BRCA2, and prevalence of other breast cancer susceptibility genes. *Journal of Clinical Oncology, 20,* 2701–2712.

Berry, D.A., Parmigiani, G., Sanchez, J., Schildkraut, J., & Winer, E. (1997). Probability of carrying a mutation of breast-ovarian cancer gene BRCA1 based on family history. *Journal of the National Cancer Institute, 89,* 227–238.

Bilimoria, M.M., & Morrow, M. (1995). The woman at increased risk for breast cancer: Evaluation and management strategies. *CA: A Cancer Journal for Clinicians, 45,* 263–278.

Bottorff, J.L., Ratner, P.A., Johnson, J.L., Lovato, C.Y., & Joab, S.A. (1998). Communicating cancer risk information: The challenges of uncertainty. *Patient Education and Counseling, 33,* 67–81.

Brewster, D.H., Stockton, D.L., Dobbie, R., Bull, D., & Beral, V. (2005). Risk of breast cancer after miscarriage or induced abortion: A Scottish record linkage case-control study. *Journal of Epidemiology and Community Health, 59,* 283–287.

Calzone, K.A., Stopfer, J., Blackwood, A., & Weber, B.L. (1997). Establishing a cancer risk evaluation program. *Cancer Practice, 5,* 228–233.

Chavez-MacGregor, M., Elias, S.G., Onland-Moret, C.O., van der Schouw, Y.T., Van Gils, C.H., Monninkhof, E., et al. (2005). Postmenopausal breast cancer risk and cumulative number of menstrual cycles. *Cancer Epidemiology, Biomarkers and Prevention, 14,* 799–804.

Claus, E.B., Risch, N., & Thompson, W.D. (1994). Autosomal dominant inheritance of early-onset breast cancer: Implications for risk prediction. *Cancer, 73,* 643–651.

Claus, E.B., Schildkraut, M.M., Thompson, W.D., & Risch, N. (1996). The genetic attributable risk of breast and ovarian cancer. *Cancer, 77,* 2318–2324.

Colditz, G.A. (2005). Epidemiology and prevention of breast cancer. *Cancer Epidemiology, Biomarkers and Prevention, 14,* 768–772.

Collaborative Group on Hormonal Factors in Breast Cancer. (2002). Breast cancer and breastfeeding: Collaborative reanalysis of individual data from 47 epidemiological studies in 30 countries, including 50,302 women with breast cancer and 96,973 women without the disease. *Lancet, 360,* 187–195.

Cornelisse, C.J., & Devilee, P. (1997). Facts in cancer genetics. *Patient Education and Counseling, 32,* 9–17.

Couch, F.J., DeShano, M.L., Blackwood, M.A., Calzone, K., Stopfer, J., Campeau, L., et al. (1997). BRCA1 mutations in women attending clinics that evaluate the risk of breast cancer. *New England Journal of Medicine, 336,* 1409–1415.

Croyle, R.T., & Lerman, C. (1999). Risk communication in genetic testing for cancer susceptibility. *Journal of the National Cancer Institute Monographs, 25,* 59–66.

Fischhoff, B. (1999). Why (cancer) risk communication can be hard. *Journal of the National Cancer Institute Monographs, 25,* 7–13.

Fisher, B., Anderson, S., Bryant, J., Margolese, R.G., Deutsch, M., Fisher, E.R., et al. (2002). Twenty-year follow-up of a randomized trial comparing total mastectomy, lumpectomy, and lumpectomy plus irradiation for the treatment of invasive breast cancer. *New England Journal of Medicine, 347,* 1233–1241.

Frank, T.S., Deffenbaugh, A.M., Reid, J.E., Hulick, M., Ward, B.E., Lingenfelter, B., et al. (2002). Clinical characteristics of individuals with germline mutations in BRCA1 and BRCA2: Analysis of 10,000 individuals. *Journal of Clinical Oncology, 20,* 1480–1490.

Frank, T.S., Manley, S.A., Olopade, O.I., Cummings, S., Garber, J.E., Bernhardt, B., et al. (1998). Sequence analysis of BRCA1 and BRCA2: Correlation of mutations with family history and ovarian cancer risk. *Journal of Clinical Oncology, 16,* 2417–2425.

Furberg, H., Newman, B., Moorman, P., & Millikan, R. (1999). Lactation and breast cancer risk. *International Journal of Epidemiology, 28,* 396–402.

Gail, M.H., Brinton, L.A., Byar, D.P., Corle, D.K., Green, S.B., Schairer, C., et al. (1989). Projecting individualized probabilities of developing breast cancer for white females who are being examined annually. *Journal of the National Cancer Institute, 81,* 1879–1886.

Ganz, P.A. (2002). Breast cancer 2002: Where do we stand? *CA: A Cancer Journal for Clinicians, 52,* 253–255.

Hamajima, N., Hirose, K., Tajima, K., Rohan, T., Calle, E.E., Heath, C.W., et al. (2002). Alcohol, tobacco and breast cancer—collaborative reanalysis of individual data from 53 epidemiological studies, including 58,515 women with breast cancer and 95,067 women without the disease. *British Journal of Cancer, 87,* 1234–1245.

Hopwood, P. (2005). Psychosocial aspects of risk communication and mutation testing in familial breast-ovarian cancer. *Current Opinion in Oncology, 17,* 340–344.

Kash, K.M., Ortega-Verdejo, K., Dabney, M.K., Holland, J.C., Miller, D.G., & Osborne, M.P. (2000). Psychosocial aspects of cancer genetics: Women at high risk for breast and ovarian cancer. *Seminars in Surgical Oncology, 18,* 333–338.

Kelly, P.T. (2000). *Assess your true risk of breast cancer.* New York: Henry Holt.

King, M.C., Marks, J.H., Mandell, J.B., & New York Breast Cancer Study Group. (2003). Breast and ovarian cancer risks due to inherited mutations in BRCA1 and BRCA2. *Science, 302,* 643–646.

Lee, S.H., Akuete, K., Fulton, J., Chelmow, D., Chung, M.A., & Cady, B. (2003). An increased risk of breast cancer after delayed parity. *American Journal of Surgery, 186,* 409–412.

Lerman, C., Lusbader, E., Rimer, B., Daly, M., Miller, S., Sands, C., et al. (1995). Effects of individualized breast cancer risk counseling: A randomized trial. *Journal of the National Cancer Institute, 87,* 286–292.

Lerman, C., Narod, S., Schulman, K., Hughes, C., Gomez-Caminero, A., Bonney, G., et al. (1996). BRCA1 testing in families with hereditary breast-ovarian cancer. A prospective study of patient decision making and outcomes. *JAMA, 275,* 1885–1892.

Lipkus, I.M., & Hollands, J.G. (1999). The visual communication of risk. *Journal of the National Cancer Institute Monographs, 25,* 149–163.

Lynch, H.T., Snyder, C.L., Lynch, J.F., Riley, B.D., & Rubinstein, W.S. (2003). Hereditary breast-ovarian cancer at the bedside: Role of the medical oncologist. *Journal of Clinical Oncology, 21,* 740–753.

Madigan, M.P., Ziegler, R.G., Benichou, J., Byrne, C., & Hoover, R.N. (1995). Proportion of breast cancer cases in the United States explained by well-established risk factors. *Journal of the National Cancer Institute, 87,* 1681–1685.

Mahon, S.M. (2003). Cancer-risk assessment: Considerations for cancer genetics. In A.S. Tranin, A. Masny, & J. Jenkins (Eds.), *Genetics in oncology practice: Cancer risk assessment* (pp. 77–138). Pittsburgh, PA: Oncology Nursing Society.

Mahue-Giangreco, M., Ursin, G., Sullivan-Halley, J., & Bernstein, L. (2003). Induced abortion, miscarriage, and breast cancer risk of young women. *Cancer Epidemiology, Biomarkers and Prevention, 12,* 209–214.

Maibach, E. (1999). Cancer risk communication—what we need to learn. *Journal of the National Cancer Institute Monographs, 25,* 179–181.

Marchbanks, P.A., McDonald, J.A., Wilson, H.G., Folger, S.G., Mandel, M.G., Daling, J.R., et al. (2002). Oral contraceptives and the risk of breast cancer. *New England Journal of Medicine, 346,* 2025–2032.

Morimoto, L.M., White, E., Chen, Z., Chlebowski, R.T., Hays, J., Kuller, L., et al. (2002). Obesity, body size, and risk of postmenopausal breast cancer: The Women's Health Initiative (United States). *Cancer Causes and Control, 13,* 741–751.

Myriad Genetic Laboratories, Inc. (2005). *Mutation prevalence tables for BRCA1/2 genes.* Retrieved May 11, 2006, from http://www.myriadtests.com/provider/mutprev.htm

National Cancer Institute. (2005). Summary report: Early reproductive events and breast cancer workshop. *Issues in Law and Medicine, 21,* 161–165.

Newcomer, L.M., Newcomb, P.A., Trentham-Dietz, A., Longnecker, M.P., & Greenberg, E.R. (2003). Oral contraceptive use and risk of breast cancer by histologic type. *International Journal of Cancer, 106,* 961–964.

Oncology Nursing Society. (2004, October). *Cancer predisposition genetic testing and risk assessment counseling* [Position statement]. Pittsburgh, PA: Author.

Press, N., Fishman, J.R., & Koenig, B.A. (2000). Collective fear, individualized risk: The social and cultural context of genetic testing for breast cancer. *Nursing Ethics, 7,* 237–249.

Rimer, B.K., Schildkraut, J.M., Lerman, C., Lin, T., & Audrain, J. (1996). Participation in women's breast cancer risk counseling trial. Who participates? Who declines? *Cancer, 77,* 2348–2355.

Rodgers, J.E. (1999). Introduction of section: Overarching considerations in risk communications: Romancing the message. *Journal of the National Cancer Institute Monographs, 25,* 21–22.

Rosser, E.M., Hurst, J.A., & Chapman, C.J. (1996). Cancer families: What risks are given and do the risks affect management? *Journal of Medical Genetics, 33,* 977–980.

Rothman, A.J., & Kiviniemi, M.T. (1999). Treating people with information: An analysis and review of approaches to communicating health risk information. *Journal of the National Cancer Institute Monographs, 25,* 44–51.

Salovey, P., Schneider, T.R., & Apanovitch, A.M. (1999). Persuasion for the purpose of cancer risk reduction: A discussion. *Journal of the National Cancer Institute Monographs, 25,* 119–122.

Sandler, G.R., Wasserman, L., Fullerton, J.T., & Romero, M. (2004). Supporting patients through genetic screening for cancer risk. *Medsurg Nursing, 13,* 233–246.

Schneider, K. (2002). *Counseling about cancer: Strategies for genetic counselors* (2nd ed.). New York: Wiley-Liss.

Shattuck-Eidens, D., Oliphant, A., McClure, M., McBride, C., Gupte, J., Rubano, T., et al. (1997). BRCA1 sequence analysis in women at high risk for susceptibility mutations. Risk factor analysis and implications for genetic testing. *JAMA, 278,* 1242–1250.

Singletary, S.E. (2003). Rating the risk factors for breast cancer. *Annals of Surgery, 237,* 474–482.

Smith-Warner, S.A., Spiegelman, D., Yaun, S.S., Adami, H.O., Beeson, W.L., van den Brandt, P.A., et al. (2001). Intake of fruits and vegetables and risk of breast cancer: A pooled analysis of cohort studies. *JAMA, 285,* 769–776.

Stopfer, J.E. (2000). Genetic counseling and clinical cancer genetics services. *Seminars in Surgical Oncology, 18,* 347–357.

Struewing, J.P., Hartge, P., Wacholder, S., Baker, B.S., Berlin, M., McAdams, M., et al. (1997). The risk of cancer associated with specific mutations of BRCA1 and BRCA2 among Ashkenazi Jews. *New England Journal of Medicine, 336,* 1401–1408.

Thompson, D., Easton, D.F., & Breast Cancer Linkage Consortium. (2002). Cancer incidence in BRCA1 mutation carriers. *Journal of the National Cancer Institute, 94,* 1358–1365.

Travis, L.B., Hill, D.A., Dores, G.M., Gospodarowicz, M., van Leeuwen, F.E., Holowaty, E., et al. (2003). Breast cancer following radiotherapy and chemotherapy among young women with Hodgkin disease. *JAMA, 290,* 465–475.

Veronesi, U., Cascinelli, N., Mariani, L., Greco, M., Saccozzi, R., Luini, A., et al. (2002). Twenty-year follow-up of a randomized study comparing breast-conserving surgery with radical mastectomy for early breast cancer. *New England Journal of Medicine, 347,* 1227–1232.

Vogel, V. (2000). Breast cancer prevention: A review of current evidence. *CA: A Cancer Journal for Clinicians, 50,* 156–170.

Weitzel, J.N. (1999). Genetic cancer risk assessment. Putting it all together. *Cancer, 86*(Suppl. 11), 2483–2492.

Women's Health Initiative Steering Committee. (2004). Effects of conjugated equine estrogen in postmenopausal women with hysterectomy: The Women's Health Initiative randomized controlled trial. *JAMA, 291,* 1701–1712.

Zhang, S., Hunter, D.J., Forman, M.R., Rosner, B.A., Speizer, F.E., Colditz, G.A., et al. (1999). Dietary carotenoids and vitamins A, C, and E and risk of breast cancer. *Journal of the National Cancer Institute, 91,* 547–556.

Zhang, S., Hunter, D.J., Hankinson, S.E., Giovannucci, E.L., Rosner, B.A., Colditz, G.A., et al. (1999). A prospective study of folate intake and the risk of breast cancer. *JAMA, 281,* 1632–1637.

CHAPTER 3

Prevention and Detection of Breast Cancer

Dianne D. Chapman, ND, APRN,BC

Introduction

In the past, breast cancer was a disease that often was detected late, associated with a poor prognosis, and not discussed in polite conversation. Today, female celebrities and politicians routinely and candidly discuss their diagnoses in the newspapers, on the Internet, and on talk shows. This public awareness of breast cancer screening and education through media announcements coupled with reinforcing support from healthcare providers encourages and motivates women to be proactive about their breast health. The routine use of screening mammography and the specialty use of other diagnostic modalities, including ultrasound and other techniques, enable physicians to identify early, nonpalpable cancers, replacing later-stage disease with a potentially curable diagnosis. The recent improvements in technology such as breast magnetic resonance imaging (MRI) allow visualization of a cancer in its earliest stage, provide important diagnostic information for treatment by identifying the absence or presence of metastatic disease, and document response to treatment.

Despite significant advances in the early detection of breast cancer, it remains the most commonly occuring cancer in women and the second leading cause of cancer deaths overall. Among women ages 20–59, it is the leading cause of cancer deaths. The death rate from breast cancer has been steadily decreasing, going from 43,844 in 1995 to 41,619 in 2003, but the incidence rate continues to show a small yearly increase (Jemal et al., 2007).

Detection Disparities

Because breast cancer accounts for approximately 26% of all new female cancers (Jemal et al., 2007), more efforts are needed to ensure that all women have access to screening. The uninsured and underinsured routinely encounter barriers to basic health care. Some cultural groups may have misconceptions about the efficacy of breast cancer screening and do not adhere to recommendations or access clinical examinations and mammography. Improving primary, secondary, and tertiary prevention methods is not the only solution to reducing incidence and death rates; improving access to clinical examinations and mammography for all cultural groups is necessary as well.

Cultural and Racial Disparities

Disparities among racial groups exist in utilization of screening mammography. These disparities stem from many factors, including misconceptions or a lack of knowledge, low income status, unemployment, and lack of insurance. Women who have not finished high school have lower rates for mammography screening than high school graduates. The mammography screening rate for low-income women is 24% lower than that for higher-income women (Bigby & Holmes, 2005). Mammography utilization rates and screening rates for African Americans are comparable to those for Caucasian women. However, non-White women are less likely to follow up on abnormal mammography results. Hispanic, American Indian, and Alaska Native women have lower rates of mammography screening than Caucasian women (Bigby & Holmes).

Disparities for Young Patients

Although breast cancer is rare in young women (approximately 1,200 annual cases in women younger than 30 [Mintzer, Glassburn, Mason, & Sataloff, 2002]), diagnostic methods often are applied inappropriately and inconsistently when a lump or mass is found in the breast. Developmentally, breast lumps are more common in this age group, and a clinician may have a low index of suspicion for breast cancer. Compounding these biases is the fact that breast cancer may be more difficult to diagnose in this age group because of normal hormonal fluctuations during the menstrual cycle that result in a nodular presentation commonly referred to as fibrocystic change. Because mammography often is not useful in young, dense breasts, ultrasound, clinical examination, and possibly a tissue sample should be performed to exclude the possibility of breast cancer (Mintzer et al.).

Conventional screening for women with a high lifetime risk of developing breast cancer often is inadequate because of increased breast density in young women, frequency of atypical imaging presentations, and the rapid growth of hereditary breast cancer, resulting in a higher rate of interval cancer (Kuhl, Schrading, et al., 2005; Robson et al., 2003). Screening recommendations differ for women with a known mutation in *BRCA1* or *BRCA2* and include mammography, ultrasound, and MRI of the breast, with imaging every six months. MRI has been shown to be more diagnostic in young women because it is not affected by breast density. Mutation carriers have a 65%–80% lifetime risk of developing breast cancer, and annual screening may not provide adequate scrutiny for these high-risk women. This screening strategy ensures that an imaging study is performed every six months, with the goal of detecting breast cancer as early as possible (Kuhl, Kuhn, & Schild, 2005; National Comprehensive Cancer Network [NCCN], 2006; Robson et al.).

Disparities for Women With Disabilities

Mammography screening for people with disabilities is fraught with physical and sociologic barriers. Most mammography facilities are ill equipped to service people using a wheelchair. Women with disabilities are living longer, and preventive measures should be available for health maintenance. Mele, Archer, and Pusch (2005) studied the breast cancer screening attitudes and beliefs of 20 women with disabilities and found that a high value was placed on clinical breast exam (CBE), breast self-examination (BSE), and mammography, but they were rarely performed. Monthly BSE was compromised by spasm, pain, lack of strength, and immobility. Women stated that lack of knowledge eroded their confidence in performing BSE, and primary providers did not give instruction or educational brochures. Despite the legal requirements for accessibility, women with disabilities continue to face barriers in finding transportation and available parking and gaining entry to providers' offices (Mele et al.).

Healthcare providers also may limit access to prevention and detection by viewing women with disabilities as not having an adequate life expectancy to warrant screening or by viewing them as asexual and therefore not requiring whole women screening, Pap tests, routine gynecologic examination, and BSE instruction (Cheng et al., 2001; Thierry, 2000).

Positioning patients for mammography is challenging for patients who are in a wheelchair or those who are unable to stand for prolonged periods. Also, women who have spinal cord injuries or muscular disease often are unable to be positioned for adequate imaging. Patients must be able to remain still, raise their arms, and rotate their shoulders as well as bend at the waist to optimize imaging. Women with disabilities also may avoid gynecologic exams and mammography because the difficulty in positioning causes discomfort and embarrassment (Cheng et al., 2001).

Very few health facilities are designed to provide necessary preventive health delivery for women with disabilities. The facility must have access for wheelchairs in every room, examination tables that can be raised and lowered, hydraulic lifts, and a staff trained in disability awareness and sensitivity as well as knowledge of the proper procedures for transferring and positioning (Schopp, Kirkpatrick, Sanford, Hagglund, & Wongvatunyu, 2002).

Disparities for Older Adults

Increasing age is a significant risk factor for developing breast cancer. The overall risk is 1 in 14 for women ages 60–79, and an estimated 35% of women are older than 70 at the time of diagnosis. Recent surveillance figures indicate that 65.3% of women older than 65 had a mammogram within the past year (Holmes & Muss, 2003). The American Cancer Society (ACS) guidelines recommend that women receive yearly screening mammography if they are in good health and would be a candidate for treatment if diagnosed (Holmes & Muss). A great deal of debate exists regarding the age at which screening mammography should be discontinued. It is a well-known fact that early detection prolongs survival, and age remains the greatest risk factor for the development of breast cancer. Factors that support screening for older adults include the increased incidence in the population, the ease of determining mammographic abnormalities in fatty-replaced breast tissue, and retrospective studies that indicate probable benefit. NCCN (www.nccn.org) and ACS (www.cancer.org) do not advocate a distinct age cutoff but recommend considering comorbidities and life expectancy. Women who have health issues that would preclude chemotherapy, hormone replacement, and surgery for breast cancer, such as severe heart disease, sedentary or bedridden lifestyle, pulmonary disease, or other organ disease that would make life expectancy less than five years, would be candidates for ceasing mammography. It is unreasonable to perform screening tests if the person has a medical condition that makes treatment inadvisable (Holmes & Muss).

Primary Prevention

Primary prevention is the act of promoting a strategy that is intended to prevent a specific condition, such as limiting fat intake to reduce the risk of heart disease or educating the public on the use of helmets for bicycle riders and seatbelts for automobile passengers. Primary prevention strategies have the potential to dramatically reduce the breast cancer incidence in high-risk women. The two most significant risk factors for breast cancer besides gender are age and the presence of a germ-line genetic mutation. The risk for developing cancer increases with age, with 50% being diagnosed after age 65 (Holmes & Muss, 2003). Women with a strong family history of breast and/or ovarian cancer may harbor a *BRCA1* or *BRCA2* genetic mutation that increases the lifetime risk of developing breast cancer to as high as 82% (King, Marks, Mandell, & New York Breast Cancer Study Group, 2003).

Until recently, having a drug that prevents or delays the development of breast cancer seemed to be an unreachable goal. The selection of tamoxifen as a prevention drug was based on results of cooperative studies conducted in the United States and Europe involving tens of thousands of women with a diagnosis of breast cancer. The National Surgical Adjuvant Breast and Bowel Project (NSABP)-P1 trial confirmed that tamoxifen could be used for chemoprevention in the primary prevention of breast cancer (Fisher et al., 1998). In addition, the NSABP-24 trial identified tamoxifen as a secondary prevention strategy for patients with estrogen-positive ductal carcinoma in situ to prevent ipsilateral and contralateral breast cancer (Fisher et al., 1999; Gasco, Argusti, Bonanni, & Decensi, 2005).The NSABP has conducted numerous studies that evaluated the efficacy of tamoxifen alone or as an adjunct to chemotherapy for treating breast cancer (Fisher et al., 1981, 1986, 1989, 1990, 1997, 1999). The NSABP studies indicated that not only was tamoxifen an effective treatment for breast cancer, but it also reduced the expected number of breast cancers that would be diagnosed in the contralateral breast.

Tamoxifen is a selective estrogen receptor modulator that binds to the estrogen receptor and acts as an agonist and antagonist, depending on the organ. Tamoxifen is an antagonist in the breast, occupying the estrogen receptor and blocking the effects of estrogen. Tamoxifen has an agonist effect in the bones, liver, and uterus by producing estrogen-like effects (Friedman, 1998). The prevention study, NSABP P-1, enrolled approximately 14,000 women in a randomized trial using either 20 mg of tamoxifen daily or a placebo (Fisher et al., 1998). Any woman 60 years of age or older was eligible to participate by virtue of age alone. Women ages 35–60 were deemed eligible for participation if their risk score using the Gail model was greater than 1.66. The Gail model is a multivariate logistic regression model using five risk factors that are given a numeric value. These factors estimate the probability of developing breast cancer over time (Gail et al., 1989). An example of an assessment tool created by the NSABP and based on the Gail model is available online at www.cancer.gov/bcrisktool/breast-cancer-risk.aspx. The NSABP P-1 trial was stopped early after it was demonstrated that the benefit from tamoxifen was statistically significant. Tamoxifen reduced the relative risk of developing breast cancer by 49%, and benefit was applicable to all age groups. The researchers also reported that tamoxifen was associated with several serious adverse effects, including endometrial cancer (3.3/1,000 versus 0.8/1,000), deep vein thrombosis (1.5/1,000 versus 0.9/1,000), stroke (2.2/1,000 versus 1.3/1,000), and

pulmonary embolism (1/1,000 versus 0.3/1,000), all occurring more frequently in women older than 50. Ultimately, the analyses suggest that the beneficial effects of tamoxifen are greatest in women younger than 50 years of age.

All women taking tamoxifen should be cautioned about the signs and symptoms of these possible complications and report any symptoms that appear, including (a) vaginal bleeding after menopause or excessive/unusual bleeding between menses, (b) pain, warmth, or swelling of calf or thigh, (c) sudden loss of extremity/facial function or sensation, and (d) chest pain, pressure, or dyspnea. Women on tamoxifen should have annual Pap tests and evaluations for any vaginal bleeding irregularities, which may include transvaginal ultrasound to evaluate the thickness of the endometrial lining and/or endometrial biopsy to assess for hyperplasia or malignant pathology (Burke, 2005; Chlebowski, 2002). Risk factors for developing a thromboembolic event are increased in those who have had surgery within the past three months, have a body mass index above 25 kg/m², a history of past or current smoking, hypertension, total cholesterol equal to or above 250, and a family history of heart disease (Duggan, Marriott, Edwards, & Cuzick, 2003; Gasco et al., 2005). A patient presenting with leg swelling, warmth, and/or pain is usually evaluated for a thrombosis with a low-invasive imaging study such as ultrasonography. A V/Q (ventilation/perfusion) scan assesses pulmonary ventilation and perfusion and is useful for diagnosing a suspected pulmonary embolism (Donnelly, Hinwood, & London, 2000). A patient with suspected stroke will have a cardiology workup with chemistries, enzymes, and electrocardiogram, as well as imaging studies such as computed tomography (CT), MRI, diffusion-weighted imaging to identify ischemia, and magnetic resonance perfusion study, to determine the diagnosis and potential prognosis for recovery (Chalela, Merino, & Warach, 2004; Frizzell, 2005; Thurnher & Castillo, 2005).

Approximately 5%–7% of women diagnosed with breast cancer have a *BRCA1* or *BRCA2* genetic mutation that predisposes them to a higher risk of developing a contralateral breast cancer and ovarian cancer (King et al., 2003). *BRCA1* and *BRCA2* mutations are associated with autosomal dominant inheritance patterns that can be inherited from the father or mother, meaning that a first-degree relative of a person with a *BRCA* mutation has a 50% likelihood of also having the mutation. Prevention strategies for carriers of a mutation vary from increased surveillance and chemoprevention to prophylactic removal of the breast and ovaries. Currently, sufficient evidence shows that prophylactic surgeries offer the best risk reduction for breast and ovarian cancers (Hartmann, Degnim, & Schaid, 2004; Hartmann et al., 2001; van Sprundel et al., 2005). A review paper by Dowdy, Stefanek, and Hartmann (2004) discussed studies that identified a quantitative risk reduction for women choosing prophylactic breast and ovarian surgeries.

Hartmann et al. (2001) conducted a retrospective study examining prophylactic mastectomy in mutation carriers and found a 100% relative risk reduction for developing breast cancer. The study group was small (26 women), and follow-up time was short (13.4 years). Although these results are dramatic, they most likely will not hold up over time (Dowdy et al., 2004; Hartmann et al., 2004). The probability of leaving breast cells behind that may become cancerous in the future is very small, but it is possible. The recommended surgery for prophylaxis is a total mastectomy that removes the breast tissue along with the nipple-areolar complex. This procedure may leave cells of breast tissue behind in the axilla, inframammary skin fold, or skin flaps (Dowdy et al.). Potential early or late complications include immediate necrosis of the skin, infection, wound dehiscence, seroma, and pain (Eisen, Rebbeck, Wood, & Weber, 2000).

The risk reduction for ovarian cancer is greater than 90% when a complete hysterectomy is performed (removal of uterus, ovaries, and fallopian tubes). The surgery also reduces the risk of breast cancer by approximately 50%. There is a risk of primary peritoneal cancer after prophylactic hysterectomy that presumably is related to the peritoneal epithelium being the same embryonic structure as the covering of the ovaries. This surgery should be performed by a gynecologic oncologist because of the potential for finding an occult ovarian cancer, and an exploration of the abdomen and pelvis usually precludes a laparoscopic approach (Dowdy et al., 2004). The complications from this surgery are few but include pain, infection, and wound dehiscence.

Women choosing a prophylactic complete hysterectomy must be counseled about the complications resulting from estrogen deprivation: bone loss, increase in serum cholesterol, vaginal dryness, and dyspareunia. If the woman has never been diagnosed with cancer, hormone replacement therapy (HRT) may be prescribed to relieve symptoms and offer protection for bone loss. Although giving HRT to carriers of the mutation is not well documented, a study by Rebbeck et al. (2005) followed women for 3.6 years and indicated that short-term HRT does not increase the risk for breast cancer. However, because little information is available about how long-term HRT may affect a mutation carrier, the healthcare team should inform patients about the possible consequences of treatment (Dowdy et al., 2004; Hartmann et al., 2001; van Sprundel et al., 2005).

Breast Examinations

Secondary cancer prevention seeks to detect cancers in the earliest possible stage. The goal of secondary prevention is to detect cancer when treatment is most likely to be effective and associated with the least morbidity. In breast cancer, secondary cancer prevention includes breast examinations and imaging modalities, especially mammography.

Breast Self-Examination

BSE has been routinely recommended by physicians, nurses, and professional organizations as an adjunct tool to fa-

cilitate the early detection of breast cancer. However, very few studies have been done to substantiate its effectiveness (i.e., decrease in mortality) or associated financial and emotional costs. The underlying rationale has been that women who perform BSE find lumps earlier than women who do not perform BSE and that the lumps are smaller and more easily treated, thereby decreasing mortality. The U.S. Preventive Services Task Force (USPSTF) issued an update on its guidelines for breast screening in 2002 through the National Guideline Clearinghouse (www.guideline.gov) (Humphrey, Helfand, Chan, & Woolf, 2002). These guidelines are still current and reflect recommendations of the recently updated NCCN guidelines (www.nccn.org). Guidelines that address recommendations for prevention or early detection differ among agencies (see Table 3-1). This often is related to the various differences in studies that each agency has chosen to review.

These recent guidelines on BSE resulted from analyses of several large trials, primarily randomized, from the United States, Europe, Russia, and China. The overall results of these studies indicated that instruction in BSE did not reduce mortality and, furthermore, led to biopsies of benign lesions (Holmberg, Ekbom, Calle, Mokdad, & Byers, 1997; Humphrey et al., 2002; Kolb, Lichy, & Newhouse, 2002; Semiglazov et al., 1999; "16-Year Mortality From Breast Cancer," 1999). The USPSTF concluded that a recommendation for monthly BSE could not be made. Hackshaw and Paul (2003) conducted a meta-analysis of 20 observational studies and three clinical trials that suggested that no decrease in mortality was associated with practicing BSE but indicated that BSE was associated with more healthcare visits and more biopsies. Healthcare providers need to understand that the statement that there is insufficient evidence to support BSE does not mean that it is ineffective but that more studies are needed to determine the effectiveness of this intervention.

Despite the recommendation, women will still choose to perform monthly BSE if they feel it is helpful or if their health practitioner actively encourages them to do so. One of the biggest benefits of BSE is that it allows women to be proactive in their breast health. Women in the United States are very aware of the prevalence of breast cancer and are taking steps to enhance early detection. Every October, which is National Breast Cancer Awareness Month, the media are saturated with breast cancer awareness information. The ACS guidelines include BSE as an option starting at age 20. Between ages 20 and 40, women should have a CBE every one to three years. Women older than age 40 are urged to have an annual CBE and mammogram and to report any breast changes promptly (Smith, Cokkinides, & Eyre, 2006).

In addition, women who choose BSE should know the proper technique and timing. Nurses often initiate and reinforce this teaching when patients come in for a routine examination or when an appointment is made to address a perceived breast problem. The best time for menstruating women to perform BSE is right after their period ends, and

Table 3-1. Overview of Selected Agency Recommendations for the Early Detection of Breast Cancer

Agency	Funding Source	Intended User	Objective	Target Population	Review Methods	Outcomes Considered	BSE Recommendations	CBE Recommendations	Mammography Recommendations	Patient Education
American Society of Clinical Oncology (ASCO) (Smith et al., 1999), medical subspecialty group	ASCO	3-page document for patients and physicians	Determine effective, evidence-based postoperative surveillance strategies for the detection and treatment of recurrent breast cancer	Patients with breast cancer	External and internal review	Overall survival, disease-free survival, quality of life, toxicity reduction, cost effectiveness	Prudent to recommend monthly practice	Every 3–6 months for the first three years after diagnosis; every 6–12 months for the next two years; then annually	Annually from time of diagnosis	Advise about symptoms of recurrence.
American Cancer Society (ACS) (Smith et al., 2006), disease-specific society	ACS	4-page document for patients, physicians, nurses, allied healthcare professionals, health plans, and managed care organizations	Determine whether new scientific findings warrant a change in ACS guidelines (reviewed annually)	Women 40 years of age or older	Peer review	Mortality caused by breast cancer in women aged 40 or older	Monthly practice offered as option	Every 1–3 years for women aged 20–39; annually beginning at age 40	Annually beginning at age 40	None stated
National Comprehensive Cancer Network (NCCN, 2006), alliance of 20 cancer centers	NCCN	38-page document for physicians	Develop guidelines to facilitate decision making	Asymptomatic women at normal risk for breast cancer	Comparison of guidelines from other groups, internal and external reviews	Breast cancer–specific survival, overall survival, net health benefit	Encourage practice.	Every 1–3 years for women aged 20–39; annually beginning at age 40	Annually beginning at age 40	None stated

(Continued on next page)

Table 3-1. Overview of Selected Agency Recommendations for the Early Detection of Breast Cancer (Continued)

Agency	Funding Source	Intended User	Objective	Target Population	Review Methods	Outcomes Considered	BSE Recommendations	CBE Recommendations	Mammography Recommendations	Patient Education
Centers for Disease Control and Prevention (CDC) (Ryerson et al., 2006)	CDC	88-page document for physicians and nurses	To present morbidity and mortality data regarding breast cancer screening recommendations, an update on National Breast and Cervical Cancer Early Detection Program	Uninsured and low-income women aged 50–64	Not stated	Morbidity and mortality of breast cancer, incidence of breast cancer, mammogram usage rates	None stated	Mentioned, not encouraged	Every 1–2 years beginning at 40. Recommend ceasing mammography at 74.	None stated
American College of Radiology (ACR, 2004), medical specialty society	ACR	7-page document for physicians	To revise screening guidelines for breast cancer in light of mounting evidence that women younger than age 50 have a shorter lead time for mammographic detection of breast cancer	Women 40 years of age or older without signs or symptoms of breast cancer; women of any age at high risk for breast cancer but without signs or symptoms of breast cancer	Peer review	Mortality rate reduction because of screening for breast cancer, cost effectiveness of screening mammography (e.g., cost per year of lives saved)	Monthly beginning at age 40	Annually beginning at age 40	Annually for women at normal risk beginning at age 40; at younger ages for asymptomatic women at high risk	None stated
U.S. Preventive Services Task Force (USPSTF, 2002), independent expert panel	United States	3-page document for physicians, nurses, and allied healthcare professionals	To summarize the current USPSTF recommendations on screening for breast cancer and the supporting scientific evidence	Women aged 40 and older	Comparison of guidelines from other groups, internal and external review	Sensitivity, specificity, and positive predictive values of screening methods; morbidity and mortality caused by breast cancer	Insufficient evidence to recommend for or against	Insufficient evidence to recommend for or against	Every 1–2 years for women starting at age 40	Insufficient evidence to recommend for or against teaching BSE

(Continued on next page)

Table 3-1. Overview of Selected Agency Recommendations for the Early Detection of Breast Cancer (Continued)

Agency	Funding Source	Intended User	Objective	Target Population	Review Methods	Outcomes Considered	BSE Recommendations	CBE Recommendations	Mammography Recommendations	Patient Education
Canadian Task Force on Preventive Health Care (CTF-PHC) (Baxter & CTF-PHC, 2001; Ringash & CTFPHC, 2001), national (non-U.S.) governmental agency	Canada	10-page document for physicians, nurses, and allied healthcare professionals	To evaluate the evidence related to the effectiveness of BSE to screen for breast cancer; to provide recommendations for teaching BSE to women as part of a periodic health examination	Asymptomatic women of all ages in the general population in Canada	External and internal peer review	Prevention of breast cancer mortality, incidence, stage detected, benign biopsy rate, number of visits for breast complaints, and psychological benefits; morbidity; to consider the available new and updated evidence regarding the effect of screening mammography on mortality among women aged 40–49 at average risk for breast cancer; to consider effects of screening mammography among women aged 40–49	For women aged 40 or younger, the risk for net harm is more likely because of the low incidence of breast cancer in this age group; for women beginning at age 70, insufficient evidence exists to make a recommendation	None stated	No recommendation for or against in women aged 40–49; every 1–2 years beginning at age 50	Women aged 50–69; for women aged 40–49, routine teaching of BSE should be excluded; for women younger than age 40, risk for net harm is more likely because of the low incidence of breast cancer; for women aged 70 and older, insufficient evidence exists; women at age 40 should be informed of potential risks and benefits to determine whether they wish to undergo mammography

BSE—breast self-examination; CBE—clinical breast examination

Note. From "Evidence-Based Practice: Recommendations for the Early Detection of Breast Cancer," by S.M. Mahon, 2003, *Clinical Journal of Oncology Nursing, 7*, pp. 694–695. Copyright 2003 by the Oncology Nursing Society. Adapted with permission.

menopausal women should choose a particular day of the month (such as when bills are paid, when the bank statement arrives, etc.) to remind them to do BSE. The current practice of BSE is a two-step activity. First, after a bath or shower, the breasts are visually examined, turning from side to side in front of a mirror with arms down, arms pressing on the hips, and arms raised overhead. These different positions alter the tension on the pectoralis muscle below the breast to best identify any puckering or change in the breast contour. The woman also notes any difference in the breast skin color or texture and any nipple changes (e.g., new evidence of inversion or protrusion, scaly or crusty appearance). The palpation examination is best performed lying down, as this allows the breast tissue to spread out evenly over the chest wall; however, many women examine their breasts in the shower. The flat pads of the first three fingers are used for the exam. Place a pillow under the shoulder and use the opposite hand of the side to be examined. First, the axilla is explored for any lumps or thickening with the arm down. Next, with the same arm raised above the shoulder, the entire breast is examined from the bra line to the collar bone and from the breastbone to the outer portion of the breast. Moving the towel to the other shoulder, the other breast is examined in the same manner. The pattern can be circular or up-and-down, according to preference (see Figure 3-1). Women who practice BSE regularly have a sense of the normal architecture of their breasts and are more aware of subtle changes that may occur.

Clinical Breast Examination

Mammography and CBE are recommended in tandem to properly screen average-risk women older than 40 years of age. Mammography has a variable false-negative rate between 10% and 30% (Bird, Wallace, & Yankaskas, 1992; Di Maggio, 2004; Elmore, Armstrong, Lehman, & Fletcher, 2005; Koomen, Pisano, Kuzmiak, Pavic, & McLelland, 2005; Majid, de Paredes, Doherty, Sharma, & Salvador, 2003), and CBE is thought to be an important adjunct procedure to detect any breast abnormalities not noted on mammography. A minority of cancers are not seen on mammography because of increased density of breast tissue, the nature of certain types of breast cancer (invasive lobular), or inexplicable reasons. An experienced breast specialist may be able to discern suspicious breast changes that are often very subtle underlying areas of thickening, mild skin changes that might include dimpling or puckering, or a slight difference in the parenchymal texture of one breast when compared to the other. Although CBE may indeed play an integral part in screening for breast cancer, no study has compared CBE alone versus no screening. The USPSTF report (Humphrey et al., 2002) reviewed clinical trials and concluded that there seems to be no difference in mortality reduction in studies that looked at CBE plus mammography versus mammography alone.

Breast Imaging

Mammography

Mammography is used for two separate indications. The first indication is a routine screening procedure for women who have no known problems and are adhering to health promotion guidelines recommended by their health provider. The second indication for mammography is when the woman or health provider notes an abnormality during monthly BSE or a routine examination. The mammogram then becomes a diagnostic imaging tool to investigate the area in question.

Screening Mammography

Mammography, along with ultrasound as an adjunct, is the primary imaging tool for breast cancer screening. Mammography is an effective and reasonable screening tool. The sensitivity of mammography can vary from 60%–90% for women with dense tissue. Younger women often have denser breasts, but breast density can remain throughout life, potentially obscuring nonpalpable abnormalities. In 2002, the USP-STF updated its guidelines for breast screening and cited the usefulness of mammography, and ACS recommended regular screening mammography beginning at age 40 (Humphrey et al., 2002; Smith, Cokkinides, & Eyre, 2005).

Some women avoid mammography because of radiation exposure concerns, ultimately delaying early detection if a problem exists (Smith & Andreopoulou, 2004). A perfect screening tool would be one that has no risk of side effects that may potentially cause harm and has 100% sensitivity and specificity; that is, it would detect all abnormalities and identify only those that need further investigation, thereby eliminating false positives and false negatives. A perfect tool is probably unattainable, though, and more effective screening tools for early detection are always under investigation. Therefore, mammography remains the "gold standard" at this time.

A mammography facility should be certified by the U.S. Food and Drug Administration (FDA) through an FDA-accrediting organization. In an effort to standardize mammography facilities, the Mammography Quality Standards Act was implemented in 1992 (due to be updated in 2007) to create performance standards for facility personnel and equipment. Surveys are conducted on a regular basis to ensure that the standards are being upheld, including properly functioning equipment, licensed/certified personnel, and documentation of continuing education. A listing of accredited facilities is available at www.fda.gov/cdrh/mammography/certified.html. The certificate of accreditation usually is posted in a readily visible area of the facility.

Currently, the mammography equipment in many facilities uses a film-screen process in which a picture or film is developed from each image and checked by a technologist and/or radiologist to assess motion, contrast, and positioning (see

---

Figure 3-1. Breast Self-Examination Instruction Card

The Rush Cancer Institute

⚓ RUSH

RUSH-PRESBYTERIAN-ST. LUKE'S
MEDICAL CENTER
1725 West Harrison Street
Chicago, Illinois 60612
(312) 563-2325

Because We Care

MONTHLY BREAST SELF-EXAM

It is important to perform your breast self-exam (BSE) the same time each month, 2-3 days after your period stops or on an appointed day for women who are no longer menstruating.

Before A Mirror

Facing a mirror with arms relaxed, look for changes in the size, shape, or skin of the breast. Changes in appearance may be puckering, dimpling, or an area of redness. Turn to the side to inspect the inner and outer portions of your breast. Repeat with arms raised over the head, with hands pressing on the hips and leaning forward from the waist with breasts suspended.

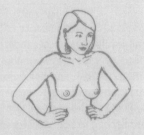

Lying Down

BSE is best performed lying on a bed. Placing a towel beneath the shoulder distributes the breast more evenly. Raise your arm and use the flat pads of the first three fingers to examine your armpit and breast with small circular motions. The area below the collarbone and beside the breastbone should be included.

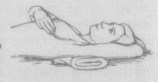

You may choose the circular or up-and-down method. Studies indicate that the up-and-down pattern may result in a more thorough exam. The important thing is to make sure all the breast tissue is examined.

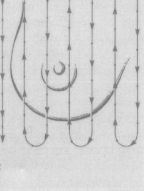

Fingers Flat

Following the pattern you choose, begin at the outermost top edge of the breast and glide the fingers along without lifting your hand away, noticing any lumps or areas of thickness.

Use light, moderate and firm pressure with each overlapping motion to ensure examining all the tissue.

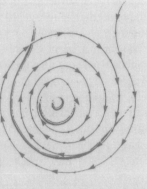

Examine the other breast in the same manner. Lubricating your hand and breast with lotion or powder helps the fingers slide over the skin.

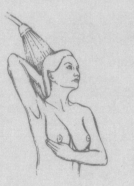

In the Shower

In addition to doing BSE lying down, you may wish to examine yourself in the shower.

This self-exam is not a substitute for periodic examinations by a qualified physician or nurse.

Note. Figure courtesy of Rush Cancer Institute, Rush-Presbyterian-St. Luke's Medical Center. Used with permission.

Figure 3-2). A new type of imaging called *digital mammography* has been developed that processes the images onto a computer (see Figure 3-3). Digital mammography is faster than conventional mammography; the image does not need to be developed because it is transferred directly to the computer screen. Initially, digital imaging was thought to be more accurate because the contrast could be manipulated, thus producing a clearer image (Elmore, Armstrong, Lehman, & Fletcher, 2005). A recent study sponsored by the American College of Radiology (ACR) Imaging Network compared digital to film-screen mammography (Digital Mammography Screening Trial (Pisano et al., 2005). The results indicate that the accuracy of film-screen mammography was similar to that of digital mammography. However, digital imaging was found to be more accurate in women younger than 50, women with radiologically dense breasts, and premenopausal or perimenopausal woman (Pisano et al.). The main drawback for the digital system is the cost. A conventional film-screen system costs approximately $90,000, whereas a digital system is $600,000. The advantages of digital over film-screen mammography are the ability to adjust the image for better definition, easy storage and retrieval, lower radiation exposure than with conventional imaging procedures, and the potential for real-time transmission to and from remote locations.

A screening mammogram is ordered annually for women, usually beginning at age 40, with average risk who are asymptomatic. Annual screening mammography is covered by Medicare and other commercial insurance companies. Medicare has certain parameters regarding annual mammography. The yearly exam must be scheduled after one calendar year

has elapsed, or Medicare will not cover the cost. The films are taken by a technologist, and cases are batched to be read by the radiologist at a later time. The standard mammogram consists of two views of each breast, four in all. One view is a cranial-caudal view that provides an image from top to bottom. The second view not only images the breast but also includes a portion of the pectoralis muscle in order to assess the axillary lymph nodes (see Figure 3-4). This view, the medial-lateral-oblique, is accomplished through a diagonal view of the breast on an angle from the armpit to the lower inner aspect of the breast (ACR, 2004). The primary purpose of a screening mammogram is to identify any new changes in the breast. If a change is detected, a diagnostic mammogram will be recommended to determine whether the change is real or artifactual. Although most cases in which patients are called back for more films result in benign findings, the process takes a significant emotional toll on patients because they often will worry about the potential diagnosis of breast cancer. This anxiety is exacerbated by the fact that most additional studies cannot be performed immediately, and it is not uncommon to wait a week for the additional workup. The financial cost for a diagnostic mammogram is approximately $200, although insurance often will cover it.

Diagnostic Mammography

Women with a history of breast cancer, women at high risk for developing breast cancer (e.g., *BRCA1* or *BRCA2* carriers), or those with a questionable finding on a screening mammogram are candidates for diagnostic mammograms. A diagnostic mammogram is performed in real time; that is, the radiologist looks at each view and determines whether additional views are needed to better evaluate a specific questionable area. The radiologist then meets with the woman immediately after the films are completed and discusses the results. If the area was an artifact or a classic benign finding, annual mammography is recommended. If the result is not completely characteristic for a benign finding but still has a finding of low suspicion, the radiologist will recommend a short-term follow-up with a repeat study in four to six months (see Figure 3-5). Any remaining questionable area usually will require an MRI of the breast and tissue sampling to determine or rule out the possibility of a malignancy (ACR, 2004). ACR uses a rating scale called BI-RADS (Breast Imaging Reporting and Data System). This system has been adopted in Europe and provides standardization for classification of a breast mass. BI-RADS rates the density of breast tissue; the presence of a mass; the shape and border appearance of the mass; the presence, type, and distribution of calcifications (macro or micro); and architectural distortion. It also rates associated findings that further clarify a mass or calcifications, such as axillary adenopathy, skin or nipple retraction, and skin thickening. The presence or absence of abnormal findings is calculated and given a number that ranges from zero (incomplete evaluation, needs more imaging) to six (known cancer) (Obenauer, Hermann, & Grabbe, 2005).

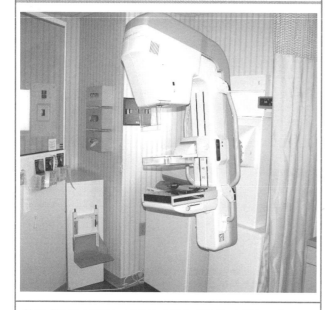

Figure 3-2. Conventional Mammography Machine

Note. Figure courtesy of Peter Jokich, MD, Rush University Medical Center. Used with permission.

Figure 3-3. Digital Mammography Machine

The equipment pictured is the Selenia™ digital mammography system.

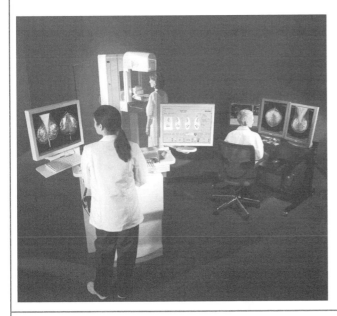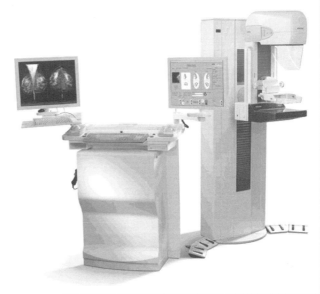

Note. Images courtesy of Hologic, Inc., Bedford, MA. Used with permission.

Figure 3-4. Cranial-Caudal and Medial-Lateral-Oblique Views of Mammogram

The image on the left is a cranial-caudal bilateral view, and the medial-lateral-oblique (MLO) view is on the right. Note the inclusion of the pectoralis muscle on the MLO view.

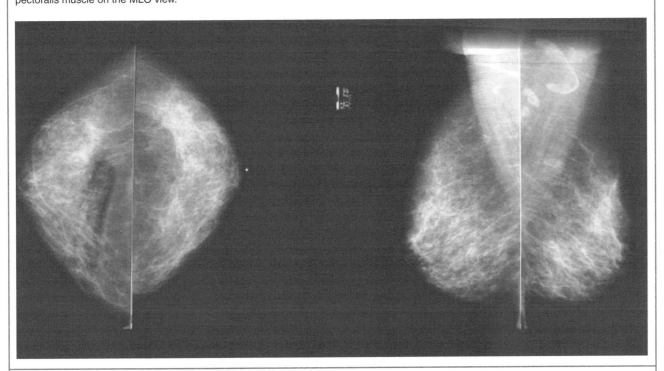

Note. Figure courtesy of Peter Jokich, MD, Rush University Medical Center. Used with permission.

Figure 3-5. Radiographic View of a Suspicious Breast Lesion

This is a magnified view of a suspicious lesion that was a cancer on biopsy. Note the irregular shape and spicules extending out from the lesion.

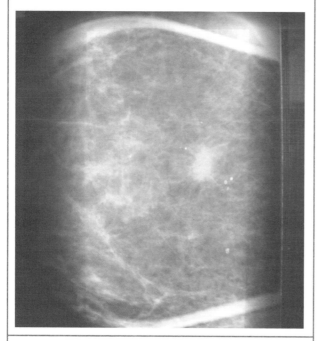

Note. Figure courtesy of Peter Jokich, MD, Rush University Medical Center. Used with permission.

Ultrasound

Ultrasound is not routinely used as a screening tool, as the sensitivity and specificity are inferior to mammography. Ultrasound is useful as an adjunct to mammography to determine whether a lesion is a cyst, a complicated cyst (fluid with cellular debris), or a solid mass. Ultrasound also is used to identify a presumed mass in young (< 35) women with very dense breasts or in pregnant or nursing women and to evaluate a suspected implant rupture (see Figures 3-6 and 3-7).

Magnetic Resonance Imaging

A breast MRI also is known as magnetic resonance mammography (MRM). MRM can be an excellent but expensive diagnostic tool for finding extremely small breast cancers or recurrences, occult breast cancers, and suspicious abnormalities in high-risk women with dense breasts and for delineating the level of suspicion for multiple questionable breast abnormalities found on mammogram. It also is often used to assess implant rupture and may be helpful in the staging of newly diagnosed breast cancers (Van Goethem et al., 2004). Preparation for the study involves an IV injection

of radioactive contrast. The radiologist examines the image for the level of enhancement within the breast that reflects changes in blood flow, capillary permeability, and extracellular volume as well as the timing of the enhancement (Smith & Andreopoulou, 2004). Malignant areas will enhance faster and appear brighter. Figures 3-8 and 3-9 are examples of how MRI changed the treatment plan for a woman with a known breast cancer. This woman presented with a diagnosed invasive lobular cancer in the right breast. Because this woman had markedly dense breasts, a bilateral MRI was ordered to exclude any other suspicious areas in the right breast and to evaluate the left breast. The MRI confirmed the presence of the right breast cancer and also indicated a suspicious enhancing area in the left breast that was a confirmed cancer on biopsy. Thus, the MRI assisted in the early detection of an unknown cancer in the left breast. The woman had bilateral mastectomies. MRI has a high sensitivity rate (95%–100%), but this modality has limitations (i.e., its ability to identify microcalcifications is not always reliable, and benign lesions may produce false-positive results and unnecessary biopsies) (Smith & Andreopoulou, 2004). Premenopausal women experience significant changes in breast volume, breast parenchyma pattern, and water content during the menstrual cycle. Conducting the MRI study at the appropriate point in the cycle minimizes the possibility of false-positive results (Muller-Schimpfle, Ohmenhauser, Stoll, Dietz, & Claussen, 1997). Therefore, women need to time the study with their menstrual cycle, between the sixth and sixteenth day (Rankin, 2000), which often postpones the test for weeks. Also, a woman may not be a candidate for MRI because of claustrophobia and/or implanted medical devices. At this time, MRI does not have

Figure 3-6. Ultrasound of the Breast

This ultrasound shows the classic presentation for a fluid-filled cyst. The borders are smooth; it is wider than it is long; and the two tails marginate the lesion.

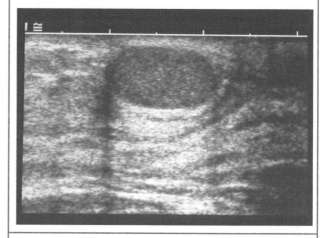

Note. Figure courtesy of Peter Jokich, MD, Rush University Medical Center. Used with permission.

adequate specificity (37%–97%) to be a useful screening tool (Orel, Schnall, LiVolsi, & Troupin, 1994), and insurance companies are reluctant to pay for MRI without documentation of specific medical necessity.

Figure 3-7. Ultrasound of the Breast Showing Indeterminate Nodule

This is an indeterminate nodule that will warrant biopsy. It is longer than it is wide. It has irregular borders and is not characteristic of a cyst.

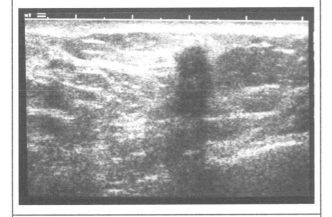

Note. Figure courtesy of Peter Jokich, MD, Rush University Medical Center. Used with permission.

Figure 3-8. Magnetic Resonance Imaging (MRI) View of Breast Cancer

This MRI image is the known cancer.

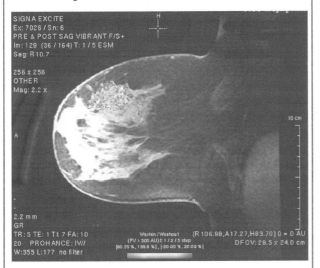

Note. Figure courtesy of Peter Jokich, MD, Rush University Medical Center. Used with permission.

Figure 3-9. Magnetic Resonance Imaging View of Bilateral Breast Cancer

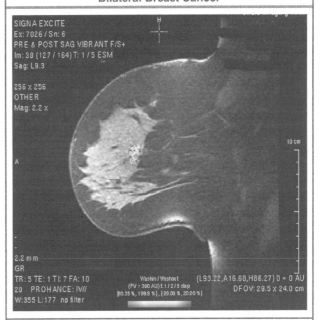

Note. Figure courtesy of Peter Jokich, MD, Rush University Medical Center. Used with permission.

Positron-Emission Tomography

Positron-emission tomography (PET) has been approved for use with many cancers and often is used to identify suspected cancers when other tests are normal. In addition, it is used to target very early-stage cancers or small metastases of approximately 5–8 mm, smaller than is visible with other imaging modalities. Prior to the actual PET scan, the patient is given an IV injection of radioactive glucose, which is used because cancer cells will absorb glucose faster than normal cells. The radiologist looks for areas of increased metabolic intensity that are referred to as *hot spots.* MRI is the usual diagnostic tool for breast lesions; PET will be used only if a diagnosis cannot be made using other techniques.

Positron-Emission Tomography/ Computed Tomography

A new imaging modality that appears promising is PET combined with CT. This method allows a more accurate assessment of the molecular uptake, thereby reducing false-positive interpretations. Usually CT is not used to diagnose breast cancers but rather to provide information regarding potential lung and liver metastases, important information used for staging. The hope is that PET/CT will improve the ability to accurately stage breast cancers preoperatively and will improve the diagnosis of primary tumors through improved characterizations (Scheidhauer, Walter, & Seemann, 2004; Zangheri et al., 2004).

Breast Biopsy

A new abnormality that has been identified either through mammography or by palpation often will need tissue sampling. This can be accomplished using various tools and decision strategies. The biopsy spectrum ranges from least invasive to more invasive, and the type of biopsy selected often depends on the suspicion and location of the finding (see Figure 3-10). The biopsy options for low to moderately suspicious findings are fine-needle aspiration (FNA) and core needle sampling that is guided by mammography (stereotactic), ultrasound, or palpation. Highly suspicious findings usually are excised.

Fine-Needle Aspiration

FNA is used when there is a palpable finding most consistent with a cyst. Breast cysts typically feel rubbery and are mobile. The healthcare provider uses a small-gauge needle (approximately 22 gauge) with a 10–20 cc syringe to pierce the mass and withdraw the fluid. Cystic contents usually are yellow to muddy colored, and the fluid can vary from thin to very turbid. If the patient has a history of benign cyst aspirations, the provider may not send the contents to cytology each time, providing that the fluid is consistent with prior aspirations. However, the patient should always have a return appointment in one to two months to confirm that the cyst has not refilled. If the area has refilled, another FNA may be done with the contents sent to cytology, or excision may be recommended (Di Maggio, 2004).

Core Needle Biopsy

Core biopsy provides a more definitive diagnosis than FNA, and many providers choose this method because a core of tissue yields a larger number of cells to examine, thereby reducing false-negative rates. Core biopsies for palpable masses are easily performed in the office. A larger gauge needle (14 gauge) is inserted into a spring-loaded device. After the area is anesthetized with a local anesthetic, the physician or advanced practice nurse pulls the trigger on the device that directs the needle into the mass. One or multiple core samples can be obtained (Di Maggio, 2004). The patient should be cautioned that a loud "pop" will be heard and not to be startled. The core or cores then are sent to pathology.

Stereotactic Biopsy

Radiology-assisted biopsies are most frequently done for nonpalpable abnormalities. The radiologist will recommend the approach that will best target the area in question, either stereotactic or ultrasound-guided. Stereotactic biopsy is performed using a specially designed table. This table is equipped with an opening through which the breast is suspended (see Figure 3-11). The mammographic equipment is

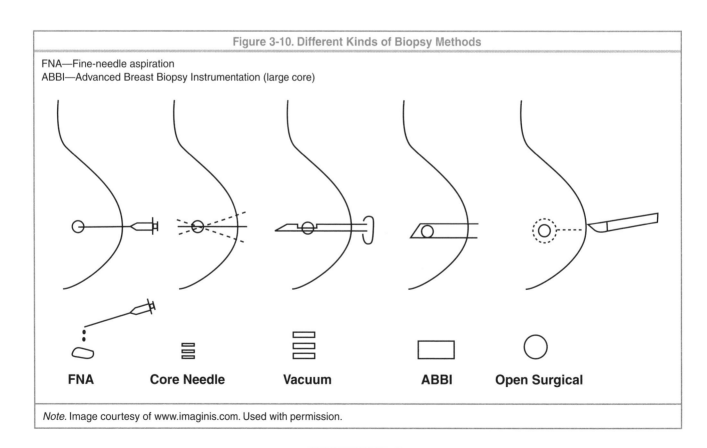

Figure 3-10. Different Kinds of Biopsy Methods

FNA—Fine-needle aspiration
ABBI—Advanced Breast Biopsy Instrumentation (large core)

FNA   **Core Needle**   **Vacuum**   **ABBI**   **Open Surgical**

Note. Image courtesy of www.imaginis.com. Used with permission.

Figure 3-11. Stereotactic Biopsy Performed in the Prone Position

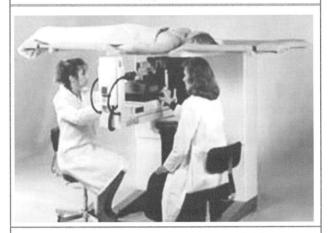

Note. Image courtesy of www.imaginis.com. Used with permission.

located beneath the table in line with the breast. The breast is compressed, and the radiologist or surgeon targets the area by obtaining a pair of images at 15° angles to calculate the exact coordinates (Kepple et al., 2004). The biopsy area then is localized with a 1 cm x 1 cm grid. The needle apparatus

(14 gauge or 8- or 11-gauge vacuum-assisted device) is lined up with the grid to ensure that the correct area is targeted (Kepple et al.). After the area is anesthetized using a local anesthetic, several core samples are obtained and sent to pathology. More than one area of the breast may be sampled. Stereotactic biopsy also may be performed in a sitting position using different equipment. This position is seldom used because of the possibility of the patient fainting. Stereotactic biopsies are recommended for abnormalities of moderate suspicion (see Figures 3-12, 3-13, and 3-14).

The radiologist may leave a small titanium clip at the biopsy site following a stereotactic biopsy. A woman with a large tumor may elect to have neoadjuvant chemotherapy to shrink the tumor and improve the surgical cosmetic outcome for later surgery. In some instances, the tumor disappears, and the target site is lost if breast preservation has been planned. The clip assists the radiologist in targeting the area of the tumor so that an adequate surgical excision can take place. A clip also may be left when calcifications are being targeted for a large-gauge needle biopsy or a wire-localized biopsy. If the pathology indicates a cancer, the area can be reexcised using the clip as a guide. The standard of care is to take a post-biopsy clip placement film to ensure the proper location. A serious complication of using a clip is migration of the clip immediately or at a later time. A new mammogram

Figure 3-12. Stereotactic Needle Placement Into Mass

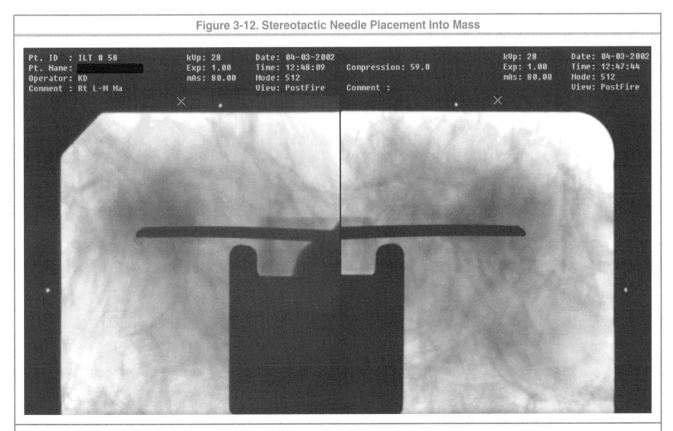

Note. Figure courtesy of Peter Jokich, MD, Rush University Medical Center. Used with permission.

Figure 3-13. Mammographic Cancer, Medial-Lateral-Oblique View

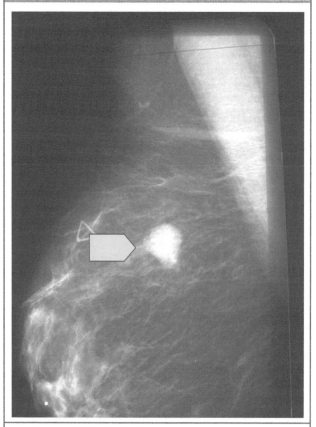

Note. Figure courtesy of Peter Jokich, MD, Rush University Medical Center. Used with permission.

Figure 3-14. Mammographic Cancer, Cranial-Caudal View

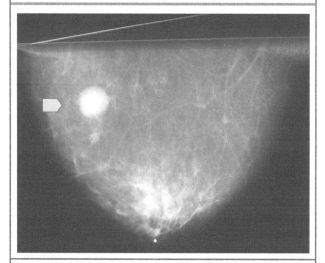

Note. Figure courtesy of Peter Jokich, MD, Rush University Medical Center. Used with permission.

and a careful assessment of the clip placement must be made prior to evaluating any patient for surgery (Esserman, Cura, & DaCosta, 2004; Gordon, 2004).

Ultrasound-Guided Biopsy

Ultrasound-guided biopsy is performed using either a biopsy gun or a vacuum-assisted device. The radiologist or surgeon locates the mass after reviewing the mammogram and ultrasound to ensure that the area correlates with both images. After a small incision is made, the abnormality is located using freehand technique with ultrasound guidance. The needle is inserted into the lesion, and samples are obtained. The sample cores then are sent to pathology (see Figure 3-15).

Wire-Localized Biopsy

A wire-localized biopsy uses breast imaging to target an area in preparation for surgical removal. A radiologist who recommends an image-guided biopsy is assured that the wire tip can be accurately placed through or alongside the lesion. A hookwire most often is used as the guide because the hook helps to keep the wire in place. Wire placement for nonpalpable lesions can be accomplished through a stereotactic method or using ultrasonography. Multiple wires can be placed either for multiple lesions or to delineate the borders of a large mass. After placement is confirmed through ultrasound or mammography, the patient is sent to the operating room with the placement films. The surgeon uses the films and guide wire to remove the target area. Once the mass is removed, the specimen is sent to mammography, where a film is taken to confirm that the area in question has been completely excised.

Excisional Biopsy

An excisional biopsy is performed when a surgeon is confident that the area in question is palpable and no other suspicious masses are identified. Scheduling the patient for an excisional biopsy indicates a reasonable suspicion that the mass may be malignant. The surgeon will make an effort to excise the area completely with a margin of normal tissue around the specimen. Often the surgeon will ink the edges of the specimen with different colors to indicate the orientation and provide histopathologic information if the lesion is malignant. The surgeon will choose to use local anesthesia or IV sedation for the procedure. Few patients need general anesthesia.

All surgical procedures, even if minor, are not without risk. The complications for breast biopsy are bleeding and infection that impairs wound healing and affects cosmesis. Nurses should instruct patients to keep the biopsy site clean and dry and to call the healthcare provider if there are any signs of bleeding or infection. Steri-Strip™ (3M Health Care, St. Paul, MN) adhesive skin closures may be used to close the biopsy wound. Patient should not bathe until these strips

Figure 3-15. Ultrasound-Guided Biopsy Technique

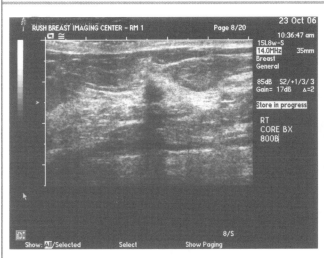

Abnormal mass on ultrasound with shadowing below

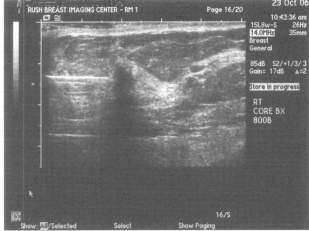

Needle approaching the center of the mass before biopsy

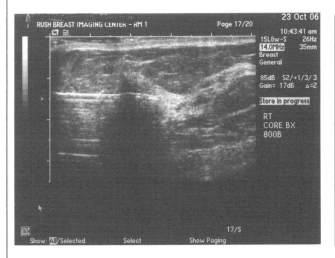

Needle through the mass after biopsy

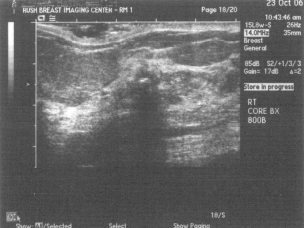

Same mass, looking straight on after removing the needle to ensure the needle was placed directly in the mass. The small white needle track was directly in the center of the mass.

Note. Figures courtesy of Kambiz Dowlat, MD, Rush University Medical Center. Used with permission.

fall off. The recommendation for showering or bathing may differ among surgeons, and specific instructions need to be communicated to patients.

Nurses will discuss the few complications associated with an excisional breast biopsy prior to the procedure. The pain usually is controlled by acetaminophen or acetaminophen with codeine. Nonsteroidal anti-inflammatory drugs are not recommended because of associated bleeding. Women should be instructed to monitor for and report typical signs of infection, including drainage, redness, or fever. Many surgeons prefer that a woman wear a bra continuously for the first week

to provide additional support and protection for the biopsy site. Nurses providing postoperative education should check on the preferences of each particular surgeon. Occasionally a seroma may develop, but it will reabsorb in a few weeks. The area quickly heals within a few weeks with a minimal scar.

Tertiary Prevention

Tertiary cancer prevention includes the ongoing surveillance and early detection of second primary malignancies and other treatment-related complications in cancer survivors. Tertiary prevention is an emerging role for oncology nurses, especially with regard to women being treated for breast cancer. The care and rehabilitation of women with breast cancer should include strategies to promote the early detection of second primary cancers, as well as strategies to reduce the risk factors for second malignancies and other long-term complications such as osteoporosis or lymphedema.

Although women are living longer after an initial diagnosis of cancer, environmental and lifestyle risk factors, treatment modalities, and the underlying genetic basis of breast cancer predispose many breast cancer survivors to developing second primary malignancies. Long-term side effects from chemotherapy that require assessment and early management include cardiotoxicity, neuropathy, ototoxicity, and renal failure. Other survivors experience complications related to surgery or radiotherapy, including paresthesias and lymphedema (see Chapter 8). Survivors also are at risk for psychosocial problems that stem from the effects of the diagnosis and/or treatment (see Chapter 9). Each of these potential problems needs to be addressed by healthcare professionals with a plan for assessment of risk, prevention, detection, and early intervention.

Definition of Second Primary Cancers

A second primary cancer is defined as the occurrence of a new cancer that is biologically independent of the original primary cancer (Neugut, Meadows, & Robinson, 1999). Second cancers may occur because of a genetic predisposition to a second cancer. Treatment with chemotherapeutic agents, especially alkylating agents, is another etiologic source. These agents have been associated with an increased risk of developing hematologic malignancies. Treatment with radiation therapy also has been associated with second primary cancers. Still other second cancers probably occur as a result of random chance. Understanding the etiology, risk factors, and subsequent development of a second cancer ultimately should result in improved screening and surveillance for survivors.

Historical Perspectives in Tertiary Prevention

The observation of multiple primary cancers was first reported in 1889 (Neugut et al., 1999). Initial criteria for classifying multiple primary cancers were first reported in the 1930s. Despite these published reports, little attention has been directed toward screening for second primary cancers. No large, prospective, randomized trials have evaluated the efficacy of monitoring patients closely to detect second cancers (Gallassi, 2000). Only recently has attention been focused on the medical and psychosocial needs of those who are long-term survivors of malignancy.

The National Cancer Institute established the Office of Cancer Survivorship in 1996. A major focus of this office is disseminating information on the risks for developing second primary cancers. As people with cancer live longer after the initial diagnosis and experience high levels of functioning after treatment, it is becoming increasingly important to provide preventive therapies and screening for the late consequences of the first diagnosis.

Incidence of Second Primary Cancers in Breast Cancer Survivors

Currently, the population of cancer survivors living longer periods of time after their initial cancer diagnosis is ever-growing. Recent estimates, according to the ACS (2005), suggest that there are more than 2.3 million women alive with a history of breast cancer. This is largely a result of improved earlier detection of malignancy and the development of more effective therapies. These improvements in treatment have created a new population of patients. The needs of these patients are unique, and healthcare providers are challenged to identify risks, detect problems early, and provide care for these patients. Tertiary prevention is aimed at this population.

Etiology of Second Cancers in Breast Cancer Survivors

The exact etiology of a second primary cancer is not always clear. Many of these cancers are thought to be treatment related. Others are related to environmental exposures. It has been recognized for some time that an individual who had cancer in one paired organ is at increased risk for developing a second cancer in the contralateral unaffected organ, especially in the case of breast cancer. The underlying premise is that whatever predisposed a person to develop the first cancer would also predispose the patient to develop the second cancer in the contralateral organ. Women with breast cancer have been reported to have three to four times the risk of developing a second breast cancer in the unaffected breast (Armstrong, Eisen, & Weber, 2000). The overall relative risk for developing a second breast cancer in the contralateral breast is estimated to be 15% (Daly & Costalas, 1999). The risk is higher in women with a family history of breast cancer, women diagnosed at an early age, and women with a history of lobular breast cancer.

Genetic Predisposition

Research advances from the Human Genome Project have demonstrated that as many as 10% of patients diagnosed with breast cancer have a germ-line hereditary predisposition to developing a second malignancy, especially with mutations in *BRCA1/2*. Genetic predisposition also plays an important etiologic role in the development of second malignancies. Many of the hereditary cancers are inherited in an autosomal dominant fashion. Germ-line mutations result in the mutated gene in all embryonic cells (the "first hit"). Further exposure to carcinogens results in loss of the second normal allele and subsequent development of cancer (the "second hit"). Thus, a germ-line mutation in all embryonic cells results in a subsequent increase in the risk of multiple cancers. A commonly occurring example is second breast and ovarian cancers, which are associated with *BRCA1* and *BRCA2* mutations. For those women with a known mutation in *BRCA1/2,* the cumulative risk is estimated to be 65% (Armstrong et al., 2000). Women who are younger at the diagnosis of their first primary breast cancer tend to have a shorter interval between malignancies.

Ovarian cancer is another common second malignancy seen in breast cancer survivors. It is estimated to occur in 5%–26% of breast cancer survivors, with a relative risk of 1.2–2.4 (Daly & Costalas, 1999; Schrag, Kuntz, Garber, & Week, 2000). The risk for developing an ovarian cancer after breast cancer often is related to mutations in *BRCA1/2.*

Second Primary Cancers as a Consequence of Treatment

It is only recently that cancer survivors have begun to understand that the very treatment that eradicated their first cancer often places them at risk for a subsequent second primary cancer. This is particularly true of radiation therapy, chemotherapy, and hormonal therapy. The use of combined therapies probably has a synergistic effect and further increases the risk (Neugut, Rheingold, & Meadows, 2004).

To date, most of the second primary cancers that are associated with radiotherapy for childhood cancers have been bone and soft tissue sarcomas and carcinomas of the thyroid gland, breast, and skin (Inskip, 1999). Factors that influence the development of second malignancies include the total dose and number of fractions, the source of energy, combinations of chemotherapeutic agents, and age at exposure (i.e., younger age increases the risk) (Rodriguez & Ash, 1996). These second cancers can occur many years to decades after the initial therapy. The organ at risk depends on the site where the radiation was delivered and how well the surrounding tissue was protected by shielding (Neugut et al., 2004). Risk may be increased in women who have received radiotherapy because of scatter radiation exposure; however, the magnitude of the risk is unknown (Neugut et al., 1999). Although data are limited in a trial of radiation therapy after lumpectomy as compared to mastectomy, results showed that there was no increased risk of second malignancies in the contralateral breast in women receiving radiation therapy (Obedian, Fischer, & Haffty, 2000).

Chemotherapeutic agents also have been associated with second primary cancers, especially hematologic malignancies. These have been reported with alkylating agents, vinca alkaloids, antimetabolites, and antitumor antibiotics (Neugut et al., 1999). Alkylating agents, in particular, have been associated with leukemias, myelodysplastic syndrome, sarcomas, and bladder cancer. These malignancies can occur within several years of the treatment (Neugut et al., 2004). (Those leukemias that occur as a consequence of treatment tend to be extremely resistant to chemotherapy when compared to de novo leukemia.) Cyclophosphamide has been associated with the development of bladder cancer (Neugut et al., 1999).

Tamoxifen frequently is used in the treatment of estrogen-dependent breast cancer. Although most clinicians use tamoxifen for only five years, the risk of endometrial cancer is increased in these women (Neugut et al., 2004). The risk is higher in those with other risk factors for the development of endometrial cancer.

Screening for Second Malignancies

Women who have been successfully treated for one breast cancer need to be informed about the risk of a second breast cancer and have appropriate screening. In general, this includes annual mammography, biannual CBE, regular self-examination, and prompt management of any change in the breast exam. For those with a known mutation in *BRCA1/2,* the efficacy of prophylactic surgery can be discussed. Prophylactic mastectomy reduces the risk of breast cancer by approximately 95% but is a major surgery with significant psychosocial issues (Schrag et al., 2000). Similarly, prophylactic oophorectomy may reduce the risk of breast cancer by as much as 50% in people with a known mutation in *BRCA1/2* (Schrag et al.).

For those women with a diagnosis of breast cancer who still have a uterus, an annual gynecologic examination is indicated. Women should be instructed regarding the early symptoms of endometrial cancer, which require prompt reporting to a healthcare provider. These include abnormal spotting, bleeding, or discharge, especially in postmenopausal women (ACS, 2007; Gallassi, 2000).

The early detection of ovarian cancer presents a significant challenge to healthcare providers. At present, no evidence exists to suggest that ultrasound, pelvic examination, or CA-125 testing decreases the morbidity and mortality associated with ovarian cancer (Schrag et al., 2000). Women need to be instructed on the limitations of these screening examinations and informed that there are few early signs or symptoms associated with ovarian cancer. For those with a known mutation in *BRCA1/2,* a prophylactic oophorectomy may be a prudent prevention strategy.

After primary treatment for breast cancer, treatment-related second primary cancers may occur. These most often include hematologic malignancies. The risk of leukemia is estimated to be 1.29% at 10 years after chemotherapy (Daly & Costalas, 1999). Two secondary leukemia syndromes have been described. Leukemias that are associated with exposure to alkylating agents may arise five to seven years after treatment, especially in regimens using cyclophosphamide. They frequently are preceded by a myelodysplastic syndrome. Anthracyclines increase the risk for developing secondary leukemias six months to five years after therapy. There are no methods of screening for these malignancies, although they should be considered in the evaluation of any woman in whom cytopenia develops after the treatment of breast cancer. This risk is relatively small when considering the benefits of chemotherapy.

Psychosocial Concerns

Anxiety and fear about cancer recurrence have been documented to be concerns in long-term survivors of cancer. Little is known about how much survivors realize they are at risk for a second primary cancer and how fearful cancer survivors are of developing one. This problem has received little attention. Every cancer survivor has a different risk of developing a second primary cancer. Clearly, efforts need to be made to better understand patients' perceptions and anxiety related to this risk.

Information about a second risk for cancer should be communicated in a nonthreatening way. Survivors need to understand that their prognosis is actually excellent when concern shifts to screening for second cancers. Healthcare providers should articulate that screening and prevention recommendations are being given to detect cancers early and further increase long-term survival and quality of life. Just as assessment of risk for second malignancies should occur in long-term follow-up, assessment of overall adjustment and quality of life should occur. For patients having difficulty adjusting to long-term survival, further intervention with a health professional with expertise in psychosocial management sometimes may be indicated.

Implications for Nurses

Healthcare providers who work with long-term survivors of cancer are well-suited to provide the comprehensive risk assessments and education that patients need regarding development of a second cancer. The process of selecting appropriate screening strategies begins with an individual risk assessment. Each cancer survivor should be considered individually. Risk factors should be documented and interpreted for the patient. The risk factor assessment should guide the selection of appropriate screening strategies.

Specific screening guidelines for second primary malignancies are vague. Currently, screening for second cancers is similar to screening for first cancers, such as following the guidelines for screening in asymptomatic persons published by ACS (2007) and a variety of other groups. These guidelines need to be tailored to the individual risks of the cancer survivor.

Cancer survivors also need to be educated about signs and symptoms of second malignancies that should be reported. This education helps to make patients better advocates for themselves and more involved in their care. Furthermore,

appropriate self-examination technique should be discussed with long-term survivors of cancer. Women should be taught proper BSE practices during the course of a professional examination. This enables women to best learn self-exam and better appreciate their own anatomic landmarks. Women who have had breast surgery should be taught how to examine the affected breast and what constitutes a normal and abnormal finding.

In addition, all survivors probably can benefit from knowledge of how to properly examine their skin. Many survivors have received photosensitizing chemotherapy and need to know how to protect their skin from further damage and how to examine for changes that might signal an early skin cancer.

Regular follow-up appointments provide an opportunity for continuity of care and to assess for long-term adjustment to the cancer diagnosis. Efforts should be made to help survivors to become active participants in their long-term follow-up. This is an opportunity to teach not only survivors about healthy lifestyles and the importance of cancer screening but also their family members. After treatment is completed, the stress level of patients and families is often lower, and they may be more receptive to this teaching.

Although the exact incidence and etiology of all second primary cancers is not completely clear, efforts should be made to identify and monitor individuals at higher risk in a consistent manner after cancer treatment completion. A recent study suggests that few healthcare providers consistently assess and recommend screening to detect second cancers. In a study of 321 oncology nurses caring for long-term survivors, the screening activities most consistently performed were mammography, professional breast examination, and Pap smear (Mahon, Spies, & Williams, 2000). Screening activities that were least likely to be recommended included colorectal cancer screening and endometrial biopsy, as well as screening for osteoporosis. These researchers also noted that when screening is recommended, it is most likely to be initiated by a physician. Because of the time that nurses spend with patients and the educational opportunity associated with these tests, nurses need to be more proactive in initiating screening and prevention strategies.

One way to ensure that screening is carried out is to develop protocols, which can be implemented at the institution. Protocols may help to ensure that recommendations are consistently discussed and recommended, especially in the realm of prevention. Protocols may include educational materials, including written materials, visual diagrams, anatomic models, and videos, and computer-aided instruction to supplement the education.

Conclusion

Prevention and early diagnosis strategies have changed dramatically in the past decade. Mammography has evolved into a recommended and accepted study for early detection of breast cancer. That has been evident through the decrease in breast cancer mortality despite slight increases in incidence. MRI of the breast has proved to be an important diagnostic tool for women with an occult breast cancer due to tissue density and other factors, as well as BRCA mutation carriers who choose close surveillance over prophylactic mastectomy. Other more-sensitive tools will continue to be developed in the future, and genetic testing will expand to include many other cancers. Nurses may understandably feel challenged by new technology and genetic advances because patients will expect them to be familiar with the intricacies and rationale for new imaging studies and to provide education regarding their cancer risk based on personal and/or family history. This task will not be easy, as nurses often do not have time to attend outside educational programs, but educational alternatives may include taking online courses and scheduling in-services within the institution.

References

American Academy of Family Physicians. (2000, August). *Screening yourself for breast cancer.* Retrieved July 24, 2006, from http://www.aafp.org/afp/20000801/605ph.html

American Cancer Society. (2005). *Breast cancer facts and figures, 2005–2006.* Atlanta, GA: Author.

American Cancer Society. (2007). *Cancer facts and figures, 2007.* Atlanta, GA: Author.

American College of Radiology. (2004, October). *ACR practice guideline for the performance of screening mammography.* Retrieved July 25, 2006, from http://www.acr.org/s_acr/bin.asp?CID=549&DID=12281&DOC=FILE.pdf

Armstrong, K., Eisen, A., & Weber, B. (2000). Assessing the risk of breast cancer. *New England Journal of Medicine, 342,* 564–571.

Assikis, V.J., Neven, P., Jordan, V.C., & Vegote, I. (1996). A realistic clinical perspective of tamoxifen and endometrial carcinogenesis. *European Journal of Cancer, 32A,* 1464–1476.

Baxter, N., & Canadian Task Force on Preventive Health Care. (2001). Preventive health care, 2001 update: Should women be routinely taught breast self-examination to screen for breast cancer? *Canadian Medical Association Journal, 164,* 1837–1846.

Bigby, J., & Holmes, M.D. (2005). Disparities across the breast cancer continuum. *Cancer Causes and Control, 16,* 35–44.

Bird, R.E., Wallace, T.W., & Yankaskas, B.C. (1992). Analysis of cancers missed at screening mammography. *Radiology, 184,* 613–617.

Burke, C. (2005). Endometrial cancer and tamoxifen. *Clinical Journal of Oncology Nursing, 9,* 247–249.

Chalela, J.A., Merino, J.G., & Warach, S. (2004). Update on stroke. *Current Opinion in Neurology, 17,* 447–451.

Cheng, E., Myers, L., Wolf, S., Shatin, D., Cui, X.P., Ellison, G., et al. (2001). Mobility impairments and use of preventive services in women with multiple sclerosis: Observational study. *BMJ, 323,* 968–969.

Chlebowski, R.T. (2002). Breast cancer risk reduction: Strategies for women at increased risk. *Annual Review of Medicine, 53,* 519–540.

Daly, M.B., & Costalas, J. (1999). Breast cancer. In A.I. Neugut, A.T. Meadows, & E. Robinson (Eds.), *Multiple primary cancers* (pp. 303–317). Philadelphia: Lippincott Williams & Wilkins.

Di Maggio, C. (2004). State of the art of current modalities for the diagnosis of breast lesions. *European Journal of Nuclear Medicine and Molecular Imaging, 31*(Suppl. 1), S56–S69.

Donnelly, R., Hinwood, D., & London, N.J. (2000). ABC of arterial and venous disease. Non-invasive methods of arterial and venous assessment. *BMJ, 320,* 698–701.

Dowdy, S.C., Stefanek, M., & Hartmann, L.C. (2004). Surgical risk reduction: Prophylactic salpingo-oophorectomy and prophylactic mastectomy. *American Journal of Obstetrics and Gynecology, 191,* 1113–1123.

Duggan, C., Marriott, K., Edwards, R., & Cuzick, J. (2003). Inherited and acquired risk factors for venous thromboembolic disease among women taking tamoxifen to prevent breast cancer. *Journal of Clinical Oncology, 21,* 3588–3593.

Eisen, A., Rebbeck, T.R., Wood, W.C., & Weber, B.L. (2000). Prophylactic surgery in women with a hereditary predisposition to breast and ovarian cancer. *Journal of Clinical Oncology, 18,* 1980–1995.

Elmore, J.G., Armstrong, K., Lehman, C.D., & Fletcher, S.W. (2005). Screening for breast cancer. *JAMA, 293,* 1245–1256.

Esserman, L.E., Cura, M.A., & DaCosta, D. (2004). Recognizing pitfalls in early and late migration of clip markers after imaging-guided directional vacuum-assisted biopsy. *Radiographics, 21,* 147–156.

Fisher, B., Costantino, J.P., Wickerham, D.L., Redmond, C.K., Kavanah, M., Cronin, W.M., et al. (1998). Tamoxifen for prevention of breast cancer: Report of the National Surgical Adjuvant Breast and Bowel Project P-1 Study. *Journal of the National Cancer Institute, 90,* 1371–1388.

Fisher, B., Dignam, J., Wolmark, N., DeCillis, A., Emir, B., Wickerham, D.L., et al. (1997). Tamoxifen and chemotherapy for lymph node-negative, estrogen receptor-positive breast cancer. *Journal of the National Cancer Institute, 19,* 1673–1682.

Fisher, B., Dignam, J., Wolmark, N., Wickerham, D.L., Fisher, E.R., Mamounas, E., et al. (1999). Tamoxifen in treatment of intraductal breast cancer: National Surgical Adjuvant Breast and Bowel Project B-24 randomised controlled trial. *Lancet, 353,* 1993–2000.

Fisher, B., Redmond, C., Brown, A., Fisher, E.R., Wolmark, N., Bowman, D., et al. (1986). Adjuvant chemotherapy with and without tamoxifen in the treatment of primary breast cancer: 5-year results from the National Surgical Adjuvant Breast and Bowel Project Trial. *Journal of Clinical Oncology, 4,* 459–471.

Fisher, B., Redmond, C., Brown, A., Wolmark, N., Wittliff, J., Fisher, E.R., et al. (1981). Treatment of primary breast cancer with chemotherapy and tamoxifen. *New England Journal of Medicine, 305,* 1–6.

Fisher, B., Redmond, C., Legault-Poisson, S., Dimitrov, N.V., Brown, A.M., Wickerham, D.L., et al. (1990). Postoperative chemotherapy and tamoxifen compared with tamoxifen alone in the treatment of positive-node breast cancer patients aged 50 years and older with tumors responsive to tamoxifen: Results from the National Surgical Adjuvant Breast and Bowel Project B-16. *Journal of Clinical Oncology, 8,* 1005–1018.

Fisher, B., Redmond, C., Wickerham, D.L., Wolmark, N., Bowman, D., Couture, J., et al. (1989). Systemic therapy in patients with node-negative breast cancer. A commentary based on two National Surgical Adjuvant Breast and Bowel Project (NSABP) clinical trials. *Annals of Internal Medicine, 111,* 703–712.

Friedman, Z.Y. (1998). Recent advances in understanding the molecular mechanisms of tamoxifen action. *Cancer Investigation, 16,* 391–396.

Frizzell, J.P. (2005). Acute stroke: Pathophysiology, diagnosis, and treatment. *AACN Clinical Issues, 16,* 421–440.

Gail, M.H., Brinton, L.A., Byar, D.P., Corle, D.K., Green, S.B., Schairer, C., et al. (1989). Projecting individualized probabilities of developing breast cancer for white females who are being examined annually. *Journal of the National Cancer Institute, 81,* 1879–1886.

Gallassi, A. (2000). Follow-up care of cancer survivors. *Lippincott's Primary Care Practice, 4,* 359–373.

Gasco, M., Argusti, A., Bonanni, B., & Decensi, A. (2005). SERMs in chemoprevention of breast cancer. *European Journal of Cancer, 41,* 1980–1989.

Gordon, P. (2004). An alternative clip-marking method for use after 14-gauge large core needle biopsy of the breast. *Canadian Association of Radiologists Journal, 55,* 75–78.

Hackshaw, A.K., & Paul, E.A. (2003). Breast self-examination and death from breast cancer: A meta-analysis. *British Journal of Cancer, 88,* 1047–1053.

Hartmann, L.C., Degnim, A., & Schaid, D.J. (2004). Prophylactic mastectomy for BRCA1/2 carriers: Progress and more questions. *Journal of Clinical Oncology, 22,* 981–983.

Hartmann, L.C., Sellers, T.A., Schaid, D.J., Frank, T.S., Soderberg, C.L., Sitta, D.L., et al. (2001). Efficacy of bilateral prophylactic mastectomy in BRCA1 and BRCA2 gene mutation carriers. *Journal of the National Cancer Institute, 93,* 1633–1637.

Holmberg, L., Ekbom, A., Calle, E., Mokdad, A., & Byers, T. (1997). Breast cancer mortality in relation to self-reported use of breast self-examination. A cohort study of 450,000 women. *Breast Cancer Research and Treatment, 43,* 137–140.

Holmes, C.E., & Muss, H.B. (2003). Diagnosis and treatment of breast cancer in the elderly. *CA: A Cancer Journal for Clinicians, 53,* 227–244.

Humphrey, L.L., Helfand, M., Chan, B.K., & Woolf, S.H. (2002). Breast cancer screening: A summary of the evidence for the U.S. Preventive Services Task Force. *Annals of Internal Medicine, 137*(5 Pt. 1), 347–360.

Inskip, P.D. (1999). Second cancers following radiotherapy. In A.I. Neugut, A.T. Meadows, & E. Robinson (Eds.), *Multiple primary cancers* (pp. 91–135). Philadelphia: Lippincott Williams & Wilkins.

Jemal, A., Siegel, R., Ward, E., Murray, T., Xu, J., & Thun, M.J. (2007). Cancer statistics, 2007. *CA: A Cancer Journal for Clinicians, 57,* 43–66.

Kepple, J., Van Zee, K.J., Dowlatshahi, K., Henry-Tillman, R.S., Israel, P.Z., & Klimberg, V.S. (2004). Minimally invasive breast surgery. *Journal of the American College of Surgeons, 199,* 961–975.

King, M.C., Marks, J.H., Mandell, J.B., & New York Breast Cancer Study Group. (2003). Breast and ovarian cancer risks due to inherited mutations in BRCA1 and BRCA2. *Science, 302,* 643–646.

Kolb, T.M., Lichy, J., & Newhouse, J.H. (2002). Comparison of the performance of screening mammography, physical examination, and breast US and evaluation of factors that influence them: An analysis of 27,825 patient evaluations. *Radiology, 225,* 165–175.

Koomen, M., Pisano, E.D., Kuzmiak, C., Pavic, D., & McLelland, R. (2005). Future directions in breast imaging. *Journal of Clinical Oncology, 23,* 1674–1677.

Kuhl, C.K., Kuhn, W., & Schild, H. (2005). Management of women at high risk for breast cancer: New imaging beyond mammography. *Breast, 14,* 480–486.

Kuhl, C.K., Schrading, S., Leutner, C.C., Morakkabati-Spitz, N., Wardelmann, E., Fimmers, R., et al. (2005). Mammography, breast ultrasound, and magnetic resonance imaging for surveillance of women at high familial risk for breast cancer. *Journal of Clinical Oncology, 23,* 8469–8476.

Mahon, S.M., Spies, M., & Williams, M. (2000). Information needs regarding menopause—results from a survey of women receiving cancer prevention and detection services. *Cancer Nursing, 23,* 176–185.

Majid, A.S., de Paredes, E.S., Doherty, R.D., Sharma, N.R., & Salvador, X. (2003). Missed breast carcinoma: Pitfalls and pearls. *Radiographics, 23,* 881–895.

Mele, N., Archer, J., & Pusch, B.D. (2005). Access to breast cancer screening services for women with disabilities. *Journal of Obstetric, Gynecologic, and Neonatal Nursing, 34,* 453–464.

Mintzer, D., Glassburn, J., Mason, B.A., & Sataloff, D. (2002). Breast cancer in the very young patient: A multidisciplinary case presentation. *Oncologist, 7,* 547–554.

Muller-Schimpfle, M., Ohmenhauser, K., Stoll, P., Dietz, K., & Claussen, C.D. (1997). Menstrual cycle and age: Influence on parenchymal contrast medium enhancement in MR imaging of the breast. *Radiology, 203,* 145–149.

National Comprehensive Cancer Network. (2006). *NCCN clinical practice guidelines in oncology: Breast cancer screening and diagnosis guidelines, version 1.2006.* Jenkintown, PA: Author.

Neugut, A.I., Meadows, A.T., & Robinson, E. (1999). Introduction. In A.I. Neugut, A.T. Meadows, & E. Robinson (Eds.), *Multiple primary cancers* (pp. 3–11). Philadelphia: Lippincott Williams & Wilkins.

Neugut, A.I., Rheingold, S.R., & Meadows, A.T. (2004). Second cancers among long-term survivors of cancer (pp. 664–668). *American Society of Clinical Oncology educational book, spring education conference.* Alexandria, VA: American Society of Clinical Oncology.

Obedian, E., Fischer, D.B., & Haffty, B.G. (2000). Second malignancies after treatment of early-stage breast cancer: Lumpectomy and radiation vs. mastectomy. *Journal of Clinical Oncology, 18,* 2406–2412.

Obenauer, S., Hermann, K.P., & Grabbe, E. (2005). Applications and literature review of the BI-RADS classification. *European Radiology, 15,* 1027–1036.

Orel, S.G., Schnall, M.D., LiVolsi, V.A., & Troupin, R.H. (1994). Suspicious breast lesions: MR imaging with radiologic-pathologic correlation *Radiology, 190,* 485–493.

Parikh, B., & Advani, S. (1996). Pattern of second primary neoplasms following breast cancer. *Journal of Surgical Oncology, 63,* 179–182.

Pisano, E.D., Gatsonis, C., Hendrick, E., Yaffe, M., Baum, J.K., Acharyya, S., et al. (2005). Diagnostic performance of digital versus film mammography for breast-cancer screening. *New England Journal of Medicine, 353,* 1773–1783.

Rankin, S.C. (2000). MRI of the breast. *British Journal of Radiology, 73,* 806–818.

Rebbeck, T.R., Friebel, T., Wagner, T., Lynch, H.T., Garber, J.E., Daly, M.B., et al. (2005). Effect of short-term hormone replacement therapy on breast cancer risk reduction after bilateral prophylactic oophorectomy in BRCA1 and BRCA2 mutation carriers: The PROSE Study Group. *Journal of Clinical Oncology, 23,* 7804–7810.

Ringash, J., & Canadian Task Force on Preventive Health Care. (2001). Preventive health care, 2001 update: Screening mammography among women aged 40–49 years at average risk of breast cancer. *Canadian Medical Association Journal, 164,* 469–476.

Robson, M.E., Morris, E., Kauff, N., Scheuer, L., Borgen, P.I., Hudis, C., et al. (2003). Breast cancer screening utilizing magnetic resonance imaging (MRI) in carriers of BRCA mutations [Abstract]. *Proceedings of the American Society of Clinical Oncology, 22,* 91.

Rodriguez, C., & Ash, C.R. (1996). Cancer therapy: Associated late effects (IV). *Cancer Nursing, 19,* 455–468.

Ryerson, A.B., Benard, V.B., & Major, A.C. (2006). *National Breast and Cervical Cancer Early Detection Program: 1991–2002 national report.* Atlanta, GA: U.S. Department of Health and Human

Services, Centers for Disease and Prevention. Retrieved from http://www.cdc.gov/cancer/nbccedp/bccpdfs/national_report.pdf

Scheidhauer, K., Walter, C., & Seemann, M.D. (2004). FDG PET and other imaging modalities in the primary diagnosis of suspicious breast lesions. *European Journal of Nuclear Medicine and Molecular Imaging, 31*(Suppl. 1), S70–S79.

Schopp, L.H., Kirkpatrick, H.A., Sanford, T.C., Hagglund, K.J., & Wongvatunyu, S. (2002). Impact of comprehensive gynecologic services on health maintenance behaviours among women with spinal cord injury. *Disability and Rehabilitation, 24,* 899–903.

Schrag, D., Kuntz, K.M., Garber, J.E., & Weeks, J.C. (2000). Life expectancy gains from cancer prevention strategies for women with breast cancer and BRCA1 or BRCA2 mutations. *JAMA, 283,* 617–624.

Semiglazov, V.F., Moiseenko, V.M., Manikhas, A.G., Protsenko, S.A., Kharikova, R.S., Popova, R.T., et al. (1999). Interim results of a prospective randomized study of self-examination for early detection of breast cancer (Russia/St. Petersburg/WHO). *Voprosy Onkologii, 45,* 265–271.

16-year mortality from breast cancer in the UK Trial of Early Detection of Breast Cancer. (1999). *Lancet, 353,* 1909–1914.

Smith, J.A., & Andreopoulou, E. (2004). An overview of the status of imaging screening technology for breast cancer. *Annals of Oncology, 15*(Suppl. 1), i18–i26.

Smith, R.A., Cokkinides, V., & Eyre, H.J. (2005). American Cancer Society guidelines for the early detection of cancer, 2005. *CA: A Cancer Journal for Clinicians, 55,* 31–44.

Smith, R.A., Cokkinides, V., & Eyre, H.J. (2006). American Cancer Society guidelines for the early detection of cancer, 2006. *CA: A Cancer Journal for Clinicians, 56,* 11–25.

Smith, T.J., Davidson, N.E., Schapira, D.V., Grunfeld, E., Muss, H.B., Vogel, V.G., 3rd, et al. (1999). 1998 update of recommended breast cancer surveillance guidelines. *Journal of Clinical Oncology, 17,* 1080–1082.

Thierry, J.M. (2000). Increasing breast and cervical cancer screening among women with disabilities. *Women's Health and Gender-Based Medicine, 9,* 9–12.

Thurnher, M.M., & Castillo, M. (2005). Imaging in acute stroke. *European Radiology, 15,* 408–415.

U.S. Preventive Services Task Force. (2002). *Recommendations and rationale: Screening for breast cancer.* Retrieved July 24, 2006, from http://www.ahcpr.gov/clinic/3rduspstf/breastcancer/brcanrr.htm

Van Goethem, M., Schelfout, K., Dijckmans, L., Van Der Auwera, J.C., Weyler, J., Verslegers, I., et al. (2004). MR mammography in the pre-operative staging of breast cancer in patients with dense breast tissue: Comparison with mammography and ultrasound. *European Radiology, 14,* 809–816.

van Sprundel, T.C., Schmidt, M.K., Rookus, M.A., Brohet, R., van Asperen, C.J., Rutgers, E.J., et al. (2005). Risk reduction of contralateral breast cancer and survival after contralateral prophylactic mastectomy in BRCA1 or BRCA2 mutation carriers. *British Journal of Cancer, 93,* 287–292.

Zangheri, B., Messa, C., Picchio, M., Gianolli, L., Landoni, C., & Fazio, F. (2004). PET/CT and breast cancer. *European Journal of Nuclear Medicine and Molecular Imaging, 31*(Suppl. 1), S135–S142.

CHAPTER 4

Pathophysiology and Staging of Breast Cancer

Susan G. Yackzan, RN, MSN, AOCN®

Introduction

Cycles of cellular proliferation and regression occur in the normal breast. These changes are a result of the influence of hormones and growth factors and are responsible for breast development, lactation, cyclic changes associated with menstruation, and eventually the involution of breast tissue that occurs after menopause (Miller, Bates, & Nabell, 2002). Figure 4-1 lists several hormones and growth factors with known or suspected influence on breast tissue. Estrogen and progesterone are the primary regulators of breast tissue growth but work in concert with many of the other hormones and growth factors (Farrar & Walker, 2002).

Because breast cancer can present in many different ways and with varied histology, a single carcinogenesis model is not easily described. As with other epithelial tumors, a presumed model includes progression from proliferative disease to atypical hyperplasia, to carcinoma in situ, to invasive cancer. On a molecular level, more than 200 genes have been implicated in the development of cellular changes that result in breast cancer (Miller et al., 2002). Table 4-1 lists some examples. Progression toward cancer may occur as a result of alterations in several different genes or as a result of a single gene

Table 4-1. Genetic Alterations in Breast Cancer	
Type of Gene	**Examples in Breast Cancer**
Oncogenes	HER2/neu, c-myc, cyclins, E-Cadherin
Tumor suppressor genes	TP53, RB
Apoptosis genes	Fas
Breast cancer susceptibility genes	BRCA1, BRCA2, TP53 (Li-Fraumeni syndrome), STK11 (Peutz-Jeghers syndrome), PTEN (Cowden syndrome)

Note. Based on information from Miller et al., 2002.

alteration that affects many cell functions (such as changes in the TP53 gene). These changes may be inherited germ-line mutations or may occur sporadically as somatic mutations. The most significant risk in the development of sporadic breast cancer appears to be hormone exposure. Risk factors for breast cancer such as age at menarche and age at menopause are based upon duration of hormone exposure.

Anatomy and Physiology of the Breast

Breasts, also known as mammary glands, function physiologically as apocrine glands in the production of milk. During fetal development, breasts develop on the ventral side of the embryo. By the fifth week of gestation, a milk line or streak develops as an ectodermal thickening and extends bilaterally from the axilla to the inguinal area (Spratt, Donegan, & Tobin, 2002). Most of this line atrophies by the sixth or seventh week of gestation, leaving a small portion bilaterally in the pectoral region. By the 10th to 16th week, the nipple and areolas have formed in those areas, followed by the downgrowth of short

Figure 4-1. Hormones and Growth Factors With Activity on Breast Tissue
• Estrogen
• Progesterone
• Oxytocin
• Prolactin
• Human placental lactogen
• Glucocorticoids
• Thyroid hormone
• Fibroblast growth factors
• Epidermal growth factors
• Transforming growth factor-beta family
• Insulin-like growth factor family

Note. Based on information from Farrar & Walker, 2002.

ducts that branch internally from the nipples. By the end of fetal development, 15–25 mammary ducts are present (Phillips & Price, 2002).

From birth until the onset of puberty, breast development is largely quiescent. With the onset of puberty, the hypothalamus secretes gonadotropin-releasing hormones, causing the release of follicle-stimulating hormone (FSH) and luteinizing hormone (LH) from the pituitary. FSH stimulates the maturation of ovarian follicles, resulting in estrogen production. Estrogen alone has no effect on breast development, but in the presence of other hormones such as prolactin, hydrocortisone, insulin, and growth factor, breast tissue responds to the presence of estrogen by development of periductal stroma and further growth of the ductal system (Farrar & Walker, 2002). Progesterone exposure, in the presence of growth hormone and insulin, stimulates development of the terminal ducts and lobuloalveolar structures, which are responsible for production of milk (Farrar & Walker; Phillips & Price, 2002). Breasts are mature but inactive after puberty. The final stage of breast development occurs with pregnancy and involves cellular proliferation and lobuloalveolar differentiation (Phillips & Price).

The adult breast is normally protuberant and circular, with a pigmented areola and nipple (see Figure 4-2). Elevated ductal openings called Montgomery tubercles normally are present on the areola. Bilaterally, the breasts lie over the pectoral fascia, may extend from the second to the sixth vertebra, and lie between the midaxillary line and the sternal edge (Phillips & Price, 2002). Cooper accessory ligaments extend from the deep layers of the breast through the lobes and attach to the overlying skin, giving shape to the breast and anchoring the gland to the skin. Breast tissue extending toward the axilla is known as the tail of Spence (Spratt et al., 2002).

Internally, the breast is made up of adipose, epithelial, and fibrous tissue (see Figure 4-3). Each breast is organized into 15–20 lobes, or segments, that are arranged radially from the nipple and are drained by a collecting duct (Farrar & Walker, 2002). Collecting ducts usually are lined with a single or double layer of simple columnar epithelium and join together so that only 5–10 open on the surface of the nipple. Within the 15–20 lobes of the breast, collecting ducts branch out and end in the functional, secretory unit of the breast known as the terminal duct lobular unit (TDLU), where milk is produced (Phillips & Price, 2002). Each TDLU is composed of alveoli or saccules that branch from the terminal ducts. The epithelial lining of these small ductal units include luminal A cells involved in milk synthesis, basal or B cells that are also known as chief cells and have stem cell activity, and myoepithelial cells that are responsible for ejection of milk (Farrar & Walker; Spratt et al., 2002).

Classification

The majority of primary breast cancers are adenocarcinomas, which can be divided into subtypes. The two major subtypes are ductal and lobular carcinomas. Based on microscopic findings, breast carcinomas are further classified as either in situ (noninvasive) or invasive (Wood, Muss, Solin, & Olopade, 2005). Other types of cancer that occur in the breast include stromal tumors, lymphomas, and metastases from other sites.

Breast Carcinomas

Carcinoma in Situ
In situ breast carcinomas are defined by the presence of malignant epithelial cells within the ducts or lobules with no extension beyond the basement membrane. In situ carcinomas do not exhibit lymphvascular invasion. They are further described as ductal carcinoma in situ (DCIS) or lobular carcinoma in situ (LCIS) (Lester, 2005; Wood et al., 2005). The distinction between the two types is not based on the presence of cancer cells within distinct ducts or lobules. In fact, most breast carcinomas of both types occur in the TDLU. Differentiation is based on the type and growth pattern of cells (Damiani & Eusebi, 2002). If left untreated and observed for more than 20 years, invasive carcinoma can be expected to occur in approximately 25%–35% of in situ carcinomas. This is a rate of about 1% per year (Lester).

Ductal carcinoma in situ (intraductal or noninvasive ductal carcinoma): DCIS most commonly presents as a nonpalpable lesion that is detected by mammography and often is found in association with microcalcifications. DCIS also may

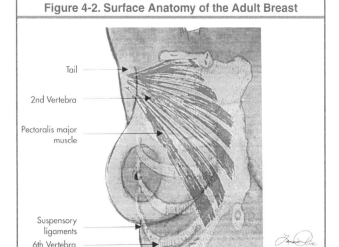

Figure 4-2. Surface Anatomy of the Adult Breast

Tail
2nd Vertebra
Pectoralis major muscle
Suspensory ligaments
6th Vertebra

Note. From "Breast Cancer Prevention and Detection: Past Progress and Future Directions" (p. 397), by J.M. Phillips and M.M. Price in K. Jennings-Dozier and S.M. Mahon (Eds.), *Cancer Prevention, Detection, and Control: A Nursing Perspective,* 2002, Pittsburgh, PA: Oncology Nursing Society. Copyright 2002 by the Oncology Nursing Society. Reprinted with permission.

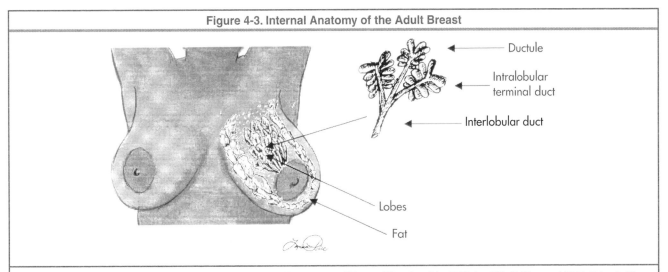

Figure 4-3. Internal Anatomy of the Adult Breast

Ductule

Intralobular terminal duct

Interlobular duct

Lobes

Fat

Note. From "Breast Cancer Prevention and Detection: Past Progress and Future Directions" (p. 397), by J.M. Phillips and M.M. Price in K. Jennings-Dozier and S.M. Mahon (Eds.), *Cancer Prevention, Detection, and Control: A Nursing Perspective,* 2002, Pittsburgh, PA: Oncology Nursing Society. Copyright 2002 by the Oncology Nursing Society. Reprinted with permission.

present as a density found on mammogram or as an incidental finding upon biopsy of other lesions. Before the advent of mammographic screening, DCIS accounted for less than 5% of all carcinomas (Lester, 2005). Approximately 62,030 new cases of in situ breast cancer are expected to be diagnosed in 2007. Eighty-five percent of these will be DCIS (American Cancer Society, 2007).

As noted previously, DCIS is defined by the existence of malignant epithelial cells with no extension beyond the basement membrane. A wide range of pathologic findings may be seen with DCIS. It may occur as a small, localized lesion or as a very extensive lesion that has spread throughout the ducts of the breast. DCIS may present as multifocal disease, occurring in separate areas of the breast. DCIS often is present as a component of invasive tumors and is thought to be a precursor lesion for invasive cancer.

Several subtypes of DCIS exist. Subtypes were traditionally defined microscopically by cell morphology and include comedocarcinoma, cribriform, papillary, micropapillary, and solid (see Table 4-2). A simpler classification system of comedo versus noncomedocarcinoma also has been suggested. Classification by cell type lacks prognostic value and is complicated by the fact that DCIS lesions may include a mixture of more than one subtype (Lester, 2005). Classification systems, including parameters for nuclear grade and cell polarization (cell orientation toward the ductal lumen), have been proposed (Damiani & Eusebi, 2002). DCIS can be categorized as nuclear grade I (low), II (intermediate), or III (high). Estrogen receptor (ER) and progesterone receptor (PR) status can be assessed on DCIS specimens.

Lobular carcinoma in situ: LCIS is typically an incidental finding. It is not commonly associated with any clinical or mammographic abnormalities. LCIS is estimated to account for 1%–4% of all cases of breast cancer and is found in 1%–2% of core biopsy specimens (Wood et al., 2005). With regard to age distribution, LCIS tends to be more prominent in younger, premenopausal women as compared with DCIS. Also, it is more frequently multifocal and bilateral as compared with DCIS. The risk of subsequent cancer occurs with nearly equal frequency in both the ipsilateral and contralateral breast after a diagnosis of LCIS. The majority of subsequent cancers are invasive ductal carcinomas. Controversy exists as to whether LCIS is a precursor lesion or simply a marker of high risk for development of future invasive lobular or ductal carcinoma (Lester, 2005; Wood et al.).

LCIS appears histologically as a proliferation of noncohesive cells. LCIS and invasive lobular carcinoma share similar cell features and genetic changes. LCIS lesions are almost uniformly ER/PR positive and are usually human epidermal growth factor receptor 2 (HER2) negative (Lester, 2005).

Invasive (Infiltrating) Carcinomas

Microscopically, invasive or infiltrating carcinomas extend beyond the basement membrane. Extension may continue through the breast parenchyma into lymphvascular spaces and may metastasize into regional lymph nodes or distant sites.

The majority of invasive breast carcinomas occur in the upper outer quadrant of the breast. When found mammographically as calcifications, invasive carcinomas are usually small, and lymph nodes are usually negative. A noted density is the most common mammographic finding for invasive carcinomas. Invasive carcinomas exhibiting this pattern are usually half the size of masses found first by palpation and have nodal metastases in less than 20% of the cases. In women

Table 4-2. Subtypes of Ductal Carcinoma in Situ (DCIS)

DCIS Subtype	Features
Comedocarcinoma	Sheets of neoplastic cells fill the terminal duct lobular unit (TDLU). Pleomorphic cells High-grade nuclei Central necrotic core (may be calcified) Periductal fibrosis and inflammation commonly present
Noncomedo DCIS	
• Cribriform	Neoplastic cells do not completely fill the TDLU. Cells that form regular fenestrations (sieve-like pattern) Smaller and more uniform cells compared to comedocarcinoma Lack of necrosis
• Papillary	Neoplastic cells arranged in fernlike pattern Papillae that project into the lumen of the duct Possibly absent myoepithelial layer of duct
• Micropapillary	Features of papillary with smaller papillae Papillae that may coalesce and appear as bulbous protrusions or bridges across the ducts
• Solid	Cancer cells completely fill the ducts. Lack of necrosis

Note. Based on information from Damiani & Eusebi, 2002; Lester, 2005.

not undergoing mammography, invasive carcinomas usually present as a palpable mass, and positive lymph nodes can be anticipated in 50% of those cases (Lester, 2005).

As with in situ carcinomas, the distinction between invasive ductal or lobular carcinoma does not actually designate a site of origin. Most carcinomas arise in the TDLU, regardless of type (Damiani & Eusebi, 2002). Components of in situ carcinoma can be found in most invasive carcinomas and often share histologic patterns with the invasive component (Schnitt & Guidi, 2004).

The cytology and growth pattern of cells determines the classification of invasive carcinomas. Subtypes reflect prognostic information and help to guide clinical decision making (Wood et al., 2005). Table 4-3 outlines several of the subtypes of invasive breast carcinoma along with significant identifying features. In some cases, histology of tumors may be mixed.

With the advent of screening mammography, several changes in the incidence and presentation of invasive breast carcinomas have developed. Increased detection of in situ carcinomas, smaller invasive cancers, lower histologic grades, and increased incidence of tubular carcinomas are among those trends (Schnitt & Guidi, 2004).

Invasive ductal carcinomas: Invasive ductal carcinomas (IDCs) comprise the majority of invasive breast cancers. Approximately 10% of IDCs exhibit special histopathologic features and tend to have more favorable prognoses. These tumor types include medullary, tubular, mucinous, papillary, and various other carcinoma subtypes. Tumors that do not meet criteria for any other category are classified by exclusion as IDCs and may be described as IDC of no special type (NST) or IDC not otherwise specified (NOS). IDCs are a group of heterogenous tumors exhibiting a range of features.

IDC usually presents as a palpable mass or abnormality found on mammogram and rarely may present as Paget disease of the nipple. Histopathology is variable within this category and may be variable within a single tumor (Schnitt & Guidi, 2004; Wood et al., 2005). Well-differentiated tumors are typically ER/PR positive and do not overexpress HER2. Poorly differentiated tumors may be ER/PR negative and HER2 positive. IDCs usually contain areas of associated DCIS. More aggressive DCIS tends to be associated with higher grade IDC, and less aggressive DCIS tends to be associated with lower grade IDC (Lester, 2005). Important prognostic features include tumor size, axillary node status, tumor grade, and lymphvascular invasion.

Gene expression profiling may be useful in identifying subtypes of IDC and is an active area of study. Relevance for prognosis and clinical decision making must be defined. In addition, usefulness of profiling will depend on widely available and consistent testing techniques (Lester, 2005).

Invasive lobular carcinomas: Invasive lobular carcinomas (ILCs) make up the second largest proportion of invasive carcinomas. The usual presentation is a mammographic density or palpable mass. ILC also may present as a vague thickening and diffuse pattern on mammogram. An increased risk of multifocal disease in the ipsilateral breast is associated with ILC. The presence of bilateral cancer also has been associated with ILC (Lester, 2005; Wood et al., 2005).

The hallmark pathology of ILC is a pattern of infiltration characterized by small cells that appear to invade the stroma in a single-file or linear strand. This is known as an Indian file pattern (Schnitt & Guidi, 2004; Wood et al., 2005). Several variant forms exist within this category, and not all ILCs exhibit the Indian file pattern. Mutation of E-cadherin has been correlated with ILC. A component of LCIS is present in most ILCs. Well-differentiated tumors are usually hormone receptor positive, and HER2 overexpression is rare. Poorly differentiated tumors are the opposite, often lacking hormone receptors and exhibiting HER2 positivity. The metastatic pattern for ILC is different than in other types of breast carcinoma and includes preferential sites such as the peritoneum, retroperitoneum, leptomeninges, gastrointestinal tract, ovaries, and uterus. ILCs rarely metastasize to the lungs and pleurae (Lester, 2005).

Medullary carcinoma: Accounting for approximately 5% of invasive cancers, medullary carcinomas usually present as

Table 4-3. Invasive Breast Carcinomas

Type	Prominent Features	Occurrence (%)
Invasive ductal	Wide variation of characteristics Usually hard, gritty mass but may be soft to firm Border usually irregular but may be distinct Gray-white tumors	65%–80%
Invasive lobular	Hallmark pattern of single-file cell infiltration (Indian file pattern) Several variant forms Consistency usually hard with irregular margins; may be rubbery Borders usually irregular Atypical metastatic pattern	10%–15%
Medullary	Well-circumscribed mass; may be lobulated Soft, fleshy tumor Prominent lymphoplasmacytic infiltrates No lymphvascular invasion	5%
Tubular	Histologically similar to benign lesions Consistency usually firm Border usually irregular	2%–3%
Mucinous (colloidal)	Well-circumscribed mass Usually soft, gelatinous tumor Large, extracellular pools of mucin Pale, gray-blue color	2%
Papillary	Well-circumscribed mass Exhibit papillae	1%–2%

Note. Based on information from Damiani & Eusebi, 2002; Lester, 2005; Schnitt & Guidi, 2004; Wood et al., 2005.

a well-circumscribed mass. Occurrence is more common in women younger than the age of 50 (Chapman & Moore, 2005). Patients may have a history of rapid, explosive growth with this tumor type (Lester, 2005). Microcalcifications are not usually found. Lymphadenopathy may be present but is most often benign and typically reveals reactive changes (Schnitt & Guidi, 2004).

Several features characterize medullary carcinomas, including poorly differentiated cells growing in a sheet-like (syncytial) pattern, lymphoplasmacytic infiltrates, and the absence of lymphvascular invasion. A component of DCIS is not uncommon. HER2 overexpression is not usually seen (Lester, 2005; Schnitt & Guidi, 2004). Also, areas of necrosis may be present (Damiani & Eusebi, 2002). Medullary carcinomas usually confer a more favorable prognosis than IDC of NST. If many but not all of the important histopathologic features are present, these tumors may be classified as atypical medullary carcinomas (Wood et al., 2005).

Tubular carcinoma: Historically, tubular carcinomas have accounted for a very small portion (1%–2%) of invasive breast carcinomas. The incidence of tubular carcinomas has increased in populations of women who undergo screening mammography. Tubular carcinomas represent up to 10% of the tumors that are less than one centimeter in diameter at diagnosis (Lester, 2005).

Tubular carcinomas may present mammographically as a mass lesion or abnormality (Schnitt & Guidi, 2004). Microcalcifications are noted in about 50% of cases (Damiani & Eusebi, 2002). Tubular carcinomas usually are small and often have an associated DCIS component. They usually are extremely well differentiated, are ER/PR positive, do not overexpress HER2, lack significant chromosomal changes, and generally exhibit good prognostic features (Schnitt & Guidi; Wood et al., 2005). Positive axillary nodes are found in less than 10% of tubular carcinoma cases (Lester, 2005).

Mucinous carcinoma (colloidal): Mucinous carcinomas (also known as colloidal cancers) usually occur in older women between 60–70 years old (Chapman & Moore, 2005). Mucinous carcinomas often present as a palpable mass and usually are well-circumscribed masses that may have grown slowly over many years (Lester, 2005; Wood et al., 2005). The incidence of mucinous carcinoma is slightly higher in the *BRCA1*-positive population (Lester). A lower incidence of positive axillary nodes and distant metastases occurs with mucinous carcinoma as compared with IDC in general.

Mucinous carcinomas are characterized by the presence of large extracellular pools of mucin in the tumor. Mucinous carcinomas usually exhibit favorable prognostic features, including low to intermediate grade, positive ER/PR status, and negative HER2 status. DCIS may be found within the tumor and may be papillary, micropapillary, cribriform, or even comedocarcinoma type (Schnitt & Guidi, 2004).

Papillary carcinoma: Papillary IDCs are very rare, accounting for less than 1%–2% of all IDCs. They usually are found in postmenopausal women (Wood et al., 2005). On mammogram, papillary carcinoma may appear as nodular densities, usually with well-circumscribed borders. On ultrasound, tumors may be multiple, lobulated, and hypoechoic (Schnitt & Guidi, 2004). A solid area within a cystic lesion may be an ultrasound presentation finding (Damiani & Eusebi, 2002).

Distinguishing in situ from invasive papillary carcinoma may be difficult. Invasive tumors often contain both. Lesions may be covered by a fibrous pseudocapsule in some cases (Damiani & Eusebi, 2002). Generalizations about prognosis should be viewed in the context of the rarity of these tumors but are generally felt to be favorable as compared with other IDCs. Tumors are often ER/PR positive and HER2 negative (Schnitt & Guidi, 2004; Wood et al., 2005).

Carcinomas of mixed histology: A small number of invasive carcinomas may share features of both IDC and ILC. In some cases, components of both histologies are present in the same tumor and may contain a transitional zone between the two patterns. In other cases, tumor cells may exhibit the cytologic features of one type but invasive characteristics of the other. Still other tumors may exhibit cytologic and invasive characteristics of both tumor types simultaneously (Schnitt & Guidi, 2004).

Other invasive breast carcinomas: Several other subtypes exist that together account for less than 1% of all invasive breast carcinomas. Adenoid cystic carcinomas are associated with an excellent prognosis, usually occur in the sixth and seventh decade, and are similar to adenoid cystic carcinomas arising in the salivary glands (Schnitt & Guidi, 2004; Wood et al., 2005). Secretory carcinomas show predominant secretory activity and usually are low-grade tumors. Cases have been recorded in children and young adults. These tumors are sometimes referred to as juvenile IDCs. Secretory carcinomas also may occur in adults and have been reported in male patients (Damiani & Eusebi, 2002). Invasive cribriform carcinoma is a well-differentiated cancer associated with a favorable prognosis (Schnitt & Guidi). Metaplastic carcinomas (carcinomas with metaplasia) are highly variant tumors and may contain elements of epithelial and mesenchymal tissues. Metaplastic carcinomas may exhibit squamous differentiation. Elements of cartilage, bone, muscle, and spindle cells, along with other cell types, have been reported in metaplastic carcinomas (Lester, 2005). Tumors may be poorly differentiated and difficult to diagnose (Schnitt & Guidi). Other subtypes include neuroendocrine tumors, invasive micropapillary carcinomas, apocrine carcinomas, invasive carcinomas with osteoclast-like giant cells or choriocarcinoma, lipid- and glycogen-rich carcinomas, and mucinous cystadenocarcinomas.

Inflammatory Breast Carcinoma

Inflammatory breast carcinoma (IBC) is defined clinically rather than by histology. IBC is a very aggressive type of breast cancer, accounting for less than 4% of cases (Chapman & Moore, 2005). Clinical characteristics mimic signs of an infection and include redness, warmth, edema (peau d'orange), breast enlargement, and tenderness. The onset of symptoms is usually quite rapid. IBC is not associated with a particular histologic subtype. Presence of cancer cells in the dermal lymphatics is indicative of IBC, although a diagnosis can be made on clinical presentation alone. A mass may or may not be palpable, and axillary nodes often are positive at the time of presentation (Cole & Kardinal, 2002; Cristofanilli, Buzdar, & Hortobagyi, 2003; Giordano & Hortobagyi, 2003).

Paget Disease

Paget disease is a rare form of breast cancer, accounting for only 1%–3% of cases. The nipple is typically involved, but extension into the areola or underlying breast is possible. The underlying pathology involves the presence of large dendritic malignant cells (Paget cells) within the epidermis. Clinical signs are caused by the disruption of normal epithelium by the malignant cells. Clinical signs are absent in up to 30% of the cases. Early clinical signs include erythema, an eczema-like appearance, and inflammation. Late signs include crusting, erosion, and bloody discharge. Nipple discharge, retraction, or inversion also may be present. A biopsy of the involved area is recommended for diagnosis (Damiani & Eusebi, 2002; Lester, 2005).

In most cases, Paget disease is associated with an underlying ductal carcinoma, either DCIS or invasive. Lesions usually are centrally located within 2 cm of the areola. In the case of associated DCIS, the malignant cells are believed to grow within the ductal system into the nipple skin without growing through the basement membrane. If associated carcinomas are palpable, a higher risk of multifocal disease and nodal metastases is present (Damiani & Eusebi, 2002).

Occult Breast Cancer

Rarely, in an estimated less than 1% of cases, breast carcinoma occurs as an occult presentation with positive axillary nodes or distant metastases without a detectable primary lesion. A thorough examination to locate the primary lesion should include physical examination and imaging studies, including mammography, ultrasound, and breast magnetic resonance imaging. Scintimammography also may be useful (Walker, 2002). Diagnoses other than breast carcinoma must be excluded, including carcinomas of other sites (lung, pancreas, gastrointestinal tract, thyroid, ovaries, renal), noncarcinomatous malignancy (melanoma, lymphoma, germ cell tumors), and nonmalignant causes (Wood et al., 2005). An appropriate biopsy technique yielding an adequate sample for study is essential to confirm the occult tumor as consistent with breast origin. When found, breast primaries are usually small or microscopic. If the tumor remains occult, staging and treatment are based on nodal or metastatic status (Walker).

Stromal Breast Tumors

Nonepithelial breast cancers arising from the breast stroma are far less common than epithelial cancers. Stromal tumors may be either benign or malignant. Fibroadenomas are benign stromal tumors. Phyllode tumors (PTs), also known as cystosarcoma phyllodes, are usually low-grade benign tumors, behaving in a manner similar to fibroadenomas (Lester, 2005). Evidence has shown that PTs actually develop from fibroadenomas, perhaps in the manner of progressive carcinogenesis (Donegan, 2002). PTs that occur as high-grade lesions exhibit marked cellular atypia and mitotic activity resembling sarcomas. In those cases, they may be referred to as phyllode sarcomas or malignant PTs. Wide excision with tumor-free margins is the treatment of choice. The behavior of PTs may be unpredictable, and both benign and malignant PTs may recur. The true malignant nature of PTs is defined by its clinical course (Donegan). Malignant PTs may recur and require reexcision with wider margins and possibly mastectomy and radiation therapy (Wood et al., 2005). Metastases to axillary lymph nodes and viscera have been reported (Donegan).

Sarcomas of the breast are very rare, accounting for about 1% of all breast malignancies. They can be distinguished from malignant PTs because of the absence of any epithelial components within the tumors (Donegan, 2002). Sarcomas of the breast can include angiosarcomas, rhabdomyosarcomas, liposarcomas, and leiomyosarcomas. Sarcomas usually present as a breast mass (Lester, 2005). Ulceration may occur with very large tumors. Breast sarcomas usually metastasize to the lungs, and spread to the lymph nodes is rare (Donegan). A slightly increased risk (0.3%–4%) of angiosarcomas after radiation therapy has been noted, most often occurring within 5–10 years following radiation therapy (Lester).

Other Breast Cancers

Lymphomas of the breast are extremely rare. Breast lymphomas usually present as painless breast masses. T-cell lymphomas may present with clinical signs similar to IBC (Wood et al., 2005). Presentation with multiple masses is also possible. Axillary nodes are involved in approximately one-third of cases, and bilateral disease may be evident. B symptoms such as fever, night sweats, anorexia, weight loss, and weakness are uncommon but present in some cases (Donegan, 2002). All histologic types of lymphoma have been reported to occur in the breast, but most are diffuse, B-cell non-Hodgkin lymphomas. Lymphomas of the breast are treated as extranodal lymphomas (Donegan; Wood et al.).

Metastasis to the breast from nonmammary sites is rare and almost never occurs in the absence of other metastases. Metastases from nonmammary cancers account for ap-

proximately 1% of breast malignancies. Metastases from melanoma, lung, prostate, and carcinoid tumors are the most frequently described. Other malignancies that can metastasize to the breast include ovarian, gastric, renal cell, thyroid, head and neck, sarcomas, colorectal, medulloblastoma, neuroblastoma, mesothelioma, bladder, endometrial, cervical, and choriocarcinoma (Schnitt & Guidi, 2004).

Staging

Staging is the process of grouping patients based on the extent of disease (Harris, 2004). Clinical staging includes a complete physical examination, imaging studies, and pathologic examination of the breast or other tissues as needed to make a diagnosis (Greene et al., 2002). Pathologic staging is particularly important in breast cancer because of the prognostic implications of tumor type, size, and extension. Breast cancer staging is incomplete without pathologic staging. All data used for clinical staging as well as the pathology from the primary site, lymph nodes, and metastatic sites are included in pathologic staging. The widely accepted staging system for breast cancer is the American Joint Committee on Cancer (AJCC) system, which is outlined in Figure 4-4. Tumor (T), node (N), and metastasis (M) form the basis of the AJCC staging system. The assigned tumor size or T may be from clinical or pathologic staging. The measurement judged to be most accurate for that case should be used. T size should be measured for the invasive component of a tumor only. Stage grouping is outlined in Table 4-4.

Breast lymphatics drain by three routes: axillary, transpectoral, and internal mammary (see Figure 4-5). For staging purposes, intramammary lymph nodes are coded as axillary. Supraclavicular nodes are classified as regional lymph nodes. Metastasis to any other lymph nodes, including cervical or contralateral internal mammary lymph nodes, is classified as distant (M1). Ipsilateral axillary lymph nodes, interpectoral lymph nodes, and lymph nodes along the axillary vein often are classified as level I, II, or III. Level I or low axillary nodes are lateral to the lateral border of the pectoralis minor muscle. Level II or mid-axillary nodes lie between the medial and lateral borders of the pectoralis minor muscle and include interpectoral (Rotter) lymph nodes. Level III or apical axillary nodes are medial to the medial margin of the pectoralis minor muscle (Greene et al., 2002).

Histologic grade should be assigned for all invasive carcinomas with the exception of medullary carcinoma (Greene et al., 2002). A pathologist completes the grading on routine sections. Scores are assigned based on three tumor features: degree of tubule formation, number of mitoses, and amount of nuclear pleomorphism (Sugg & Donegan, 2002). The Nottingham combined histologic grade or Elston-Ellis modification of the Scarff-Bloom-Richardson grading system is currently recommended

Figure 4-4. American Joint Committee on Cancer Tumor, Node, Metastasis (TNM) Staging System for Breast Cancer

Definition of TNM

Primary Tumor (T)

Definitions for classifying the primary tumor (T) are the same for clinical and pathologic classification. If the measurement is made by physical examination, the examiner will use the major headings (T1, T2, or T3). If other measurements, such as mammographic or pathologic measurements, are used, the subsets of T1 can be used. Tumors should be measured to the nearest 0.1 cm increment.

TX	Primary tumor cannot be assessed
T0	No evidence of primary tumor
Tis	Carcinoma *in situ*
Tis (DCIS)	Ductal carcinoma *in situ*
Tis (LCIS)	Lobular carcinoma *in situ*
Tis (Paget's)	Paget's disease of the nipple with no tumor

Note: Paget's disease associated with a tumor is classified according to the size of the tumor.

T1	Tumor 2 cm or less in greatest dimension
T1mic	Microinvasion 0.1 cm or less in greatest dimension
T1a	Tumor more than 0.1 cm but not more than 0.5 cm in greatest dimension
T1b	Tumor more than 0.5 cm but not more than 1 cm in greatest dimension
T1c	Tumor more than 1 cm but not more than 2 cm in greatest dimension
T2	Tumor more than 2 cm but not more than 5 cm in greatest dimension
T3	Tumor more than 5 cm in greatest dimension
T4	Tumor of any size with direct extension to (a) chest wall or (b) skin, only as described below
T4a	Extension to chest wall, not including pectoralis muscle
T4b	Edema (including peau d'orange) or ulceration of the skin of the breast, or satellite skin nodules confined to the same breast
T4c	Both T4a and T4b
T4d	Inflammatory carcinoma

Regional Lymph Nodes (N)

Clinical

NX	Regional lymph nodes cannot be assessed (e.g., previously removed)
N0	No regional lymph node metastasis
N1	Metastasis to moveable ipsilateral axillary lymph nodes
N2	Metastases in ipsilateral axillary lymph nodes fixed or matted, or in clinically apparent* ipsilateral internal mammary nodes in the *absence* of clinically evident axillary lymph node metastasis
N2a	Metastasis in ipsilateral axillary lymph nodes fixed to one another (matted) or to other structures
N2b	Metastasis only in clinically apparent* ipsilateral internal mammary nodes and in the *absence* of clinically evident axillary lymph node metastasis
N3	Metastasis in ipsilateral infraclavicular lymph node(s) with or without axillary lymph node involvement, or in clinically apparent* ipsilateral internal mammary lymph node(s) and in the *presence* of clinically evident axillary lymph node metastasis; or metastasis in ipsilateral supraclavicular lymph node(s) with or without axillary or internal mammary lymph node involvement
N3a	Metastasis in ipsilateral infraclavicular lymph node(s)
N3b	Metastasis in ipsilateral internal mammary lymph node(s) and axillary lymph node(s)
N3c	Metastasis in ipsilateral supraclavicular lymph node(s)

Clinically apparent is defined as detected by imaging studies (excluding lymphoscintigraphy) or by clinical examination or grossly visible pathologically.

Pathologic (pN)[a]

pNX	Regional lymph nodes cannot be assessed (e.g., previously removed, or not removed for pathologic study)
pN0	No regional lymph node metastasis histologically, no additional examination for isolated tumor cells (ITC)

Note: Isolated tumor cells (ITC) are defined as single tumor cells or small cell clusters not greater than 0.2 mm, usually detected only by immunohistochemical (IHC) or molecular methods but which may be verified on H&E stains. ITCs do not usually show evidence of malignant activity e.g., proliferation or stromal reaction.

(Continued on next page)

Figure 4-4. American Joint Committee on Cancer Tumor, Node, Metastasis (TNM) Staging System for Breast Cancer
(Continued)

pN0(i–)	No regional lymph node metastasis histologically, negative IHC
pN0(i+)	No regional lymph node metastasis histologically, positive IHC, no IHC cluster greater than 0.2 mm
pN0(mol–)	No regional lymph node metastasis histologically, negative molecular findings (RT-PCR)[b]
pN0(mol+)	No regional lymph node metastasis histologically, positive molecular findings (RT-PCR)[b]

[a] Classification is based on axillary lymph node dissection with or without sentinel lymph node dissection. Classification based solely on sentinel lymph node dissection without subsequent axillary lymph node dissection is designated (sn) for "sentinel node," e.g., pN0(i+) (sn).

[b] RT-PCR: reverse transcriptase/polymerase chain reaction.

pN1	Metastasis in 1 to 3 axillary lymph nodes, and/or internal mammary nodes with microscopic disease detected by sentinel lymph node dissection but not clinically apparent**
pN1mi	Micrometastasis (greater than 0.2 mm, none greater than 2.0 mm)
pN1a	Metastasis in 1 to 3 axillary lymph nodes
pN1b	Metastasis in internal mammary nodes with microscopic disease detected by sentinel lymph node dissection but not clinically apparent**
pN1c	Metastasis in 1 to 3 axillary lymph nodes and in internal mammary lymph nodes with microscopic disease detected by sentinel lymph node dissection but not clinically apparent.** (If associated with greater than 3 positive axillary lymph nodes, the internal mammary nodes are classified as pN3b to reflect increased tumor burden)
pN2	Metastasis in 4 to 9 axillary lymph nodes, or in clinically apparent* internal mammary lymph nodes in the *absence* of axillary lymph node metastasis
pN2a	Metastasis in 4 to 9 axillary lymph nodes (at least one tumor deposit greater than 2.0 mm)
pN2b	Metastasis in clinically apparent* internal mammary lymph nodes in the *absence* of axillary lymph node metastasis
pN3	Metastasis in 10 or more axillary lymph nodes, or in infraclavicular lymph nodes, or in clinically apparent* ipsilateral internal mammary lymph nodes in the *presence* of 1 or more positive axillary lymph nodes; or in more than 3 axillary lymph nodes with clinically negative microscopic metastasis in internal mammary lymph nodes; or in ipsilateral supraclavicular lymph nodes
pN3a	Metastasis in 10 or more axillary lymph nodes (at least one tumor deposit greater than 2.0 mm), or metastasis to the infraclavicular lymph nodes
pN3b	Metastasis in clinically apparent* ipsilateral internal mammary lymph nodes in the *presence* of 1 or more positive axillary lymph nodes; or in more than 3 axillary lymph nodes and in internal mammary lymph nodes with microscopic disease detected by sentinel lymph node dissection but not clinically apparent**
pN3c	Metastasis in ipsilateral supraclavicular lymph nodes

* *Clinically apparent* is defined as detected by imaging studies (excluding lymphoscintigraphy) or by clinical examination.
** *Not clinically apparent* is defined as not detected by imaging studies (excluding lymphoscintigraphy) or by clinical examination.

Distant Metastasis (M)

MX	Distant metastasis cannot be assessed
M0	No distant metastasis
M1	Distant metastasis

DCIS—ductal carcinoma in situ; LCIS—lobular carcinoma in situ

Note. Used with permission of the American Joint Committee on Cancer (AJCC), Chicago, Illinois. From *AJCC Cancer Staging Manual, Sixth Edition* (pp. 227–228), by F.L. Greene, D.L. Page, I.D. Fleming, A. Fritz, C.M. Balch, D.G. Haller, et al. (Eds.), 2002, New York: Springer, www.springeronline.com.

(Greene et al.). In this system, each of the three features is reviewed and receives a score of one to three points, according to severity (with one being favorable and three being more severe). Scores are summed to calculate a final total score, which can range from three to nine. Totals of three to five indicate a well-differentiated or low-grade tumor (grade 1), totals of six to seven indicate a moderately differentiated or intermediate-grade tumor (grade 2), and totals of eight to nine indicate a poorly differentiated or high-grade tumor (grade 3) (Sugg & Donegan).

Prognostic and Predictive Factors

Prognostic factors include patient or tumor characteristics that are taken at the time of surgery or diagnosis and are used

Table 4-4. Breast Cancer Stage Grouping			
Stage	**T**	**N**	**M**
Stage 0	Tis	N0	M0
Stage I	T1*	N0	M0
Stage IIA	T0	N1	M0
	T1*	N1	M0
	T2	N0	M0
Stage IIB	T2	N1	M0
	T3	N0	M0
Stage IIIA	T0	N2	M0
	T1*	N2	M0
	T2	N2	M0
	T3	N1	M0
	T3	N2	M0
Stage IIIB	T4	N0	M0
	T4	N1	M0
	T4	N2	M0
Stage IIIC	Any T	N3	M0
Stage IV	Any T	Any N	M1

*T1 includes T1mic

Note. Stage designation may be changed if post-surgical imaging studies reveal the presence of distant metastases, provided that the studies are carried out within four months of diagnosis in the absence of disease progression and provided that the patient has not received neoadjuvant therapy.

Note. Used with permission of the American Joint Committee on Cancer (AJCC), Chicago, Illinois. From *AJCC Cancer Staging Manual, Sixth Edition* (p. 228), by F.L. Greene, D.L. Page, I.D. Fleming, A. Fritz, C.M. Balch, D.G. Haller, et al. (Eds.), 2002, New York: Springer, www.springeronline.com.

confined and not metastatic. In the AJCC staging system, in situ carcinoma is designated as *Tis* and subclassified by type. *Microinvasion* refers to the extension of cancer cells beyond the basement membrane but with no focus more than 0.1 cm in greatest dimension. When multiple foci of microinvasion exist, the size of the largest is used for classification (Greene et al., 2002).

Nodal Status

Lymph node status continues to be the single most important prognostic factor in breast cancer. Histologic examination of lymph nodes is necessary for reliable staging. Clinical staging alone can result in unacceptable false-positive and false-negative status (Lester, 2005; Sheldon, 2005). With negative lymph nodes, the 10-year disease-free survival rate is approximately 70%–80%. One to three positive nodes decreases the rate to 35%–40%, and more than 10 positive nodes decreases the 10-year disease-free survival rate to 10%–15% (Lester).

Lymph node dissection can be used to determine both the presence of lymph node metastases and the total number of nodes with metastases. The objective determines the extent of dissection. A complete axillary dissection is desirable if lymph nodes are positive for metastases. Complete dissections allow for an accurate count of positive nodes and decrease the risk of progressive growth and regional recurrence in the axilla (Sugg & Donegan, 2002). If the objective is to determine whether lymph node metastasis is present, axillary node sampling can be done. Sentinel node biopsy involves the identification and sampling of the first draining node from the breast cancer. Radiotracer, colored dye, or both are used to identify the sentinel node. Sentinel nodes have been identified most often in level I nodes but also in level II or III. In the absence of lymph node mapping and sentinel lymph node biopsy, removal of nodes from levels I and II is considered the minimum accepted procedure (Sugg & Donegan). Controversy exists over the clinical significance of micrometastases detected solely by immunohistochemistry or reverse transcriptase-polymerase chain reaction (Lester, 2005).

Lymph node sampling or dissection is not without risks. Lymphedema occurs in 15%–20% of breast cancer cases. The extent of axillary dissection affects the risk of lymphedema (Chapman & Moore, 2005). Sentinel lymph node biopsy has decreased the risk of lymphedema significantly but has not entirely eliminated the risk (Sheldon, 2005).

Tumor Size

Tumor size also appears to be a reliable prognostic factor. Larger tumor sizes increase the likelihood of positive axillary nodes and decrease the likelihood of disease-free survival. Tumors less than one centimeter in diameter with node-negative disease have a five-year survival rate of nearly 99% and a

to estimate outcomes (Sheldon, 2005; Wood et al., 2005) (see Table 4-5). Important prognostic factors such as invasive disease, nodal status, extension, and tumor size are incorporated into the TNM staging system. Predictive factors are clinical or pathologic characteristics that are used to determine the likelihood of response to treatment (Lester, 2005; Sheldon). Some are well established, whereas others are still under study.

Extent of Invasion

Pathologic examination of a tumor is necessary to determine the extent of invasion. In situ carcinoma by definition is

Figure 4-5. Breast and Regional Lymph Nodes

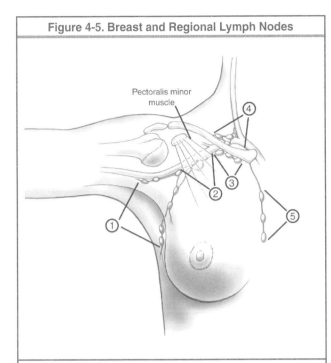

Pectoralis minor muscle

Schematic diagram of the breast and regional lymph nodes. (1) Low axillary, Level I; (2) Mid-axillary, Level II; (3) High axillary, apical, Level III; (4) Supraclavicular; (5) Internal mammary nodes.

Note. Used with permission of the American Joint Committee on Cancer (AJCC), Chicago, Illinois. From *AJCC Cancer Staging Manual, Sixth Edition* (p. 224), by F.L. Greene, D.L. Page, I.D. Fleming, A. Fritz, C.M. Balch, D.G. Haller, et al. (Eds.), 2002, New York: Springer, www.springeronline.com.

10-year survival rate approaching 90% (Chapman & Moore, 2005; Lester, 2005). More than 50% of women with tumors larger than two centimeters in diameter will eventually die of the disease (Lester).

Histologic Grade

Survival statistics described in terms of histologic grade show that 85% of women with well-differentiated grade I tumors, 60% of women with moderately differentiated grade II tumors, and 15% of women with poorly differentiated grade III tumors are alive at 10 years (Lester, 2005). Well-differentiated tumors are a minority. Histologic grade may be useful in identifying potential response to chemotherapy and therefore is useful as both a prognostic and predictive factor. Higher-grade tumors may exhibit greater responsiveness to adjuvant chemotherapy (Schnitt & Guidi, 2004; Sugg & Donegan, 2002).

Hormone Receptor Status

The ER/PR status of tumors is both prognostic and predictive. The majority of invasive breast cancers (50%–85%)

retain ERs, allowing estrogen to stimulate tumor cell growth (Chapman & Moore, 2005; Sugg & Donegan, 2002). Patients with ER-/PR-positive tumors show better disease-free and overall survival and longer survival after recurrence. Tumors that are ER positive usually exhibit other favorable features such as low-grade histology and lower proliferative rates (Sugg & Donegan). Positive ER status also is predictive of response to hormonal therapy (Sheldon, 2005).

HER2 Status

The proto-oncogene *erb*-b2, also known as HER2/*neu,* is a transmembrane growth factor receptor and a member of the human epidermal growth factor receptor (HER) family. It is normally present on breast epithelium and is overexpressed in approximately 20%–30% of breast cancers as a result of gene amplification (Sheldon, 2005; Sugg & Donegan, 2002; Wood et al., 2005). Tumors that overexpress HER2 are associated with higher grade, ER-negative status, higher proliferative indices, and poorer prognosis (Wood et al.). As a predictive factor, HER2 overexpression is a predictor of response to trastuzumab. HER2 overexpression also may predict responsiveness to chemotherapy and resistance to endocrine therapy (Chapman & Moore, 2005).

Proliferative Rate

Several indices of tumor proliferative rate can be assessed. Flow cytometry can be used to assess ploidy and S-phase fraction. *Ploidy* refers to the amount of DNA in a tumor. Diploid is normal. Aneuploid is abnormal and can result from either increased or decreased DNA content. The *S-phase fraction* refers to the number of cells in the S phase of the cell cycle. The mitotic index assesses the number of tumor cells undergoing

Table 4-5. Prognostic Factors for Breast Cancer

Prognostic Factor	Favorable Findings
Invasion	In situ disease
Lymph node status	Negative
Tumor size	Smaller size
Histologic grade	Grade 1, well-differentiated
Lymphvascular invasion	Negative
Distant metastasis	Negative
Histologic type	Tubular, invasive cribriform, papillary, mucinous, and medullary carcinoma

Note. Based on information from Chapman & Moore, 2005; Schnitt & Guidi, 2004; Sugg & Donegan, 2002; Wood et al., 2005.

mitosis and is assessed by reviewing tumors using high-power microscopic fields. Ki-67 and MIB are antibodies that identify antigens expressed by cells in proliferative phases of the cell cycle. Thymidine labeling index measures cells in the S phase of the cell cycle (Sugg & Donegan, 2002; Wood et al., 2005). Higher proliferative rates correlate with poor tumor grades, younger age of patients, ER-/PR-negative status, and HER2 overexpression. As a predictive factor, tumors exhibiting high proliferative rates may be more responsive to chemotherapy (Wood et al.).

Other Factors

Tumor invasion of the lymph and vascular systems appears to be a negative prognostic finding and is strongly associated with the presence of lymph node metastasis. A finding of tumor cells in the dermal lymphatics is associated with inflammatory carcinoma and indicates a poor prognosis (Lester, 2005). Perineural invasion, the extent of DCIS, and tumor angiogenesis also have been suggested as prognostic factors (Lester; Schnitt & Guidi, 2004; Sugg & Donegan, 2002). Some histologic types of invasive breast cancer are associated with a better prognosis than others. Favorable diagnoses include tubular, invasive cribriform, and papillary carcinomas. Assessing the molecular markers of tumors is a growing area of interest (Duffy, 2005). Microarray analysis is a technique that can be used to look for genes within a tumor that confer favorable or unfavorable prognosis. Risk scores from assays may be used to assist with decision making regarding adjuvant therapy (Wood et al., 2005).

Nursing Implications

Patient education about breast cancer pathophysiology, staging, and prognosis is a very complex and essential nursing process. Education usually begins with a positive biopsy result and includes basic breast cancer information as well as information on the importance of complete pathologic staging. In the presurgical setting, staging education is necessary as shared decisions are made regarding surgical treatments, such as the choice between mastectomy and lumpectomy and the lymph node sampling procedure that will be used. Presurgical information also is important to help to set the stage for a better postsurgical visit when a multidisciplinary team of surgical, medical, and radiation oncology professionals may present treatment options based on staging and predicted benefit.

References

American Cancer Society. (2007). *Cancer facts and figures, 2007.* Atlanta, GA: Author.

Chapman, D.D., & Moore, S. (2005). Breast cancer. In C.H. Yarbro, M.H. Frogge, & M. Goodman (Eds.), *Cancer nursing: Principles and practice* (6th ed., pp. 1022–1088). Sudbury, MA: Jones and Bartlett.

Cole, J., & Kardinal, C.G. (2002). Locally advanced and inflammatory breast cancer. In W.L. Donegan & J.S. Spratt (Eds.), *Cancer of the breast* (5th ed., pp. 579–595). Philadelphia: Saunders.

Cristofanilli, M., Buzdar, A.U., & Hortobagyi, G.N. (2003). Update on the management of inflammatory breast cancer. *Oncologist, 8,* 141–148.

Damiani, S., & Eusebi, V. (2002). Gross and microscopic pathology. In W.L. Donegan & J.S. Spratt (Eds.), *Cancer of the breast* (5th ed., pp. 347–375). Philadelphia: Saunders.

Donegan, W.L. (2002). Sarcomas of the breast. In W.L. Donegan & J.S. Spratt (Eds.), *Cancer of the breast* (5th ed., pp. 917–944). Philadelphia: Saunders.

Duffy, M.J. (2005). Predictive markers in breast and other cancers: A review. *Clinical Chemistry, 51,* 494–503.

Farrar, W.B., & Walker, M.J. (2002). Physiology and function of the breast. In W.L. Donegan & J.S. Spratt (Eds.), *Cancer of the breast* (5th ed., pp. 45–55). Philadelphia: Saunders.

Giordano, S.H., & Hortobagyi, G.N. (2003). Inflammatory breast cancer. Clinical progress and the main problems that must be addressed. *Breast Cancer Research, 5,* 284–288.

Greene, F.L., Page, D.L., Fleming, I.D., Fritz, A., Balch, C.M., Haller, D.G., et al. (Eds.). (2002). *AJCC cancer staging manual* (6th ed.). New York: Springer.

Harris, J.R. (2004). Staging of breast cancer. In J.R. Harris, M.E. Lippman, M. Morrow, & C.K. Osborne (Eds.), *Diseases of the breast* (3rd ed., pp. 653–667). Philadelphia: Lippincott Williams & Wilkins.

Lester, S. (2005). The breast. In V. Kumar, A.K. Abbas, & N. Fausto (Eds.), *Robbins and Cotran's pathologic basis of disease* (7th ed., pp. 1119–1154). Philadelphia: Saunders.

Miller, D.M., Bates, P.J., & Nabell, L. (2002). Molecular biology of breast cancer. In W.L. Donegan & J.S. Spratt (Eds.), *Cancer of the breast* (5th ed., pp. 181–198). Philadelphia: Saunders.

Phillips, J.M., & Price, M.M. (2002). Breast cancer prevention and detection: Past progress and future directions. In K. Jennings-Dozier & S.M. Mahon (Eds.), *Cancer prevention, detection, and control: A nursing perspective* (pp. 389–444). Pittsburgh, PA: Oncology Nursing Society.

Schnitt, S.J., & Guidi, A.J. (2004). Pathology of invasive breast cancer. In J.R. Harris, M.E. Lippman, M. Morrow, & C.K. Osborne (Eds.), *Diseases of the breast* (3rd ed., pp. 541–579). Philadelphia: Lippincott Williams & Wilkins.

Sheldon, D.G. (2005). Beyond lymph node staging: Molecular predictors of outcome in breast cancer. *Surgical Oncology Clinics of North America, 14,* 69–84.

Spratt, J.S., Donegan, W.L., & Tobin, G. (2002). Gross anatomy of the breast. In W.L. Donegan & J.S. Spratt (Eds.), *Cancer of the breast* (5th ed., pp. 29–44). Philadelphia: Saunders.

Sugg, S.L., & Donegan, W.L. (2002). Staging and prognosis. In W.L. Donegan & J.S. Spratt (Eds.), *Cancer of the breast* (5th ed., pp. 477–506). Philadelphia: Saunders.

Walker, A. (2002). Diagnosis and management of occult primary breast cancer. In W.L. Donegan & J.S. Spratt (Eds.), *Cancer of the breast* (5th ed., pp. 945–949). Philadelphia: Saunders.

Wood, W.C., Muss, H.B., Solin, L.J., & Olopade, O.I. (2005). Malignant tumors of the breast. In V.T. DeVita, Jr., S. Hellman, & S.A. Rosenberg (Eds.), *Cancer: Principles and practice of oncology* (7th ed., pp. 1415–1477). Philadelphia: Lippincott Williams & Wilkins.

CHAPTER 5

Local and Regional Control

Dianne D. Chapman, ND, APRN,BC

Introduction

A woman who receives a diagnosis of breast cancer is understandably upset, anxious, and fearful. The time until the final pathology is available is often 24–48 agonizing hours, and health providers relaying the news should be aware of this anxiety. The process of delivering the results can be done in several ways. If a biopsy has been performed in the office, a reading often can be returned within an hour, and the patient/family and physician can have a face-to-face conversation. More often, however, the biopsy is done in a radiology suite or an operating room, and the patient must wait a day or two for the results. Because patients prefer to hear the results as soon as they are available, results frequently are given to patients over the telephone. The particular aspects of the call should be discussed with patients beforehand, as some women have no privacy at work or do not want the results conveyed to them at an inopportune time. Usually, the preferred place for the call is at home, and the provider who delivers the news should be compassionate and understanding. However, the availability of various technologic devices may find women answering calls at inappropriate times, such as during a meeting, while shopping, or while driving a car. It is not helpful to discuss treatment options at the same time as giving the diagnosis because most women react to hearing the word *cancer* and will hear very little else.

Once the diagnosis is made, healthcare professionals should discuss treatment options with both patients and their family members. This discussion is a very important component of treatment planning. When information about the diagnosis, prognostic factors, additional testing, and treatment options is given, it is advisable for women to bring a supportive significant other not only to provide support but also so that another person hears the information. Furthermore, patients should obtain a second opinion that will serve as either a conclusive opinion or a differing opinion. A differing opinion is often confusing for patients and should be explained in terms of evidence-based medicine. If this is

the case, patients will be encouraged to seek another opinion as a "tie breaker." Opinions rendered for invasive or in situ cancer can differ dramatically regarding surgical and medical treatment options. Some surgeons adhere to strict lumpectomy and mastectomy parameters, whereas others are more willing to relax the parameters if patients understand that they are requesting and agreeing to a surgery that is not the standard of care. An example of this would be doing a large lumpectomy that would severely compromise the cosmetic outcome, leaving the woman with a deformed breast. The surgeon and patient need to come to an agreement after a complete discussion of the options, and this conversation should be well documented in the chart.

Women must consider not only the research data available about various treatment options but also their own personal preferences, which often are influenced by the experiences of friends and family. The treatment decision is based on the woman's feelings about her breasts and may be influenced by her partner's feelings. For women considering breast restoration, a consultation with both a plastic surgeon and a prosthetic fitter might clarify the best choice in her particular situation. These consultations allow women to better understand what a reconstructed breast might look like (by seeing pictures from a plastic surgeon) or by seeing what prosthetic options are available. Women considering breast restoration need to be assured that no "correct" decision exists, but that she needs to consider her options and then choose what is best for her. This usually results in more confidence and increased satisfaction with the long-term outcome.

Nurses are invaluable to patients during this trying and uncertain time. Social supports are important for meeting the emotional and physical needs of patients in difficult situations. Evaluating patients' coping styles will help nurses to better understand their needs and reactions during treatment. Iwamitsu et al. (2005) conducted a study and found that those who suppressed negative emotions had a higher level of anxiety than those who expressed negative feelings. The study also reported that these patients experienced more emotional distress, manifested in depression and fatigue. Assessing patients' social support network will allow nurses to assist patients in scheduling tangible supports such as child care or transportation if needed. People who have and use social supports feel better during treatment and have better interactions with healthcare providers (Han et al., 2005; Iwamitsu et al.). Oncology nurses serve as educators, informing patients about the potential complications of surgery and the side effects of treatment, as well as addressing their questions. Oncology nurses also are coaches who provide encouragement when patients do not feel well or are depressed, and they serve as counselors who acknowledge, discuss, and share good and bad news. For those women struggling to make treatment decisions, oncology nurses using evidence-based medicine might recommend the National Comprehensive Cancer Network and American Cancer Society's *Breast Cancer Treatment Guidelines for Patients,* available for free at www.nccn.org or by calling 888-909-NCCN.

Today, the treatment of breast cancer involves a team of doctors who discuss surgical, hormonal, chemotherapeutic, and radiation therapy options. A breast center provides a setting that is designed to address the needs of women and their families in providing a patient-friendly environment to discuss treatment options with a team of experts. Regardless of the setting, a surgeon or the breast cancer team has a responsibility to thoroughly explain the characteristics of the breast cancer (histopathology and clinical presentation) and the rationale for the options being presented.

The following lists potential discussion topics to address during the treatment consultation. Keep in mind that a detailed discussion regarding chemotherapy will likely need to occur after the definitive surgery is completed, when the exact stage of disease is known.

- Surgery
  - What are the risks/benefits of surgery (lumpectomy versus mastectomy and sentinel node biopsy versus axillary node dissection)?
  - Does my survival differ with the type of surgery?
  - What is the risk of lymphedema?
  - Will I be hospitalized?
  - Will I have drains to care for?
  - Will I need someone to stay with me if I live alone?
  - What is my recovery time?
- Radiation
  - Will I need radiation?
  - How often is it given?
  - What is the difference between whole-breast radiation and partial-breast radiation?
  - What are the side effects?
- Chemotherapy
  - Is chemotherapy or hormonal therapy recommended?
  - What are the side effects?
  - Are there clinical trials for my cancer?

Surgery

Patients usually present to the team after a biopsy has been completed and the diagnosis has been given. The initial discussion with the team involves the type of surgery to be done (mastectomy versus lumpectomy with or without axillary node sampling, the probability of chemotherapy and/or hormone therapy, and radiation therapy), if indicated. The surgeon assesses and discusses the technical and biologic rationale, including potential complications of each of the surgical options presented. The medical oncologist also is a participant, consulting with the other physicians and advising patients about the likelihood of chemotherapy or hormonal therapy, although a thorough discussion of future chemotherapy/hormonal therapy does not take place until all the pathology is reviewed. If patients are recommended to and elect to receive neoadjuvant chemotherapy before surgery, the medical oncologist will request a small incisional biopsy for estrogen receptor (ER), progesterone receptor (PR), and HER2/*neu* status, if not previously done. The radiation oncologist discusses the radiation treatment plan and side effects of radiation therapy.

Women also need to be given the opportunity to participate in a clinical trial if it is appropriate and available. The National Surgical Adjuvant Breast and Bowel Project (NSABP) has conducted cooperative landmark studies investigating the effectiveness of surgical options, chemotherapy/hormone treatment, and radiation treatment that have determined the current treatment of breast cancer. Among other things, these trials have presented evidence that lumpectomy with radiation is equal to mastectomy in overall survival (Fisher & Anderson, 1994; Fisher et al., 1995; Fisher, Bauer, et al., 1985; Fisher et al., 1993; Fisher, Costantino, et al., 1989; Fisher et al., 2002; Fisher et al., 1977; Fisher, Redmond, et al., 1985; Fisher, Redmond, Poisson, et al., 1989); that chemotherapy improves survival (Fisher, 1999; Fisher, Anderson, et al., 2001; Fisher, Dignam, Bryant, & Wolmark, 2001; Fisher et al., 1997; Fisher & Redmond, 1992; Fisher et al., 1986; Fisher et al., 1981; Fisher, Redmond, Dimitrov, et al., 1989); and that tamoxifen provides risk reduction for cancer in high-risk women older than age 35 (Fisher et al., 2005; Fisher et al., 1998). Thus, women should be made aware of trials for surgery, radiation therapy, hormonal therapy, chemotherapy, quality of life, symptom management, or combination trials. These trials may be available through the National Cancer Institute, NSABP, other cooperative groups, or investigator-developed protocols from an individual institution. Additional consents will be necessary, which often are managed by a research nurse. Women need to be informed that such trials are a reasonable approach to therapy in many cases and should be reminded that much of what is now known about breast cancer and its treatment has been made possible because of the numerous women who participated in clinical trials.

Surgical treatment options for breast cancer should begin by frankly discussing the survival outcomes of lumpectomy versus mastectomy and listening as patients express their feelings and biases. Lumpectomy does carry a higher risk of recurrence over time, but after the completion mastectomy is performed, no survival differences are seen compared to the women who initially choose mastectomy (Fisher, Bauer, et al., 1985; Fisher et al., 1977). Some clinical considerations exist that will sway a surgeon to recommend mastectomy, which include cosmetic deficits that result from a large tumor in a small breast, extensive noninvasive cancer, or multiple cancers within the same breast. Mastectomy is never a wrong choice for the treatment of breast cancer, but women may choose it over breast-conserving treatment if they are not well informed about the aforementioned studies. The potential complications of the surgery are discussed at this time, too, and include wound infection, seroma, and flap necrosis.

Historical Perspective

Surgery for breast cancer is based on one outcome—removal of the cancer with a margin of normal tissue surrounding the malignancy. Until approximately 25 years ago, removing the cancer was accomplished solely through mastectomy. William Halsted, MD, initiated the first standard of care for mastectomy in the late 19th century. This procedure removed the breast, all the lymph nodes, and the pectoralis major and minor muscles and is more commonly known as a radical mastectomy (Halsted, 1907). This procedure prevailed until a study in the 1970s compared the radical mastectomy with an alternative approach that spared the pectoralis major muscle (known as a modified radical mastectomy) and showed comparable survival (Fisher et al., 1977). By the 1980s, modified radical mastectomy was the common choice for surgery (Sakorafas, 2001). Modified radical mastectomy was less disfiguring; however, losing a breast still caused many women to suffer emotional and psychological distress. At this time, lumpectomy was not a consideration because of the fear of increased local recurrence and decreased survival. Advances in the science of breast cancer treatment began to demonstrate that disease-free survival improved with cytotoxic drugs and/or hormone therapy, and a large cooperative study showed no difference in survival between mastectomy and breast conservation treatment (lumpectomy, axillary node dissection, and radiation therapy) when adjuvant treatment was included (Fisher, Redmond, Wickerham, et al., 1989). Figures 5-1, 5-2, and 5-3 show a modified radical mastectomy, a total mastectomy (with or without lymph node sampling), and a lumpectomy.

Sentinel Node Biopsy

Sentinel lymph node (SLN) biopsy was introduced approximately 10 years ago to provide an alternative to the standard

Figure 5-1. Modified Radical Mastectomy

Modified radical mastectomy includes removal of breast tissue, removal of a skin ellipse that includes the tumor site and nipple areola complex, and axillary node sampling.

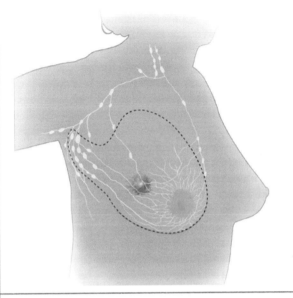

Note. From *What You Need to Know About Breast Cancer* (NIH Publication No. 05-1556) (p. 28), by the National Cancer Institute, 2005, Bethesda, MD: Author. Used with permission.

Figure 5-2. Total Mastectomy

Total mastectomy includes removal of breast tissue only; it most often is used for ductal carcinoma in situ. There may or may not be axillary sampling.

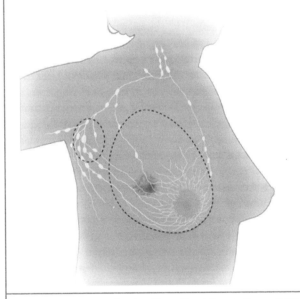

Note. From *What You Need to Know About Breast Cancer* (NIH Publication No. 05-1556) (p. 27), by the National Cancer Institute, 2005, Bethesda, MD: Author. Used with permission.

Figure 5-3. Lumpectomy

Lumpectomy with axillary sampling involves removal of the tumor with surrounding normal tissue.

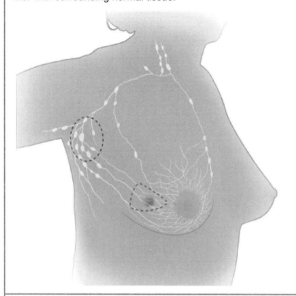

Note. From *What You Need to Know About Breast Cancer* (NIH Publication No. 05-1556) (p. 27), by the National Cancer Institute, 2005, Bethesda, MD: Author. Used with permission.

Figures 5-5, 5-6, and 5-7 show the injection at the tumor site, location of the sentinel node, and excision of the tumor and node(s). The sentinel node removal is completed first, followed by removal of the tumor. There is a break between the surgeries to clean the immediate area, and the patient is cleaned and redraped. This sequence reduces the potential contamination of the axilla with malignant cells.

Surgery and node evaluation are important for staging the cancer. The tumor (T), node involvement (N), and evidence of distant metastasis (M) are standard considerations used to determine the type of therapy that will be given. The American Joint Committee on Cancer has issued a sixth edition of its manual for staging various cancers to evaluate the disease. Stage I breast cancer is a tumor less than 2 cm with no posi-

---

Figure 5-4. Lymphatics of the Breast

Lymphatics of the breast leading to (A) axillary nodes, which are distributed over a large area from the lateral aspects of the breast proper to the axillary vessels; (B) interpectoral chain leading to interpectoral node (circle detail) and to high nodes in the axilla; and (C) chain of the internal mammary leading frequently to nodes in second interspace and to supraclavicular and cervical nodes. The levels of lymph nodes (I, II, III) are defined by the pectoralis minor muscle.

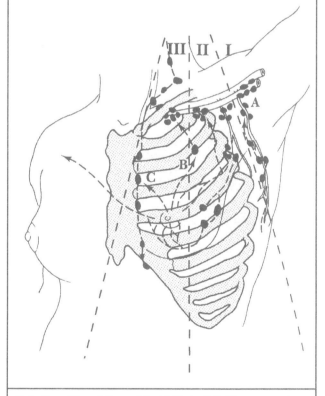

Note. From "Breast Cancer" (p. 1048), by D.D. Chapman and S. Moore in C.H. Yarbro, M.H. Frogge, and M. Goodman (Eds.), *Cancer Nursing: Principles and Practice* (6th ed.), 2005, Sudbury, MA: Jones and Bartlett. Copyright 2005 by Jones and Bartlett. Reprinted with permission.

---

axillary node dissection, removing level I and often level II nodes (see Figure 5-4). The American Society of Clinical Oncology (ASCO) recently published guidelines for SLN biopsy (Lyman et al., 2005). This procedure is appropriate for women with early-stage breast cancer who have clinically negative axillary nodes. Because the risk of leaving residual disease in the axilla is 10%–40% when a sentinel node is positive, a completion axillary dissection is recommended when a positive sentinel node is identified (Hwang et al., 2003; Kepple et al., 2004; Kuerer & Newman, 2005; Van Zee et al., 2003). There has been discussion as to whether a finding of micrometastasis in the sentinel node warrants a completion axillary dissection. Some believe that these cells result from the immediate dislodging of the tumor, rather than from metastasis (Bold, 2002). Nevertheless, the ASCO guidelines recommend that axillary lymph node dissection be performed on anyone with metastatic disease greater than 2 mm (Lyman et al.).

The breast, being a gland, drains into the axillary lymph nodes, and the first node (or nodes) to receive the drainage is known as the sentinel node. The sentinel node is identified through an injection of blue dye, radiocolloid injection, or both (Bold, 2002; Mamounas, 2005). The breast usually is injected either at the subareolar or peritumoral site, and the node(s) is targeted visually (with blue dye) or by using a probe (i.e., radiocolloid). The identification rate for the sentinel node is 90% (Kepple et al., 2004).

**Figure 5-5. Sentinel Lymph Node Biopsy:
Injection at the Tumor Site**

Radioactive substance and/or blue dye is injected near the tumor.

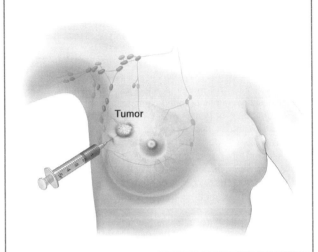

Note. From *Breast Cancer PDQ®: Treatment,* by the National Cancer Institute, 2005. Retrieved August 11, 2006, from http://www.cancer.gov/cancertopics/pdq/treatment/breast/Patient/page5

**Figure 5-7. Sentinel Lymph Node Biopsy:
Removal of Nodes**

The first lymph nodes to take up the material are removed and checked for cancer cells.

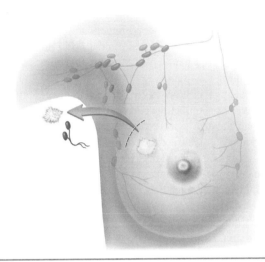

Note. From *Breast Cancer PDQ®: Treatment,* by the National Cancer Institute, 2005. Retrieved August 11, 2006, from http://www.cancer.gov/cancertopics/pdq/treatment/breast/Patient/page5

**Figure 5-6. Sentinel Lymph Node Biopsy:
Location of Nodes**

The probe locates the nodes receiving the injected radioisotope. Note that two nodes are identified.

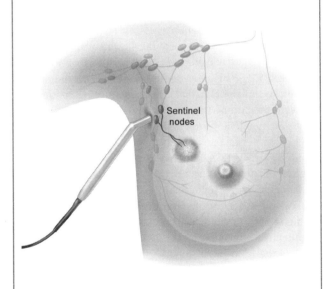

Note. From *Breast Cancer PDQ®: Treatment,* by the National Cancer Institute, 2005. Retrieved August 11, 2006, from http://www.cancer.gov/cancertopics/pdq/treatment/breast/Patient/page5

tive nodes and no sign of distant metastasis. Stage II disease consists of tumors 2–4.99 cm large with one to three positive axillary nodes and no sign of distant metastasis, or tumors greater than 5 cm with no positive nodes and no sign of distant metastasis. Stage III disease consists of more extensive local/regional disease with suspected but unproven distant metastasis, and stage IV breast cancer is described as the presence of distant metastasis (Greene et al., 2002).

The surgeon and oncology nurse participate in the patient/family education in preparation for breast surgery. The surgeon addresses the technical aspects of the surgery, and the nurse discusses what to expect the day of the surgery, postoperative hand/arm limitations, beginning exercises, drain care, and follow-up after the surgery.

The pain and arm/shoulder dysfunction occur mainly because of the standard axillary dissection surgery and are less of an issue with the more widespread implementation of SLN biopsy. Pain can be alleviated through a patient-controlled analgesia pump or oral analgesics, depending on the type of surgery. A woman who has undergone immediate reconstruction will have different pain issues than one who has a mastectomy alone. Depending on the type of surgery performed, patients will have up to two drains. The nurses in the hospital will instruct patients on emptying and measuring the contents and recording the amount drainage. Usually the drain is attached to a bulb that maintains low suction through collapsing the bulb prior to drain connection. The bulb should be emptied periodically (usually two to three times a day). Patients also should be attentive to the function of the drain, noting if it becomes blocked (drainage ceases). A blocked drain can result in a hematoma or seroma and potentially can cause infection. If the drain appears to be blocked, it can be milked to restore function. Milking is done by holding the drain with a hemostat or pinched fingers and moving down from the proximal end of the drain to the distal end. This is done while the other hand holds the proximal end firmly to avoid dislodging the drain.

Early postsurgery exercises are confined to raising the arm no higher than the shoulder and consist of hair care and shoulder touches with the arm extended at 90 degrees. The American Cancer Society has published the booklet *Exercises After Breast Surgery* that can be ordered or downloaded from its Web site (www.cancer.org). This booklet addresses exercises that can be done immediately after surgery as well as those to be done when the physician indicates that more strenuous exercises may begin (see Figures 8-1, 8-2, and 8-3 in Chapter 8).

The potential for infection in the hand and arm is increased when lymph nodes have been removed. Patients should be instructed to avoid any potential for infection. They should wear a protective glove during cooking, cleaning, and gardening. A manicure may cause slight nicks in the skin, but if it is desired, the manicurist should be cautioned about clipping cuticles and should ensure that the instruments are clean (see Chapter 7 for lymphedema precautions). Taking blood drawings and blood pressures on the affected arm should be avoided. Any injury to the skin should be addressed immediately and washed thoroughly and an antibiotic ointment applied. Any area that appears to be inflamed or infected should be reported to the nurse or physician. Infection can result in lymphedema that is transitory or permanent. Avoiding lymphedema is not always possible, but certain precautions should be taken, such as avoiding lifting heavy, inert objects with the affected arm. In addition, any repetitive exertion, such as raking leaves, shoveling snow, and working out with heavy weights, has the potential to cause arm swelling. This is because of the increased blood flow to the area, which challenges a compromised lymph system. A person who has been very active is advised to return to her normal activities with caution, noting any activity that causes arm or hand swelling. If swelling is noted, raising and resting the arm above the level of the heart should facilitate drainage. Figure 5-8 and Table 5-1 address infection precautions and postmastectomy exercises.

Minimally Invasive Surgery

Lumpectomy and mastectomy continue to be considered standard surgery for breast cancer, but as surgeons strive to improve the cosmetic outcome and reduce morbidity, minimally invasive surgical options are under investigation. Ablation surgery has been used for metastatic hepatic tumors for years, and the utilization of ablative techniques for benign

---

Figure 5-8. Patient Information: Hand and Arm Procedures

- Do not permit injections (chemotherapy), blood samples, or vaccinations to be done on your affected arm unless approved by your physician.
- When trimming cuticles, take extra care not to tear hangnails. Professional manicures are recommended.
- Wear heavy gloves when gardening and digging or handling thorny plants.
- Always use a thimble when sewing to avoid pinpricks, and wear rubber gloves while washing dishes.
- Protect your arm from burns, especially from small appliances such as irons or frying pans, and from the sun.
- Be sure that your hand and arm are well protected with an elbow-length mitt when reaching into a hot oven.
- Always have blood pressure measurements taken on the opposite arm.
- Avoid arm constriction from tight elastic, sleeves, or jewelry.
- Do not carry a heavy purse or other objects—especially grocery bags or luggage—with your affected arm.
- Avoid strenuous upper body aerobics unless arm is supported by a properly fitted antilymphedema compression sleeve. Lifting weights of any kind is not recommended.
- Apply a good lanolin cream several times daily if your skin appears dry.
- Treat cuts and scratches by washing the area well and applying an antiseptic. Contact your physician if signs of infection, redness, warmth, or swelling occur.

Note. From "Breast Cancer" (p. 1053), by D.D. Chapman and S. Moore in C.H. Yarbro, M.H. Frogge, and M. Goodman (Eds.), *Cancer Nursing: Principles and Practice* (6th ed.), 2005, Sudbury, MA: Jones and Bartlett. Copyright 2005 by Jones and Bartlett. Reprinted with permission.

---

and malignant breast lesions reflects the trend toward less-invasive procedures (Simmons, 2003). These procedures all cause tumor destruction, meaning that margins cannot be assessed and that any prognostic tissue information (tumor grade, ER, PR, HER2/*neu* status) must be retrieved prior to ablation (Kepple et al., 2004). These surgical techniques are under investigation, and more research is needed to better understand the long-term results.

Laser Ablation

Laser ablation uses heat to damage the tumor and destroy cancer cells. Imprecise targeting has been a drawback in the past, but placement of the laser probe guided by stereotactic mammography or magnetic resonance imaging has improved accuracy (Dowlatshahi et al., 2001; Simmons, 2003). The lesion is heated to 100°C for 15–20 minutes (Simmons). The photographs shown in Figures 5-9 through 5-12 depict the process of a laser ablation. Dowlatshahi et al. studied the effect of laser ablation, eradicating the tumor by performing the laser ablation and also surgically excising the tumor conventionally for histopathic review. Figure 5-9 shows the biopsy-proven mammographic cancer. Figure 5-10 shows the heat probe in

Table 5-1. Postmastectomy Exercises

When to Begin	Purpose	Exercises: Perform Exercises 5–10 Times Each, Three Times a Day
Postoperatively days 1–5	Prevent and/or reduce swelling	• Position arm against your side in a relaxed position. Elbow should be level with your heart, and the wrist just above the elbow when resting. • Rotate wrist in a circular fashion. • Touch fingers to shoulder and extend arm fully.
After drains are removed	Promote muscle movement without stretching	• While standing, brace yourself with your other arm and bend over slightly, allowing your affected arm to hang freely. Swing the arm in small circles and gradually increase in size. Make 10 circles—rest—repeat in the opposite direction. • Swing arm forward and back as far as you can without pulling on the incision. • While standing, bend over slightly and swing arms across the chest in each direction. • While sitting in a chair, rest both arms at your side. Shrug both shoulders, then relax. • While sitting or standing, pull shoulders back, bring the shoulder blades together.
After sutures are removed	Stretch and regain full range of motion; to gain mobility of your shoulder, you must move it in *all* directions, several times a day	• While lying in bed with arm extended, raise arm over your head and extend backward. • While lying in bed, grasp a cane or short pole with both hands across your lap. Extend arms straight up and over your head and return. • Repeat, rotating the cane clockwise and then counterclockwise while over your head. • While standing, extend arm straight over your head and down. • Extend your elbow out from your side at a 90° angle—hold it for 10 seconds—relax. • Extend your arm straight out from your side even with your shoulder—extend arm straight up toward the ceiling. • Stand at arm's length facing a wall. Extend arms so your fingertips touch the wall. Creep fingers up the side of the wall, stepping forward as necessary. Repeat the procedure going down the wall—keep arms extended. • Stand sideways to the wall. Extend arm out so fingers touch the wall. Creep up the wall a little more each day.
After six weeks	Strengthen arm and shoulder and regain total use of arm and shoulder	• Use hand and arm normally. • Begin water aerobics. • Begin overall fitness program. • Begin aerobics, Jazzercise, or other resistive exercises. • Avoid using weights, as these may increase arm edema and subsequent swelling.

Note. From "Breast Cancer" (p. 1054), by D.D. Chapman and S. Moore in C.H. Yarbro, M.H. Frogge, and M. Goodman (Eds.), *Cancer Nursing: Principles and Practice* (6th ed.), 2005, Sudbury, MA: Jones and Bartlett. Copyright 2005 by Jones and Bartlett. Reprinted with permission.

the tumor and the other sensor monitoring the temperature of the surrounding tissue. Figure 5-11 is a cross-section of the excised tumor, and Figure 5-12 shows the sequential improvement in the mammogram. Note the two clips to demarcate the area for future imaging.

Cryoablation

Cryoablation also has been used in hepatic tumors, using extreme cold to kill cancer cells by disrupting the cell membrane. The only U.S. Food and Drug Administration (FDA)-approved indication is for core-biopsy–proven fibroadenoma. Ultrasound guidance is used for correct placement, and the tumor is subjected to multiple freeze-thaw cycles at temperatures of –160°C to –196°C. The time required for each cycle depends on the size of the lesion. As with laser ablation, prognostic tumor information must be gathered before the procedure, because the procedure destroys the tumor (Dowlatshahi et al., 2001; Simmons, 2003).

Radiofrequency Ablation

Radiofrequency ablation uses friction heat generated by high-frequency alternating current that causes ion movement in the tissue. The cell kill is achieved by altering the cell membrane, the structure of the nucleus, and DNA replication.

Figure 5-9. Mammographically Detected Breast Cancer

Image used in treatment planning for laser ablation.

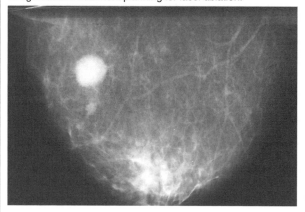

Note. Image courtesy of Kambiz Dowlat, MD, Professor of Surgery, Rush University Medical Center. Used with permission.

Figure 5-10. Laser Therapy

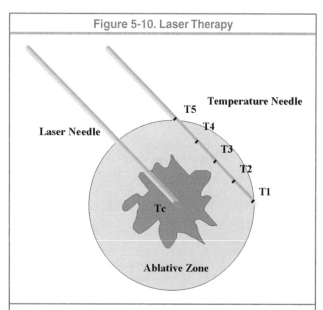

Note. Image courtesy of Kambiz Dowlat, MD, Professor of Surgery, Rush University Medical Center. Used with permission.

The probe is placed using stereotactic or ultrasound guidance, and electrodes are deployed through the tip of the probe. The target temperature is 95°C and is maintained for 15 minutes (Dowlatshahi et al., 2001; Simmons, 2003).

Radiation Therapy

External Beam Radiation Therapy

Until a few years ago, external beam radiation therapy (EBRT) following treatment for breast cancer consisted of

Figure 5-11. Post-Interstitial Laser Therapy Lumpectomy Section

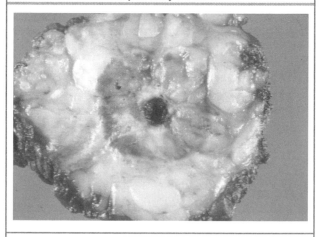

Note. Image courtesy of Kambiz Dowlat, MD, Professor of Surgery, Rush University Medical Center. Used with permission.

treating the entire breast and lumpectomy bed for 6–6½ weeks, beginning a few weeks after surgery or one month after completion of chemotherapy (Gordils-Perez, Rawlins-Duell, & Kelvin, 2003). The goal of radiation to the breast is to eradicate any microscopic disease that may remain in the breast, reducing the recurrence of local/regional disease. Before therapy begins, patients present for a planning session, during which the proper dose to be delivered is calculated by a physicist and discussed with the physician. Radiation planning uses a series of radiographs or a computed tomography (CT) scan with special software to ensure that the angle and dose are accurate, thereby sparing the heart and lung as well as other normal tissues. Although treatment in a prone position may be done, most patients are treated in a supine position, with the arm raised above the shoulder and resting on an immobilizing device to ensure proper positioning for each treatment (Gordils-Perez et al.) (see Figure 5-13).

EBRT usually is associated with minor side effects, including skin changes and breast, axillary, and possible arm swelling. Skin changes include erythema, itching, and tenderness, thickening, telangiectasia, and slight darkening of the skin. Some breast swelling may occur, but it is usually transient and occurs more in large-breasted women than smaller-breasted women. A 5%–11% risk of lymphedema exists if the axilla is radiated (Coen, Taghian, Kachnic, Assaad, & Powell, 2003). Fatigue also may occur during treatment, usually beginning during the third or fourth week.

Local skin reactions need to be monitored to prevent progression to dry and wet desquamation that can lead to infection and temporarily delay treatment. Although fair-skinned women are more susceptible to skin problems, all women need to be checked for changes and cautioned to stay out of the sun during treatment. Because some skin products

Figure 5-12. Laser-Treated Breast Cancer

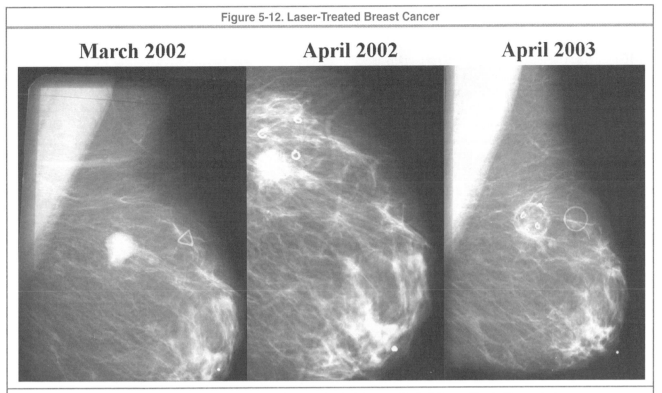

March 2002 **April 2002** **April 2003**

Note. Image courtesy of Kambiz Dowlat, MD, Professor of Surgery, Rush University Medical Center. Used with permission.

may contain ingredients that interfere with delivering the correct radiation dose, nurses must educate patients about acceptable products. Many skin care products, including deodorants, contain metals or alcohol that will interfere with the delivery of the radiation or exacerbate skin toxicity. Nurses often will have a variety of products for patients to try before deciding which to purchase. Women may be more comfortable wearing cotton bras or soft camisoles during this time. Most women complete EBRT without any significant problems.

A decade ago, women who were unable to commit to the time frame of six weeks or who had travel difficulties were advised to have a mastectomy because no other radiation options were available. Scientists and physicists began exploring alternative methods to deliver adequate radiation to the breast in a shorter time frame (four to five days), and various types of accelerated partial-breast irradiation (APBI) modalities are being used and continue to be studied.

Accelerated Partial-Breast Irradiation

Interstitial Multicatheter

Interstitial catheters have been used for decades as a method of providing a treatment boost following standard breast radiation. This system involves the placement of a series of catheters at specific intervals surrounding the

Figure 5-13. Positioning for External Beam Radiation Therapy

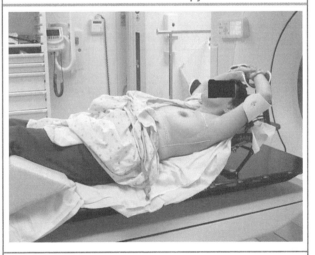

Note. Figure courtesy of Adam Dickler, MD, Rush University Medical Center. Used with permission.

biopsy cavity after surgery is completed. Correct placement of the catheters is critical. Before the advent of image-guidance techniques, proper catheter placement was extremely operator-dependent, but now optimal placement of the radiation source is ensured using stereotactic, ultrasound, or CT guidance with three-dimensional planning. This treatment usually is given over five days, twice a day for 30 minutes. This technique of radiation therapy is well tolerated, but patients may be upset by the appearance of the breast with the catheters in place (Arthur & Vicini, 2005). This treatment usually is offered to patients who are older than 40 years of age because of an increased risk of multifocal disease in younger women, occurring outside the radiation field, providing inadequate treatment. Candidates also usually have early-stage breast cancer (stage I or II) with a tumor size no larger than 3 cm and negative nodes on biopsy (Chen et al., 2006). Figures 5-14 and 5-15 demonstrate catheters placed in the breast and catheters attached to the radiation source.

Figure 5-14. Catheters Placed in the Breast

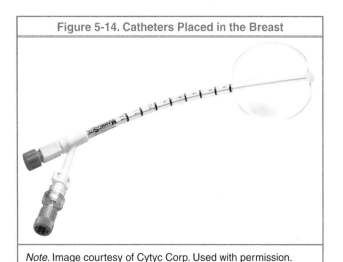

Note. Image courtesy of Cytyc Corp. Used with permission.

Figure 5-15. Catheters Attached to the Radiation Source

Note. Image courtesy of Cytyc Corp. Used with permission.

MammoSite

The MammoSite® (Cytyc Corp., Palo Alto, CA) technique was created in response to the complaints surrounding interstitial multicatheter radiation. The MammoSite process of APBI delivers the radiation dose through a balloon with a tube attachment that is inserted into the biopsy cavity either during or after surgery (Zannis et al., 2005). Once the proper placement is confirmed, sterile water is infused to inflate the balloon, and the dose is delivered in a single circumferential source, 1 cm from the surface of the balloon. The manufacturer claims this method provides an improved dosimetric coverage. MammoSite is the preferred method used in the United States (Arthur & Vicini, 2005). Vicini et al. (2005) discussed the results of the American Society of Breast Surgeons MammoSite Brachytherapy Registry Trial. Eighty-seven institutions enrolled 1,237 patients with early-stage breast cancer. The patient eligibility criteria were age older than 45 years, tumor size equal to or greater than 2 cm, invasive histology, and clear margin status with negative lymph nodes. The technical criteria for enrollment were a distance of 5 mm between the skin and applicator, although 7 mm was preferred; balloon conformance of 1 cm around the biopsy cavity; and biopsy cavity of at least 3 cm in one dimension. CT scan was recommended after device placement (Vicini et al.). The results of this study indicated that good cosmesis was achieved in 92% of the patients, device-related infections occurred in 5.3%, and radiation recall events with subsequent chemotherapy happened with 13.5% of the patients. At 12-month follow-up, cosmetic results were comparable to whole-breast radiation therapy and the toxicity of infection and radiation recall were acceptable to patients.

Nursing Implications for Radiation Therapy

Prior to starting therapy, patients meet with the physician and nurse to plan treatment. This is an appropriate time for the nurse to address any concerns and provide additional education about the treatment process. Although no set standards exist for APBI, the American Brachytherapy Society (www.americanbrachytherapysociety.org) recommends that women should be 45 years of age or older, tumor size should be less than 3 cm, margins must be negative for disease, and patients must have no positive lymph nodes (Arthur & Vicini, 2005). The American Society of Breast Surgeons (www.breastsurgeons.org) reissued guidelines in December 2005 that agree with the American Brachytherapy Society. Complications with this procedure are not well documented. Shah et al. (2004) compared skin complications of interstitial brachytherapy and MammoSite partial-breast irradiation and found little difference in cosmesis. Skin erythema equal to grade I was higher with MammoSite (17.3% versus 42.9%), but skin erythema greater than grade I was higher with interstitial (5.3% versus 0%). Interstitial also resulted in more subcutaneous fibrosis, but symptomatic fat necrosis was not significantly different between the two modalities (Shah et al.).

Nursing care of patients undergoing brachytherapy focuses on catheter and skin care. The site should be cleansed with half-strength hydrogen peroxide, antibiotic ointment applied, and the area covered with a sterile gauze pad. The dressing is changed once a day, and the site is assessed for signs of infection (pain, increased erythema, drainage). Women should be instructed to check oral temperature three times a day and report fever greater than 101°F. Patients also are instructed to avoid swimming or submerging the device in water (Hogle, Quinn, & Heron, 2003).

Breast Reconstruction

Women who choose a mastectomy will need some type of breast restoration. This is important for weight replacement as well as for cosmetic and self-esteem issues. Each woman needs to choose the restoration option that fits her lifestyle and desires. Women choose breast reconstruction for a variety of reasons. The American Society of Plastic Surgeons (2006) estimated that during 2005, 57,778 women underwent some type of breast reconstruction. Of these women, 11,631 chose an implant; 34,660 chose a tissue expander with an implant; 9,578 chose a transverse rectus abdominis myocutaneous (TRAM) flap; and 1,909 chose a deep inferior epigastric perforator flap.

Silicone Implants

The advent of silicone implants in the 1960s dramatically changed the treatment of breast cancer. Mastectomy remained the curative treatment, but now women had the option to choose a permanent prosthesis implanted in the breast rather than a removable external prosthesis inside a bra. Silicone implants, first introduced in 1963, produced a natural contour and suppleness for reconstructed and augmented breasts. In 1992, the FDA restricted the use of silicone implants because of concerns regarding
- Possible obscuration of a breast cancer on mammography (at that time, implants for augmentation were inserted into the parenchyma)
- Development of breast cancer or other soft tissue tumors
- Implant longevity
- Silicone gel leakage and the resulting local and systemic effects
- A possible connection with autoimmune disease.

However, a large retrospective study failed to confirm any correlation between breast cancer and autoimmune disease, and subsequent studies have not confirmed the other concerns (Blackburn & Everson, 1997; Janowsky, Kupper, & Hulka, 2000; Tugwell et al., 2001).

As of the time of this printing, the FDA has approved two silicone implants for use in breast reconstruction and augmentation (FDA, 2006). Studies of the long-term safety of the silicone implants are ongoing.

Saline Expanders and Implants

Almost every woman who chooses mastectomy is a candidate for an expander or implant. The optimal candidate has a breast volume of 500 g or less and has minimal ptosis. Women with marked ptosis (greater than 2 cm) often will require alteration of the contralateral breast to achieve an acceptable symmetrical result (Spear & Spittler, 2001). Saline expanders may be implanted immediately or anytime after mastectomy. The advantage of immediate reconstruction is combining two surgeries, thereby avoiding the need for an additional anesthetic. Although there has been a debate that immediate reconstruction delays the start of chemotherapy, several studies have determined that immediate reconstruction is an acceptable option with few oncologic effects (Knottenbelt, Spauwen, & Wobbes, 2004; Rey et al., 2005; Taylor & Kumar, 2005; Yeh, Lyle, Wei, & Sherry, 1998). Additionally, immediate reconstruction lessens the psychological distress related to the loss of the breast (Al-Ghazal, Sully, Fallowfield, & Blamey, 2000). Women may choose delayed reconstruction for personal reasons related to longer convalescence or uncertainty about wanting the procedure. Medical reasons also can cause delayed reconstruction. The patient may have comorbid conditions that preclude the length of time needed for surgery, or the patient may have advanced disease that will require more extensive postchemotherapy radiation treatments (Schechter et al., 2005).

After the surgeon removes the breast, the plastic surgeon begins the reconstructive surgery, placing the expander behind the pectoralis muscle. If the reconstruction is delayed, the operation begins with the plastic surgeon opening the skin along the mastectomy scar. The purpose of the expander is to gradually stretch the skin to the desired size to match the other breast. Some large-breasted women may elect to have breast reduction on the contralateral side to achieve better symmetry. The expander resembles a pocket with a tube and a port attached on the lateral side that is placed near the axilla. Approximately two to three weeks after insertion of the expander, the saline injections begin (Malata, McIntosh, & Purushotham, 2000). The implant port is injected every one to two weeks until the desired effect is achieved, usually three to four months (see Figure 5-16). If a patient has mildly ptotic breasts, the implant is overfilled at first, then slightly deflated months later, achieving the desired cosmetic effect (Spear & Spittler, 2001). The amount of saline injected at one sitting depends on the amount of skin tension and the comfort of the patient. The saline expander is then surgically removed and a permanent prosthesis is placed (Malata et al.; Moran, Herceg, Kurtelawicz, & Serletti, 2000). Complications of permanent prostheses include capsular contraction, ranging from minimal to severe, and visible skin ripples, more com-

---

Figure 5-16. Tissue Expansion

This illustration shows the process of stretching the chest skin and soft tissue to accommodate the permanent breast implant.

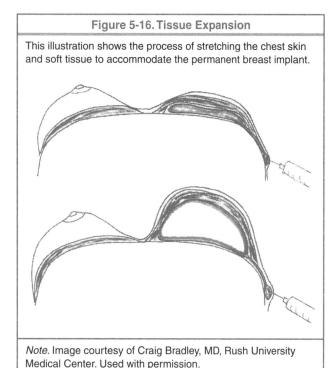

Note. Image courtesy of Craig Bradley, MD, Rush University Medical Center. Used with permission.

---

mon in thin women. Some degree of capsular contraction is expected and usually is minimal, but severe contraction may necessitate removing the expander or implant (Malata et al.). Collis, Coleman, Foo, and Sharpe (2000) reported that the incidence of capsular contraction has been historically estimated to be as high as 50%, but using textured rather than smooth implants has reduced it to approximately 10%.

Following placement of the implant, patients usually have a large postoperative dressing and often one or more surgical drains. Women resume normal activities gradually as tolerated. Patients must avoid vigorous exercise in the first six to eight weeks; however, walking for exercise generally is acceptable by the second week. Lifting anything heavier than five to seven pounds is contraindicated in the first six weeks. Postoperatively, women may experience numbness, tingling, or tightness, with more pronounced symptoms in thin women. These symptoms typically decrease gradually over six to eight weeks.

Part of the informed consent regarding implants is a discussion of their associated risks. The risk of leakage or rupture always exists. If an implant is placed in a young woman who has a good prognosis, the implant may eventually wear out and need to be replaced, although there is no consensus as to when this will occur. Women need to be aware of whether their health insurance will pay for additional procedures that may be needed or for corrections to provide symmetric cosmesis in the other breast. Following both implant and flap procedures, the plastic surgeon may recommend additional procedures on the unaffected side.

This may include mastopexy, reduction mammaplasty, or augmentation mammaplasty. Women need to discuss these procedures with their oncology team because postoperative scarring can interfere with mammography and subsequent screening.

Autologous Flaps

Some women are averse to synthetic material being implanted into their bodies and will seek other reconstructive methods. Autologous breast reconstruction surgeries are more extensive because the donor site must be harvested first and then implanted, requiring a longer operating time and more anesthesia. The recovery time is significantly longer than with implant surgery, ranging from six to eight weeks instead of three to four weeks. The cosmetic outcome appears more natural than with implant surgery, but autologous flaps have more potential complications.

Transverse Rectus Abdominis Myocutaneous Flap

The TRAM flap is a common autologous surgery that involves removing all or part of the rectus abdominis muscle with an ellipse of skin (see Figures 5-17 and 5-18). The TRAM flap can be implanted as a pedicled or free flap. A pedicled flap retains its own blood supply and is tunneled under the skin to the breast. A free flap is disconnected from its blood supply and reattached using blood vessels of the axilla and chest wall (Malata et al., 2000; Sandau, 2002). Patients who are potentially ineligible for the TRAM flap are those with conditions that may compromise vascular integrity, such as prior abdominal surgery, prior irradiation, a body weight greater than 25% over their ideal body weight, smoking, and a history of diabetes, collagen vascular disease, or hypertension (Chang, Reece, et al., 2000; Chang, Wang, et al., 2000; Malata et al.). The surgeon also may evaluate the patient for psychological issues that preclude eligibility, including a history of mental illness or unrealistic expectations of the surgery. Complications include abdominal bulge and hernia, upper fullness, and upper bulge.

Deep Inferior Epigastric Perforator Flap

The deep inferior epigastric perforator flap is a newer reconstruction technique that preserves the muscle, utilizing the skin and fat. The integrity of the muscle is maintained, resulting in less morbidity and less postoperative pain (Blondeel et al., 2000; Grotting, Beckenstein, & Arkoulakis, 2003; Keller, 2001; Malata et al., 2000). One disappointing complication has been an initial increased incidence of fat necrosis resulting in partial flap loss. This complication was reduced by changing the selection process to exclude smokers, avoiding harvesting large flaps, and revising the method of assessing vascular integrity (Kroll, 2000).

Figure 5-17. TRAM Flap Procedure

These illustrations show how the abdominal muscles (rectus abdominus) are used to reconstruct the breast.

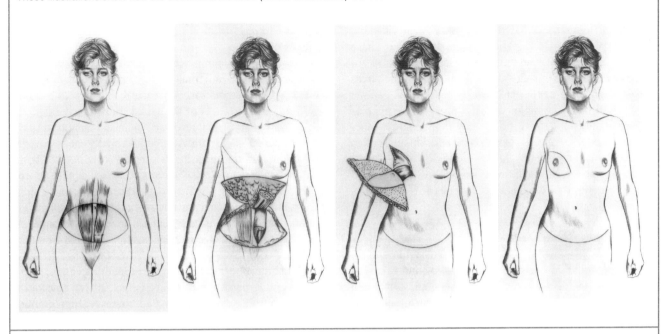

Note. Figures courtesy of the National Cancer Institute.

Figure 5-18. Cosmesis Achieved With TRAM Procedure

Photo A shows the patient post mastectomy and prior to the TRAM flap procedure. Following the surgery, the patient's newly formed breast mound and abdominal incision show the surgical scars (B), which will fade over time.

A

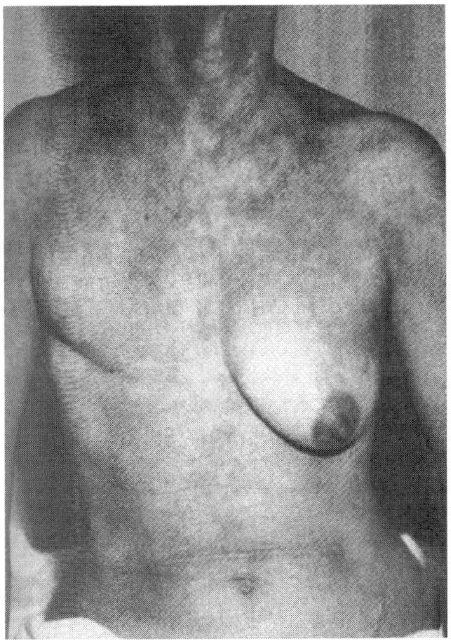

B

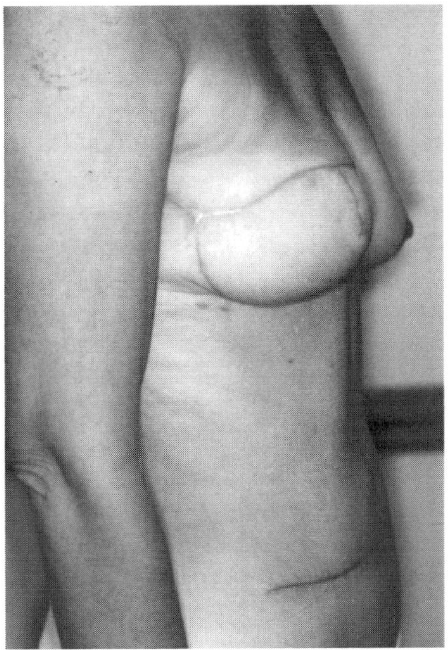

Note. Photos courtesy of Craig Bradley, MD, Rush University Medical Center. Used with permission.

Latissimus Dorsi Flap

The latissimus dorsi flap can be used in combination with an implant or as an autologous flap when other sites are unavailable (Clough, Louis-Sylvestre, Fitoussi, Couturaud, & Nos, 2002; Heitmann, 2003; Malata et al., 2000; Rainsbury, 2002). Autologous-alone flaps often are larger than those used with an implant, and more tissue is harvested. All of the fat overlying the muscle is used. In addition, other areas may be used, such as the fat above the iliac crest and the scapular fat pad. The major complications of this type of reconstruction are seroma and alteration of shoulder function and strength. Patients also are at risk for infection, flap necrosis, or incomplete attachment of the skin graft—all of which may necessitate additional surgical procedures and ultimately compromise cosmesis (Clough et al.) (see Figures 5-19 and 5-20).

Gluteal Flaps

Two types of gluteal flap reconstructive techniques exist: superior and inferior. The superior gluteus maximus flap has a shorter pedicle than the inferior, making the insertion and anastomosis more challenging. The inferior flap often is chosen over the superior flap because of the longer pedicle and the availability of more tissue. This procedure is technically more difficult and requires the use of microsurgery as well as vein grafts to establish adequate vascularization at the chest wall. Both of these procedures may be converted to perforator flaps, using skin and fat while sparing muscle. Seroma

and sciatica are complications associated with this procedure (Serletti & Moran, 2000).

Postoperative Care

Postoperative care for reconstruction differs between implant and autologous reconstruction. Women who have implants require judicious monitoring for hematoma and infection. Hematoma causes greater than expected bruising, swelling, and firmness of the breast. Infection is suspected with signs of erythema, fever, and unusual amounts of swelling, tenderness, and pain. Antibiotics usually can resolve the infection, but in rare cases, the implant may need to be removed (Handel, Cordray, Gutierrez, & Jensen, 2000). Patients also will be wearing a binder to keep the breast in line with the contralateral breast and prevent migration of the implant. The plastic surgery team usually replaces the binder, changes the initial dressing, and observes patients for any of the previously described changes. Nurses may be asked to change dressings later and must be instructed in the proper procedure.

Attentive postoperative care is crucial for autologous flaps, especially during the first 72 hours. A Doppler monitor is usually placed on the breast to monitor blood flow and detect any signs of thrombosis. Nurses must assess the site for discoloration, firmness, and change in temperature, all of which may indicate a loss of blood flow to the flap. Presence of any of these signs must be reported immediately to the surgeon.

Figure 5-19. Latissimus Dorsi Flap Procedure

These illustrations depict lifting the latissimus muscle to create a breast mound.

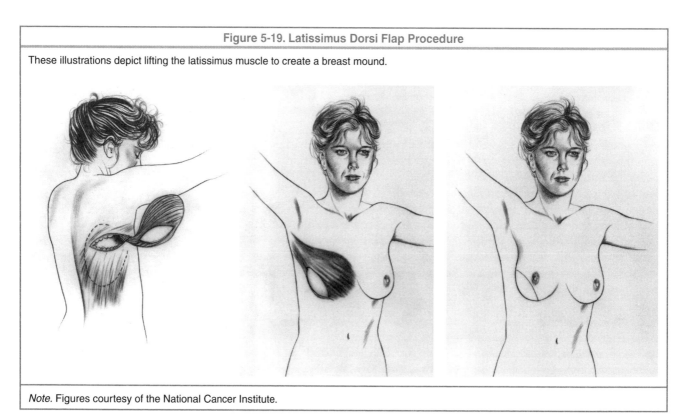

Note. Figures courtesy of the National Cancer Institute.

Figure 5-20. Cosmesis Achieved With Latissimus Dorsi Flap Procedure

Photo A shows the patient presurgery. Following the mastectomy and latissimus dorsi flap procedures, the patient's breasts are not symmetrical (B). Mastopexy is performed on the healthy breast, and a nipple is tattooed on the breast mound (C).

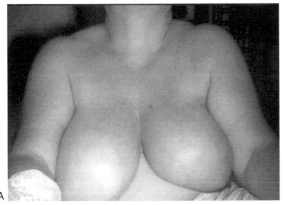

A

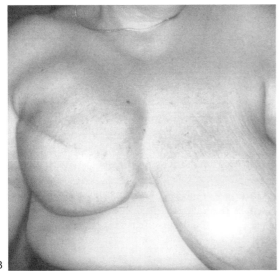

B

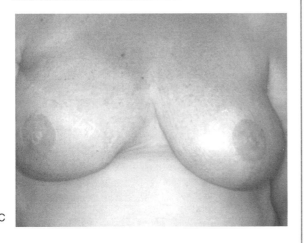

C

Note. Photos courtesy of Craig Bradley, MD, Rush University Medical Center. Used with permission.

Once the reconstruction has been completed, patients may elect to have a nipple created with breast tissue (most common) or grafted onto the breast. The nipple construction is performed through an incision that creates a permanent projection of tissue. Care is taken to match the placement of the nipple through vertical and horizontal caliper measurements of the nipple and areola to achieve symmetry (Losken, Mackay, & Bostwick, 2001). Many women choose this because of the psychological and aesthetic benefit to feel more complete and have a more natural look when undressed. After the incision is well healed, the nipple/areola complex is tattooed intradermally to match pigmentation (see Figure 5-21). Overall, most women are satisfied with the cosmetic appearance of the reconstruction, although the major source of dissatisfaction is the projection of the nipple (Jabor, Shayani, Collins, Karas, & Cohen, 2002; Losken et al.).

Postoperative care after reconstruction of the nipple requires changing dressings for approximately 7–14 days. The tattooing requires fewer days of dressing changes. Pa-

Figure 5-21. Bilateral Nipple Reconstruction

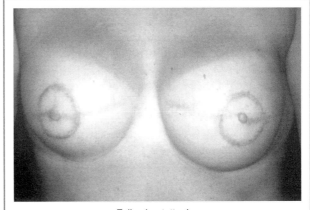

Following tattooing

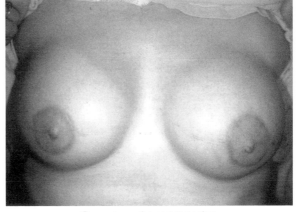

Several months post-tattooing

Note. Photos courtesy of Craig Bradley, MD, Rush University Medical Center. Used with permission.

tients must assess for signs and symptoms of infection and notify the plastic surgeon immediately if the wound opens or bleeding occurs.

Nurses need to help women throughout the reconstructive process. This begins with helping women in seeking several opinions prior to making a decision. Figure 5-22 lists questions for patients to ask plastic surgeons. Women also need to understand that reconstruction will not replace the breast and will not be perfect. For many, however, it will be a significant improvement and worth the time invested in the process.

Prophylactic Surgery

For women with a known mutation in *BRCA1* or *BRCA2*, prophylactic mastectomy is often an appropriate risk-reduction strategy. These women may have a prior diagnosis of breast cancer or may be unaffected. They often will receive care in the oncology setting. For those who choose prophylactic mastectomy, an axillary lymph node dissection is not indicated if there is no diagnosis of malignancy. However, these women must make a choice about breast restoration. For those who choose reconstruction, immediate reconstruction generally is planned. The education and nursing care required is similar to that required for women who have a diagnosis of cancer. These women require more emotional support as they decide whether to have a significant surgery for breast cancer prevention.

Conclusion

The treatment of breast cancer has changed dramatically in the past 40 years. Initially there was one treatment for breast cancer, a radical surgery that was emotionally and physically disfiguring. Research in breast cancer has introduced therapies that are less invasive and more curative, now offering

---

Figure 5-22. Questions to Ask When Considering Breast Reconstructive Surgery

- What are the possible surgical options?
- What are the benefits of the recommended procedure?
- What are the risks of the recommended procedure?
- What are the limitations of the recommended procedure?
- How many times has the surgeon done this particular procedure?
- Does the surgeon have pictures of women he or she has done this procedure on?
- What type of anesthesia will be used?
- How long will the surgery take?
- What follow-up procedures will be needed?
- Where will the incisions be placed?
- What is the anticipated recovery?
- When is it recommended that reconstruction begin?
- What is the cost? How much will insurance cover?

---

lumpectomy when appropriate and radiation therapy that will treat only the disease site. For those who choose mastectomy, breast restoration is greatly improved. The continuing research of new therapies and strategies in breast cancer management will help women to obtain good local/regional control of the malignancy. When combined with appropriate adjuvant systemic therapy, the long-term outlook for many women is excellent.

References

Al-Ghazal, S.K., Sully, L., Fallowfield, L., & Blamey, R.W. (2000). The psychological impact of immediate rather than delayed breast reconstruction. *European Journal of Surgical Oncology, 26,* 17–19.

American Society of Plastic Surgeons. (2006). *2005 reconstructive breast surgery: Age distribution.* Arlington Heights, IL: Author.

Arthur, D.W., & Vicini, F.A. (2005). Accelerated partial breast irradiation as a part of breast conservation therapy. *Journal of Clinical Oncology, 23,* 1726–1735.

Blackburn, W.D., Jr., & Everson, M.P. (1997). Silicone-associated rheumatic disease: An unsupported myth. *Plastic and Reconstructive Surgery, 99,* 1362–1367.

Blondeel, P.N., Arnstein, M., Verstraete, K.M., Depuydt, K., Van Landuyt, K.H., Monstrey, S.J., et al. (2000). Venous congestion and blood flow in free transverse rectus abdominis myocutaneous and deep inferior epigastric perforator flaps. *Plastic and Reconstructive Surgery, 106,* 1295–1299.

Bold, R. (2002). Surgical management of breast cancer: Today and tomorrow. *Cancer Biotherapy and Radiopharmaceuticals, 17,* 1–9.

Chang, D.W., Reece, G.P., Wang, B., Robb, G.L., Miller, M.J., Evans, G.R., et al. (2000). Effect of smoking on complications in patients undergoing free TRAM flap breast reconstruction. *Plastic and Reconstructive Surgery, 105,* 2374–2380.

Chang, D.W., Wang, B.G., Robb, G.L., Reece, G.P., Miller, M.J., Evans, G.R., et al. (2000). Effect of obesity on flap and donor-site complications in free transverse rectus abdominis myocutaneous flap breast reconstruction. *Plastic and Reconstructive Surgery, 105,* 1640–1648.

Chen, P.Y., Vicini, F.A., Benitez, P., Kestin, L.L., Wallace, M., Mitchell, C., et al. (2006). Long-term cosmetic results and toxicity after accelerated partial-breast irradiation. *Cancer, 106,* 991–999.

Clough, K.B., Louis-Sylvestre, C., Fitoussi, A., Couturaud, B., & Nos, C. (2002). Donor site sequelae after autologous breast reconstruction with an extended latissimus dorsi flap. *Plastic and Reconstructive Surgery, 109,* 1904–1911.

Coen, J.J., Taghian, A.G., Kachnic, L.A., Assaad, S.I., & Powell, S.N. (2003). Risk of lymphedema after regional nodal irradiation with breast conservation therapy. *International Journal of Radiation Oncology, Biology, Physics, 55,* 1209–1215.

Collis, N., Coleman, D., Foo, I.T., & Sharpe, D.T. (2000). Ten-year review of a prospective randomized controlled trial of textured versus smooth subglandular silicone gel breast implants. *Plastic and Reconstructive Surgery, 106,* 786–791.

Dowlatshahi, K., Francescatti, D., Bloom, K., Jewell, W.R., Schwartzberg, B.S., Singletary, S.E., et al. (2001). Image-guided surgery of small breast cancers. *American Journal of Surgery, 182,* 419–425.

Fisher, B. (1999). Highlights from recent National Surgical Adjuvant Breast and Bowel Project studies in the treatment and prevention of breast cancer. *CA: A Cancer Journal for Clinicians, 49,* 159–177.

Fisher, B., & Anderson, S. (1994). Conservative surgery for the management of invasive and noninvasive carcinoma of the breast: NSABP trials. National Surgical Adjuvant Breast and Bowel Project. *World Journal of Surgery, 18,* 63–69.

Fisher, B., Anderson, S., Redmond, C.K., Wolmark, N., Wickerham, D.L., & Cronin, W.M. (1995). Reanalysis and results after 12 years of follow-up in a randomized clinical trial comparing total mastectomy with lumpectomy with or without irradiation in the treatment of breast cancer. *New England Journal of Medicine, 333,* 1456–1461.

Fisher, B., Anderson, S., Tan-Chiu, E., Wolmark, N., Wickerham, D.L., Fisher, E.R., et al. (2001). Tamoxifen and chemotherapy for axillary node-negative, estrogen receptor-negative breast cancer: Findings from National Surgical Adjuvant Breast and Bowel Project B-23. *Journal of Clinical Oncology, 19,* 931–942.

Fisher, B., Bauer, M., Margolese, R., Poisson, R., Pilch, Y., Redmond, C., et al. (1985). Five-year results of a randomized clinical trial comparing total mastectomy and segmental mastectomy with or without radiation in the treatment of breast cancer. *New England Journal of Medicine, 312,* 665–673.

Fisher, B., Costantino, J., Redmond, C., Fisher, E., Margolese, R., Dimitrov, N., et al. (1993). Lumpectomy compared with lumpectomy and radiation therapy for the treatment of intraductal breast cancer. *New England Journal of Medicine, 328,* 1581–1586.

Fisher, B., Costantino, J., Redmond, C., Poisson, R., Bowman, D., Couture, J., et al. (1989). A randomized clinical trial evaluating tamoxifen in the treatment of patients with node-negative breast cancer who have estrogen-receptor-positive tumors. *New England Journal of Medicine, 320,* 479–484.

Fisher, B., Costantino, J.P., Wickerham, D.L., Cecchini, R.S., Cronin, W.M., Robidoux, A., et al. (2005). Tamoxifen for the prevention of breast cancer: Current status of the National Surgical Adjuvant Breast and Bowel Project P-1 Study. *Journal of the National Cancer Institute, 97,* 1652–1662.

Fisher, B., Costantino, J.P., Wickerham, D.L., Redmond, C.K., Kavanah, M., Cronin, W.M., et al. (1998). Tamoxifen for prevention of breast cancer: Report of the National Surgical Adjuvant Breast and Bowel Project P-1 Study. *Journal of the National Cancer Institute, 90,* 1371–1388.

Fisher, B., Dignam, J., Bryant, J., & Wolmark, N. (2001). Five versus more than five years of tamoxifen for lymph node-negative breast cancer: Updated findings from the National Surgical Adjuvant Breast and Bowel Project B-14 Randomized Trial. *Journal of the National Cancer Institute, 93,* 684–690.

Fisher, B., Dignam, J., Wolmark, N., DeCillis, A., Emir, B., Wickerham, D.L., et al. (1997). Tamoxifen and chemotherapy for lymph node-negative, estrogen receptor-positive breast cancer. *Journal of the National Cancer Institute, 89,* 1673–1682.

Fisher, B., Jeong, J.H., Anderson, S., Bryant, J., Fisher, E.R., & Wolmark, N. (2002). Twenty-five-year follow-up of a randomized trial comparing radical mastectomy, total mastectomy, and total mastectomy followed by irradiation. *New England Journal of Medicine, 347,* 567–575.

Fisher, B., Montague, E., Redmond, C., Barton, B., Borland, D., Fisher, E.R., et al. (1977). Comparison of radical mastectomy with alternative treatments for primary breast cancer. A first report of results from a prospective randomized clinical trial. *Cancer, 39*(Suppl. 6), 2827–2839.

Fisher, B., & Redmond, C. (1992). Systemic therapy in node-negative patients: Updated findings from NSABP clinical trials. National Surgical Adjuvant Breast and Bowel Project. *Journal of the National Cancer Institute Monographs, 11,* 105–116.

Fisher, B., Redmond, C., Brown, A., Fisher, E.R., Wolmark, N., Bowman, D., et al. (1986). Adjuvant chemotherapy with and without tamoxifen in the treatment of primary breast cancer: 5-year results from the National Surgical Adjuvant Breast and Bowel Project Trial. *Journal of Clinical Oncology, 4,* 459–471.

Fisher, B., Redmond, C., Brown, A., Wolmark, N., Wittliff, J., Fisher, E.R., et al. (1981). Treatment of primary breast cancer with chemotherapy and tamoxifen. *New England Journal of Medicine, 305,* 1–6.

Fisher, B., Redmond, C., Dimitrov, N.V., Bowman, D., Legault-Poisson, S., Wickerham, D.L., et al. (1989). A randomized clinical trial evaluating sequential methotrexate and fluorouracil in the treatment of patients with node-negative breast cancer who have estrogen-receptor-negative tumors. *New England Journal of Medicine, 320,* 473–478.

Fisher, B., Redmond, C., Fisher, E.R., Bauer, M., Wolmark, N., Wickerham, D.L., et al. (1985). Ten-year results of a randomized clinical trial comparing radical mastectomy and total mastectomy with or without radiation. *New England Journal of Medicine, 312,* 674–681.

Fisher, B., Redmond, C., Poisson, R., Margolese, R., Wolmark, N., Wickerham, L., et al. (1989). Eight-year results of a randomized clinical trial comparing total mastectomy and lumpectomy with or without irradiation in the treatment of breast cancer. *New England Journal of Medicine, 320,* 822–828.

Fisher, B., Redmond, C., Wickerham, D.L., Wolmark, N., Bowman, D., Couture, J., et al. (1989). Systemic therapy in patients with node-negative breast cancer. A commentary based on two National Surgical Adjuvant Breast and Bowel Project (NSABP) clinical trials. *Annals of Internal Medicine, 111,* 703–712.

Gordils-Perez, J., Rawlins-Duell, R., & Kelvin, J.F. (2003). Advances in radiation treatment of patients with breast cancer. *Clinical Journal of Oncology Nursing, 7,* 629–636.

Greene, F.L., Page, D.L., Fleming, I.D., Fritz, A., Balch, C.M., Haller, D.G., et al. (Eds.). (2002). *AJCC cancer staging manual* (6th ed.). New York: Springer.

Grotting, J.C., Beckenstein, M.S., & Arkoulakis, N.S. (2003). The art and science of autologous breast reconstruction. *Breast Journal, 9,* 350–360.

Halsted, W.H. (1907). The results of radical operations for the cure of carcinoma of the breast. *Surgery, 66,* 1.

Han, W.T., Collie, K., Koopman, C., Azarow, J., Classen, C., Morrow, G.R., et al. (2005). Breast cancer and problems with medical interactions: Relationships with traumatic stress, emotional self-efficacy, and social support. *Psycho-Oncology, 14,* 318–330.

Handel, N., Cordray, T., Gutierrez, J., & Jensen, J.A. (2000). A long-term study of outcomes, complications, and patient satisfaction with breast implants. *Plastic and Reconstructive Surgery, 117,* 757–767.

Heitmann, C.M. (2003). The extended latissimus flap revisited. *Plastic and Reconstructive Surgery, 111,* 1697–1701.

Hogle, W.P., Quinn, A.E., & Heron, D.E. (2003). Advances in brachytherapy: New approaches to target breast cancer. *Clinical Journal of Oncology Nursing, 7,* 324–328.

Hwang, R.F., Krishnamurthy, S., Hunt, K.K., Mirza, N., Ames, F.C., Feig, B., et al. (2003). Clinicopathologic factors predicting involvement of nonsentinel axillary nodes in women with breast cancer. *Annals of Surgical Oncology, 10,* 248–254.

Iwamitsu, Y., Shimoda, K., Abe, H., Tani, T., Okawa, M., & Buck, R. (2005). Anxiety, emotional suppression, and psychological distress before and after breast cancer diagnosis. *Psychosomatics, 46,* 19–24.

Jabor, M.A., Shayani, P.M., Collins, D.R., Karas, T., & Cohen, B.E. (2002). Nipple-areola reconstruction: Satisfaction and clinical determinants. *Plastic and Reconstructive Surgery, 110,* 457–463.

Janowsky, E.C., Kupper, L.L., & Hulka, B.S. (2000). Meta-analyses of the relation between silicone breast implants and the risk of connective-tissue diseases. *New England Journal of Medicine, 342,* 781–790.

Keller, A. (2001). The deep inferior epigastric free flap for breast reconstruction. *Annals of Plastic Surgery, 46,* 474–480.

Kepple, J., Van Zee, K.J., Dowlatshahi, K., Henry-Tillman, R.S., Israel, P.Z., & Klimberg, V.S. (2004). Minimally invasive breast surgery. *Journal of the American College of Surgeons, 199,* 961–975.

Knottenbelt, A., Spauwen, P.H.M., & Wobbes, T. (2004). The onco-logical implications of immediate breast reconstruction. *European Journal of Surgical Oncology, 30,* 829–833.

Kroll, S.S. (2000). Fat necrosis in free transverse rectus abdominis myocutaneous and deep inferior epigastric perforator flaps. *Plastic and Reconstructive Surgery, 106,* 576–583.

Kuerer, H.M., & Newman, L.A. (2005). Lymphatic mapping and sentinel lymph node biopsy for breast cancer: Developments and resolving controversies. *Journal of Clinical Oncology, 23,* 1698–1705.

Losken, A., Mackay, G.J., & Bostwick, J.I. (2001). Nipple reconstruc-tion using the C-V flap technique: A long-term evaluation. *Plastic and Reconstructive Surgery, 108,* 361–369.

Lyman, G.H., Giuliano, A.E., Somerfield, M.R., Benson, A.B., III, Bodurka, D.C., Burstein, H.J., et al. (2005). American Society of Clinical Oncology guideline recommendations for sentinel lymph node biopsy in early-stage breast cancer. *Journal of Clinical On-cology, 23,* 7703–7720.

Malata, C.M., McIntosh, S.A., & Purushotham, A.D. (2000). Im-mediate breast reconstruction after mastectomy for cancer. *British Journal of Surgery, 87,* 1455–1472.

Mamounas, E.P. (2005). Continuing evolution in breast cancer surgi-cal management. *Journal of Clinical Oncology, 23,* 1603–1606.

Moran, S.L., Herceg, S., Kurtelawicz, K., & Serletti, J.M. (2000). TRAM flap breast reconstruction with expanders and implants. *AORN Journal, 71,* 354–362.

Rainsbury, R.M. (2002). Breast-sparing reconstruction with latis-simus dorsi miniflaps. *European Journal of Surgical Oncology, 28,* 891–895.

Rey, P., Martinelli, G., Petit, J.Y., Youssef, O., De Lorenzi, F., Rietjens, M., et al. (2005). Immediate breast reconstruction and high-dose chemotherapy. *Annals of Plastic Surgery, 55,* 250–254.

Sakorafas, G.H. (2001). Breast cancer surgery. Historical evolu-tion, current status, and future perspectives. *Acta Oncologica, 40,* 5–18.

Sandau, K.E. (2002). Free TRAM flap breast reconstruction [Re-view]. *American Journal of Nursing, 102*(4), 36–43.

Schechter, N.R., Strom, E.A., Perkins, G.H., Arzu, I., McNeese, M.D., Langstein, H.N., et al. (2005). Immediate breast reconstruc-tion can impact postmastectomy irradiation. *American Journal of Clinical Oncology, 28,* 485–494.

Serletti, J.M., & Moran, S.L. (2000). Microvascular reconstruction of the breast. *Seminars in Surgical Oncology, 19,* 264–271.

Shah, N.M., Tenenholz, T., Arthur, D., DiPetrillo, T., Bornstein, B., Cardarelli, G., et al. (2004). MammoSite and interstitial brachy-therapy for accelerated partial breast irradiation: Factors that affect toxicity and cosmesis. *Cancer, 101,* 727–734.

Simmons, R.M. (2003). Ablative techniques in the treatment of benign and malignant breast disease. *Journal of the American College of Surgeons, 197,* 334–338.

Spear, S.L., & Spittler, C.J. (2001). Breast reconstruction with im-plants and expanders. *Plastic and Reconstructive Surgery, 101,* 1964–1972.

Taylor, C.W., & Kumar, S. (2005). The effect of immediate breast reconstruction on adjuvant chemotherapy. *Breast, 14,* 18–21.

Tugwell, P., Wells, G., Peterson, J., Welch, V., Page, J., Davison, C., et al. (2001). Do silicone breast implants cause rheu-matologic disorders? A systematic review for a Court-Ap-pointed National Science Panel. *Arthritis and Rheumatism, 44,* 2477–2484.

U.S. Food and Drug Administration. (2006). *Breast implant questions and answers.* Retrieved February 13, 2007, from http://www.fda.gov/cdrh/breastimplants/qa2006.html#2

Van Zee, K.J., Manasseh, D.M., Bevilacqua, J.L., Boolbol, S.K., Fey, J.V., Tan, L.K., et al. (2003). A nomogram for predicting the likelihood of additional nodal metastases in breast cancer patients with a positive sentinel node biopsy. *Annals of Surgical Oncology, 10,* 1140–1151.

Vicini, F.A., Beitsch, P.D., Quiet, C.A., Keleher, A., Garcia, D., Snider, H.C., et al. (2005). First analysis of patient demographics, technical reproducibility, cosmesis, and early toxicity: Results of the American Society of Breast Surgeons MammoSite breast brachytherapy trial. *Cancer, 104,* 1138–1148.

Yeh, K.A., Lyle, G., Wei, J.P., & Sherry, R. (1998). Immediate breast reconstruction in breast cancer: Morbidity and outcome. *American Surgeon, 64,* 1195–1199.

Zannis, V., Beitsch, P., Vicini, F., Quiet, C., Keleher, A., Garcia, D., et al. (2005). Descriptions and outcomes of insertion techniques of a breast brachytherapy balloon catheter in 1403 patients enrolled in the American Society of Breast Surgeons MammoSite breast brachytherapy registry trial. *American Journal of Surgery, 190,* 530–538.

CHAPTER 6

Breast Restoration With Prostheses

Michelle Casey, CFA, and Suzanne M. Mahon, RN, DNSc, AOCN®, APNG

Introduction

Restoration of the breast is an important aspect in the care and rehabilitation of women with breast cancer. For most women diagnosed with breast cancer, some surgical treatment is usually necessary. Many of these women will require at least some degree of breast restoration to improve body image and prevent physical problems.

Breast restoration might include surgical procedures to reconstruct a breast (see Chapter 5) as well as the use of prostheses. Prostheses are also extremely useful in correcting breast disparities that result because of extensive or multiple surgical biopsies or atrophy occurring long-term following lumpectomy and radiation. In some cases, they are useful for improving the outcome of reconstructive surgery. Along with prostheses, many women achieve improved cosmesis through the use of expertly fitted bras and camisoles.

Body Image

Breast restoration is central to restoring and improving body image after the surgical management of breast cancer. Issues related to breast surgery and body image often are discussed in nursing and medical literature (Cohen, Kahn, & Steeves, 1998; Rees & Bath, 2000). Adjustment to changes or disturbances in body image contributes to the quality of life in those diagnosed with cancer (Wang, Cosby, Harris, & Liu, 1999). Nurses who provide education and information about breast restoration ultimately can help to improve the quality of life for breast cancer survivors and, in many cases, women who have undergone breast biopsy.

The concept of body image has several dimensions. Cohen et al. (1998) noted that body image includes not only the mental picture of the physical self but also who that person believes she is and how she feels about herself. When a woman looks in the mirror and perceives herself to be attractive, she can be more confident. Breast restoration also helps to reduce or remove the constant reminder that a woman has faced a life-threatening diagnosis. It can allow a woman to wear attractive clothes comfortably, which ultimately results in improved self-image.

Treatment for breast cancer includes not only treatment for the cancer but treatment of the person as well. Women need instruction, encouragement, and support as they pursue options for breast restoration and need to be reminded that this is important to their long-term well-being and recovery. Often, in the midst of active treatment with chemotherapy and radiation therapy, women neglect this aspect of their care or feel that it is an inappropriate concern. Conversely, pursuing breast restoration should improve self-image and well-being and ultimately will make other aspects of care easier to tolerate. Reaby (1998) noted that most women benefit significantly from having a knowledgeable healthcare provider helping them to better understand the options available for breast restoration, including the use of a prosthesis and/or reconstructive surgery.

Prostheses

Selecting a Fitter

Nursing responsibility begins with supporting women in their decision to explore breast restoration options and referring them to reputable providers. Many more options are currently available for breast prostheses than in the past. It is no longer satisfactory to "send" women to a place to "get" a prosthesis. Oncology nurses who discuss the need for breast prostheses with patients must be able to understand what the experience of having a prosthesis fitted is like for patients. Using this information, nurses can provide anticipatory guidance for patients so that they will know what to expect during the fitting and how they can prepare for it. It is recommended that nurses meet with prosthetic providers in the setting where care is provided. This will allow the nurses to specifically describe how, when, and where the fitting will occur and guide women through the process. In many cases, fitters can provide nurses with a few samples of prostheses and fancy bras to show patients prior to a fitting. This can give them some idea of what to expect and some hope that it is still possible to wear beautiful undergarments.

It takes a tremendous amount of courage for women to have a breast prosthesis fitted, and oncology nurses are well suited to provide support and encouragement for women as they go through the fitting process. Research suggests that the fitting for a prosthesis can be as difficult and emotionally upsetting as the surgical procedure or diagnosis of cancer itself (Roberts, Livingston, White, & Gibbs, 2003).

Nurses need to emphasize that the fitting is a process, probably for life, and not a single, isolated event. It may take several fittings initially, and ideally women will have the fit checked on an annual basis. For this reason, it is critical that the women be comfortable working with the fitter. As a woman's body changes because of treatment or the normal effects of aging, different prostheses or bras might be needed. Nurses who care for women during long-term follow-up can facilitate long-term adjustment to body image by encouraging women to be reevaluated and refitted when changes are needed. Often, these women are not aware of the need for continued evaluation of a prosthesis, particularly if their surgery was done many years ago when choices were extremely limited.

Although research is limited, as many as 30% of women are dissatisfied with the external prosthesis for which they have been fitted (Roberts et al., 2003). Dissatisfaction often is linked to the fitting experience, including insufficient time, lack of privacy, fitting by a man, incorrect fit, and attitude of the fitter. Dissatisfaction also occurs when the prosthesis is uncomfortable to wear or if clothing and lingerie choices are extremely limited.

Prosthetic Centers

Oncology nurses often are the first to initiate a referral to a prosthetic center. These nurses must be familiar with the resources in their community and geographic area to make appropriate referrals. Being fitted for any type of breast prosthesis can be a very emotional experience for women, and it is important to ensure that they receive not only a well-fitted prosthesis but also a caring and personal environment for the fitting.

Nurses must learn who will be providing the fitting for their patients. Certification for fitters is available through each individual breast prosthesis manufacturer. This type of certification typically involves a one-day seminar. In these seminars, content usually includes the principles of taking measurements, the shapes of prostheses, and various bra styles. These seminars are presented by the manufacturers of these items. At the end of the day, participants usually take

an open-book test on the content. This training is aimed at familiarizing the fitters with the manufacturer's products and, ultimately, promoting their sale.

Certification by a manufacturer is probably not adequate to ensure the expertise of a fitter. Apprenticeship with an experienced, competent fitter is paramount. Typically, this period of training takes several months. Fitters can come from various educational backgrounds. These might include degrees in education, medical subspecialties, or a social sciences background, or sometimes fitters are long-term survivors of cancer.

Because prosthesis fitters can come from so many different backgrounds, it is important to ensure that women are referred to a fitter who is empathetic, caring, and adequately trained, preferably through an apprenticeship. Excellent interpersonal skills are extremely important to ensure that the fitting process is as easy as possible for patients. Whenever possible, it is best if the nurse can tell a patient the name of the person who will be providing the fitting so that the experience is a more personal one.

The actual setting where the fitting occurs is another important consideration. Prostheses can be purchased from many different places. Many times, the prosthesis fitting occurs at a durable medical equipment (DME) company; therefore, it is helpful to inform patients that there will be people needing other DME at the location in addition to those needing breast prostheses. Women should be assured that the fitting will occur in a private area. Optimally, the area where the fitting occurs should be feminine and nonclinical in nature. Prostheses also are sometimes distributed and fitted through lingerie stores.

Prosthetic Needs and Services Available at the Time of Diagnosis

At the time of diagnosis, some women find it beneficial to learn about the various prosthetic options. Although this is a busy time for patients, especially prior to surgery, nurses should encourage women to learn about what options are available. Women who are having difficulty deciding between mastectomy and breast-sparing surgery may find it helpful to understand the options for permanent prostheses or reconstruction available following mastectomy. For women considering whether to have immediate reconstruction, education about the various prosthetic options, both temporary and long-term, can facilitate decision making. Most reputable fitters are willing to see women during this time frame.

Seeing the fitter prior to surgery helps women to establish a relationship with the fitter as well as to begin to realistically anticipate what will happen in the future. A visit prior to surgery also provides the fitter with an opportunity to provide women with a temporary prosthesis to use in the immediate postoperative period. For many women, this can alleviate a significant amount of worry about the immediate postoperative period.

If it is not possible for patients to see the fitter prior to surgery (which is frequently the case), some prosthetic centers will make a few different types of prostheses and bras available for nurses to show patients in the office. Although this is not a replacement for seeing the fitter, it can give women a much more tangible idea of what to expect and what a prosthesis actually looks and feels like.

Regardless of whether patients see the fitter preoperatively, a discussion regarding prosthesis and bra options can help women to begin to understand and assimilate the process of breast restoration. This anticipatory guidance also will help women to realize that it is normal and appropriate to be concerned about their appearance, despite many other significant treatment issues and decisions that must be dealt with during this time.

Temporary Prostheses

Although it is optimal for women to see the fitter prior to surgery, in reality, this is difficult to achieve. It is, however, important for all women undergoing breast surgery to have a temporary prosthesis. A temporary prosthesis is a lightweight fiber-filled prosthesis that can be worn immediately following surgery. These should be shaped and pinned to the bra to prevent movement. Figure 6-1 shows examples of several types of temporary prostheses. They come in a wide variety of sizes, shapes, and colors.

Most temporary prostheses are generically sized. Some, such as those provided through the American Cancer Society (ACS), have an opening through which excess fiber can be removed to achieve a more symmetric appearance in the bra. It is important to assure the woman receiving the prosthesis that almost all women remove some of the filling and that there is nothing wrong with her because she needs to adjust the size. She should be assured that the temporary prosthesis tends to be sized large. It is even more important to assure the woman that a temporary prosthesis is much different from the one she will eventually use. The permanent prosthesis will stay in place and will therapeutically replace the weight of the breast lost in surgery. A permanent prosthesis will not need continual adjustments.

A temporary prosthesis may be given to patients through ACS's Reach to Recovery program, which also typically includes literature and a visit from a breast cancer survivor (ACS, 2006). Nurses need to become familiar with how the program is administered in their geographic region. This referral usually requires a physician's order. The volunteers receive special training and do not administer medical advice. They will show patients how to use the temporary prosthesis. In some cases, temporary prostheses also may be distributed through a prosthetic center. Nurses working in breast care need to explore what options are readily available in their geographic area and provide assistance to patients in accessing these resources.

Some of the temporary prostheses, such as those shown in Figure 6-1, can range in cost from $70–$80. When available, the Reach to Recovery program provides the temporary prosthesis free of charge. The availability of free or low-cost temporary prostheses makes it unnecessary for women to try to camouflage the physical effects of the surgery in the immediate postoperative period with socks, cotton, washcloths, sanitary pads, shoulder pads, or other novel means.

The temporary prosthesis can be worn in a front-hook leisure bra, prosthetic camisole, or the woman's own bra. The bra straps can be adjusted to obtain a more symmetric appearance. A leisure bra is a soft, comfortable, front-hook, pocketed bra (see Figure 6-2). It gives support to the unaffected breast and contains the temporary prosthesis. A disadvantage of temporary prostheses is that they tend to move up the chest wall, especially with movement. A leisure bra or the woman's own bra can help to anchor the prosthesis.

A prosthetic camisole is a soft, pocketed camisole that can be tucked into pants or skirts and helps to prevent the prosthesis from moving up the chest wall. This camisole also may be useful for women who have drains in place or who find wearing a bra uncomfortable, especially in the immediate postoperative period. Camisoles are available with cotton drain pouches that attach with Velcro® (Velcro Industries, Manchester, NH) to the interior band and can be cleaned regularly and easily.

Figure 6-1. Temporary Prostheses

Temporary prostheses are sized based on the woman's bra cup size and, to a smaller extent, the band size. They are available in a variety of shades and sizes. Most require some adjustment and need to be pinned in the bra.

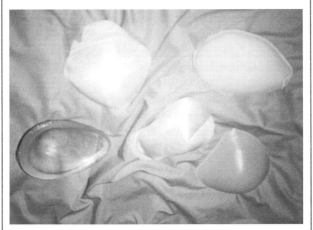

Note. From "Patient Education for Women Being Fitted for Breast Prostheses," by S.M. Mahon and M. Casey, 2003, *Clinical Journal of Oncology Nursing, 7,* p. 195. Copyright 2003 by the Oncology Nursing Society. Reprinted with permission.

Figure 6-2. Temporary Prosthesis With a Leisure Bra

A leisure bra is a bra with front hooks. It can be especially helpful for women with limited mobility in the early postoperative period or because of arthritic or other conditions. A temporary prosthesis can be pinned inside this bra.

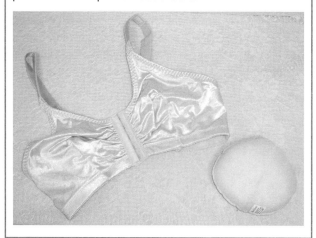

Figure 6-3. Questions to Ask About Insurance Coverage

- Is the fitter an approved provider in the insurance network?
- How much are benefits changed if the woman chooses an out-of-network provider?
- What are the preauthorization requirements?
- Is a prescription adequate, or is a letter of medical necessity required?
- Is there a deductible?
- What percentage of the cost of a form is covered?
- What forms (brands/types) are covered?
- Are replacement forms covered? Under what circumstances are replacements covered? How often can forms be replaced?
- Is there a charge to see the fitter?
- Are bras covered? Do they need to be a specific type?
- How many bras are covered per year?
- How frequently can bras be replaced?
- Are other garments, such as camisoles, covered?
- Are swim forms covered?

Some insurance companies will pay for a portion of the costs for a leisure bra or prosthetic camisole. Sometimes, however, it is in the woman's best interest to not use all of her benefits for a temporary prosthesis and to save the coverage for a permanent prosthesis. Clarification of benefits is extremely important. Some women will choose to buy the bra or camisole and pay out of pocket. Leisure bras and prosthetic camisoles can be used both in the immediate postoperative period and also long term. Many women wear them while sleeping or relaxing at home.

Permanent Prostheses

Most women are ready to be fitted for a permanent prosthesis four to six weeks following a mastectomy. This waiting period allows for postoperative swelling and skin sensitivity to resolve. Prior to the fitting, it is important to determine insurance coverage and obtain preauthorization (see Figure 6-3). This may take a few days to a week or more depending on the amount of information that is needed and the letters of medical necessity that may be required. The prosthetic center usually can assist women in finding out this information and completing the necessary paperwork. Women also should ascertain that the prosthetic provider is a recognized provider for their insurance company, or the benefits could be significantly reduced or eliminated for prosthetic coverage.

Fitting a permanent prosthesis usually takes at least one to two hours. Some helpful reminders for a woman going to a fitting are included in Figure 6-4. Many prosthetic centers prefer that clients make an appointment to ensure that a fitter will be available. It takes a lot of courage for patients to come for a fitting. It is optimal for the woman to bring a supportive

person along for the fitting, such as a sister, spouse, relative, or friend. She also should bring a solid-color form-fitting shirt or sweater or some other piece of clothing that she did not think she would be able to wear again, along with any bras she had liked to wear in the past, because often it is possible to continue to use those bras.

At the fitting, the woman should be taken into a private room. The fitter usually will begin by getting acquainted with the woman. This includes conversing about her surgery, a little about her experiences to date, anticipated treatment, and lifestyle. This conversation will help to relax the woman and, more importantly, will provide the fitter with important information about the patient so that she will receive the prosthesis and other items that will best meet her needs and, ultimately, improve her quality of life. The fitter also can tell the woman about what the fitting process will entail.

Next, the woman will be asked to unbutton or pull up a top so that the fitter can take some general measurements

Figure 6-4. Things to Do When Going to a Prosthetic Fitting

- Make an appointment with a fitter.
- Ascertain that the fitter is an approved provider for insurance and that insurance benefits have been verified.
- Bring an objective, supportive person.
- Bring bras that have been previously worn to determine whether they still can be used.
- Bring a tight-fitting solid-color top to help to assess for symmetry.
- Bring any items of clothing that the woman desires to wear but is concerned that it may no longer be possible.
- Plan on spending at least two hours at the initial fitting, and understand that several fittings may be necessary to obtain an optimal fit. Realize that the fit of the prosthesis should be assessed on a regular (usually annual) basis.
- Bring an open mind and be willing to try different bras and forms.

and see what type of bra the woman has chosen in the past. Many women are surprised to learn of the importance of the bra fitting and that a bra is fitted prior to fitting the prosthesis. Fitting the bra first is important because the bra shapes the unaffected breast and has a big impact on the woman's ultimate comfort.

Typically, the fitter will bring a wide variety of styles of bras into the room. The woman will be asked to remove her top and bra and will try on a variety of bras. Often these bras will have pockets to secure the prosthesis. When both the fitter and the woman are satisfied with the bra in terms of appearance and comfort, a selection of prostheses is introduced.

Permanent prostheses come in a variety of shapes and sizes (see Figure 6-5). These include nonattachable prostheses traditionally used in the pocket of a bra. At this point in the fitting, the fitter should talk to the patient about the importance of replacing the weight lost with the surgery. It is extremely important to correctly replace the weight to prevent long-term complications to the back, neck, and shoulder areas. If the weight is not replaced, the body will compensate by shoulder drop on the affected side. Often, in trying to conceal asymmetry, women will curve and drop the affected shoulder. The weight of the permanent prosthesis also keeps the prosthesis in place on the chest wall. Some women, especially older adults, state that the weight is important to restore balance. Insurance companies actually cover the costs associated with a prosthesis because of the need for weight replacement, not for cosmetic reasons.

Traditional prostheses are made from silicone encased in polyurethane. They are molded into various shapes, densities, weights, and sizes. After the first prosthesis is placed in the bra, a measurement from the center seam to an outer seam is

taken and compared with the unaffected side. This helps to guide the fitter on sizing. A measurement is taken from the collarbone to the nipple area to ensure that projection is equal and there is symmetry. Optimally, a fitting drape is applied (see Figure 6-6). This is a solid silk-like piece of fabric that ties at the neck and around the back. It is pulled tightly to check that symmetry has been achieved. Symmetry also can

---

Figure 6-6. Fitting Drape

Some fitters use a fitting drape such as this to make asymmetry more obvious. This drape demonstrates how the left side is fuller than the right. Some fitters use a tight-fitting shirt that the woman brings to the fitting to also check for asymmetry.

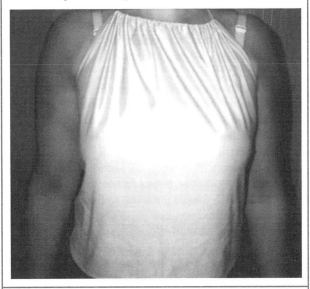

Note. From "Patient Education for Women Being Fitted for Breast Prostheses," by S.M. Mahon and M. Casey, 2003, *Clinical Journal of Oncology Nursing, 7,* p. 196. Copyright 2003 by the Oncology Nursing Society. Reprinted with permission.

---

be checked by having the woman wear a tight-fitting top. The fitter can check whether all points of fullness are identical on each side. The woman also is observed moving her arms and shoulders. The woman is questioned about comfort and the general feel. Often it takes trying 7–15 different prostheses before a proper fit is achieved. The fitter always should listen to the woman because, ultimately, the woman will select what is best for her. The fitter considers the shape and size of the remaining breast, as well as the amount of tissue on the chest wall and under the arm.

Prostheses are available in many different shapes. Some prostheses are designed for more radical surgeries. These tend to be fuller and have a tail that extends under the arm. Those designed for modified mastectomies taper more gradually to the chest wall and do not extend as far under the arm (see Figure 6-5).

Figure 6-5. Permanent Prostheses

Permanent prostheses come in many different skin tones and sizes.

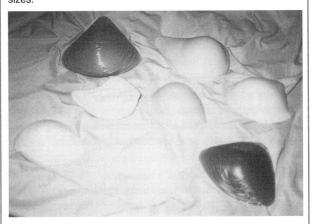

Note. From "Patient Education for Women Being Fitted for Breast Prostheses," by S.M. Mahon and M. Casey, 2003, *Clinical Journal of Oncology Nursing, 7,* p. 197. Copyright 2003 by the Oncology Nursing Society. Reprinted with permission.

The prosthesis can be made out of different densities of silicone to simulate the density of the natural breast. If the woman has more ptosis, which occurs naturally with aging, a soft, dual-layer prosthesis might be best. This prosthesis has a firm back and a very soft conformable front, which can simulate a pendulous breast.

The weight of the prosthesis is an extremely important consideration. Some manufacturers whip air into the silicone before it is molded to reduce the weight of the prostheses by 15%–20%. Thus, prostheses come in many different weights, and there is an optimal weight for each woman. To determine the weight, the woman needs to try on at least 5–10 different weights. Most women will know which feels the best and is balanced. The fitter has to be responsible in this area. It is important not to fit a prosthesis that is too light because therapeutic weight replacement will not be achieved, and the woman will be at risk for developing shoulder drop. The fitter also needs to let the woman help in making this determination. It is best for the fitter not to describe a prosthesis as light or heavy because it may prejudice the decision. Many women will be more comfortable with their decision if they take a prosthesis home and wear it to determine whether it is the right fit. If it truly is uncomfortable, it can be exchanged for a different one. Women also need to reacclimate their body to the weight from the prosthesis. A typical schedule is for the woman to wear it for two to three hours the first day and then add two hours each day. This helps to reduce minor body aches.

Attachable prostheses come in two types. One attachable version of breast prosthesis can be applied with the use of Velcro and ostomy tape (see Figure 6-7). This form typically is worn during the first four to six months after surgery with a piece of fabric attached to the Velcro to allow the skin to heal postoperatively. Once the skin is healed, a piece of ostomy tape is applied to the chest wall, which has Velcro attached to it. The prosthesis is attached by the Velcro to the chest wall and can be worn with any fitted bra. Women can wear this prosthesis while swimming and during strenuous athletic activities, and they can shower with the ostomy tape in place because it dries quickly. The ostomy tape is replaced as needed. Generally, women must change the tape every two to four weeks. Ostomy skin supplies can be used to enhance how long the tape lasts and prevent skin damage. Some women, for a variety of reasons, prefer this prosthesis. In addition to feeling more secure when participating in some activities, it can be worn to bed, as well as with bras and swimsuits the women wore prior to surgery. This type also can be a good choice in terms of weight replacement because the weight of the prosthesis is supported by the chest wall and not the bra.

An even newer type of prosthesis is a breast form with rejuvenating silicone on the back of the prosthesis (see Figure 6-8). This prosthesis must be supported by a bra. The silicone

Figure 6-7. Attachable Prostheses

One type of attachable prosthesis utilizes ostomy tape that is applied to a healed chest wall. The ostomy tape has Velcro loop fasteners. The back of the prosthesis also has Velcro fasteners that attach the prosthesis to the chest wall.

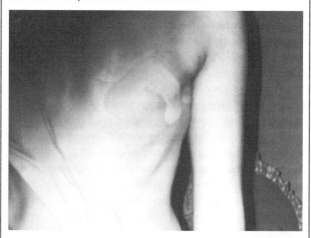

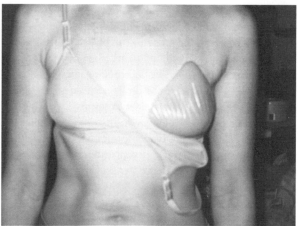

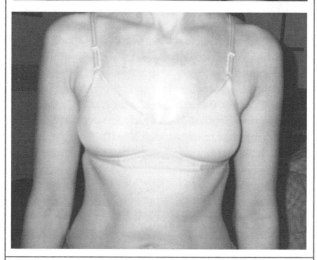

Note. From "Patient Education for Women Being Fitted for Breast Prostheses," by S.M. Mahon and M. Casey, 2003, *Clinical Journal of Oncology Nursing, 7,* p. 198. Copyright 2003 by the Oncology Nursing Society. Reprinted with permission.

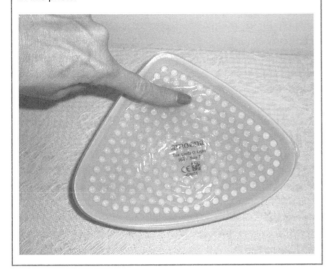

is critical. A cast also is made of the nipple. This form has a nipple, fits the chest wall, and is worn directly against the body, not in a pocket (see Figure 6-9). The woman needs to be at a stable weight. Benefits include that many women like the personalization and that it can be worn when swimming. The approximate cost is $3,000, and it sometimes is covered by insurance. It takes specialized training to fit a custom prosthesis.

Figure 6-9. Custom Prosthesis With Nipple

sticks directly to the chest wall. The woman must be willing to meticulously care for this prosthesis on a daily basis. At night, the prosthesis must be scrubbed with a cleansing solution and a scrub brush to reactivate the silicone. Several restrictions accompany this prosthesis. For example, it does not work well for women with a lot of perspiration or those experiencing hot flashes. In addition, it cannot be worn while swimming.

Today, prostheses are made in a few different shades to better match the skin color of women of different ethnicities. Most manufacturers have prostheses in ivory, blush, and tawny for African American women. This includes both the attachable and nonattachable types.

Also, some general care instructions exist for all women who wear a permanent prosthesis. The prosthesis should be washed with a mild soap and water and towel-dried on a daily basis. Ideally, they are stored in a cradle, which comes with the prosthesis. This cradle supports the shape of the silicone prosthesis and increases its longevity. Most silicone breast prostheses have a two-year warranty against defects, such as gel separation or peeling finish.

For some women, a custom prosthesis is an appropriate choice. This may be the case if they have an uneven or irregular chest wall. In addition, some women will be comfortable only if they have an aesthetic reproduction of their breast. A custom prosthesis may allow the woman to choose the exact skin tone and size. A cast is made of the chest wall, the other breast, and a bra with a prosthesis. A custom prosthesis is bra-specific, so careful bra selection

Restoration to Correct Lumpectomy, Reconstruction, and Surgical Disparities

Partial prostheses are available for women who have had lumpectomies, reconstruction, or multiple biopsies or those with congenital disparities. These come in varying shapes, thicknesses, and sizes (see Figure 6-10). Some fitters will custom design prostheses with fiber-filled pads or foam breast cups. Many times, a well-fitted, supportive bra can disguise the disparity and is all that is needed. These principles also are helpful to women undergoing reconstruction using expanders, during which time their prosthesis needs to be changed. Occasionally, after surgical reconstruction, some disparity or asymmetry still is evident and can be camouflaged with a well-fitted bra and a partial prosthesis.

These disparities often are very simple to correct, but women fail to receive these corrective options. Many women expend a lot of energy and experience much frustration as they try to correct these problems with home remedies. Insurance companies are mandated to provide prosthetics and bras for any woman undergoing breast surgery, and many women are not aware of this. Nurses must educate women about this service to help them to avoid the frustration and discouragement associated with this problem.

The best way to educate women about these options is often unclear. Many women believe that the sole pur-

Figure 6-10. Partial Prostheses

Partial prostheses come in a variety of shapes and thicknesses to correct many different breast disparities or asymmetry. They are typically worn in a bra.

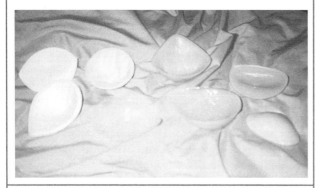

Note. From "Patient Education for Women Being Fitted for Breast Prostheses," by S.M. Mahon and M. Casey, 2003, *Clinical Journal of Oncology Nursing, 7,* p. 197. Copyright 2003 by the Oncology Nursing Society. Reprinted with permission.

pose of a lumpectomy or reconstruction is to completely eliminate the need for prosthetic services. However, it is impossible, even with the most talented surgeons, to completely eliminate disparities. For many women being treated with lumpectomy and radiation, the disparities magnify with time. Often, refitting the bra will eliminate many problems.

An underserved group in breast prosthetics is women who have had multiple breast biopsies or who have had a large biopsy resulting in breast disparities. Although they do not have a cancer diagnosis, they may benefit from a better-fitted bra and, in some cases, a partial prosthesis.

Healthcare providers need to develop strategies and approaches to discuss these issues with women. Often, asking women whether they have had any trouble with wearing clothes or if they are satisfied with the surgical outcome of the lumpectomy or reconstruction will open the door to providing this education. This needs to be done in a caring, nonjudgmental, nonthreatening, and unhurried manner.

Insurance Issues

Federal law now mandates that insurance cover the initial breast prosthesis or breast reconstruction. This includes partial-breast prosthesis for women who go through reconstruction and do not desire to have surgery on the unaffected breast. This law also provides for women who have had lumpectomies and need a partial prosthesis to correct disparity. Insurance companies cover different prostheses at varying amounts. Some insurance companies dictate what prostheses will be covered or mandate that a specific provider be used.

Medicare covers 80% of each state's allowable amount for the permanent prosthesis every two years, a leisure prosthesis every six months, and a portion of up to six bras per year. Most supplemental policies will cover the remaining portion of the allowable amount.

Optimally, women should consult their insurance policy before being fitted to be sure that the fitter is an approved provider. Figure 6-3 provides a list of questions to help women to better understand their benefits. Most reputable fitters will precertify or verify benefits prior to the fitting to provide optimal coverage and choice in forms and other accessories. Often, women will need preauthorization, a prescription, and/or a letter of medical necessity prior to a fitting. Fitters usually will help women in obtaining the proper paperwork from their oncologist or surgeon.

Replacement prosthesis frequently will be covered when the proper documentation of need is submitted for medical review. Most prosthetics have two-year warranties, and few last beyond that time. Weight gain or loss (often as little as 5–10 pounds) also may necessitate a replacement prosthesis. Furthermore, women who were diagnosed many years ago may not be aware of the laws and benefits that may be available to them.

Accessories

At the time of diagnosis, women frequently think they will have to give up many things because of surgery. This might include activities such as swimming or being able to wear beautiful bras or other lingerie. Pockets can be sewn into bras with adequate support for the prosthesis and for coverage of the breast. This allows women to continue to wear bras that they had selected prior to surgery. Additionally, swimsuits are available with pocket(s). These suits typically are more conservatively cut with higher coverage and more material under the arm. Pockets also can be sewn into swimsuits that provide adequate coverage of the surgical area. Different types of swimming and exercise forms are available and often are covered by insurance under a separate billing code. These can be made of fiberfill or a firm, durable type of silicone. These forms also are appropriate for women who want to exercise vigorously. Insurance often will pay for these prostheses as well.

Prosthetic camisoles can be worn immediately during the postoperative period. These camisoles have a pocket to hold a fiber-filled breast form. Most camisoles do not offer much support for the remaining breast; however, they are useful in the immediate postoperative period, during radiation therapy, or for women with difficulties healing or tolerating a bra.

Front-hook leisure bras are another option (see Figure 6-2). These can be worn postoperatively with a fiber-filled prosthesis throughout the healing period. This provides some support for the natural breast. Some women also like to wear these in the evening with a nightgown or other lingerie.

Conclusion

Providing women with comprehensive education about breast prostheses and other restoration accessories is a very important but often overlooked responsibility of nurses. Nurses can assist patients with adjusting to body image changes and can facilitate coping by offering encouragement and education about prostheses and what to anticipate during the fitting process. To provide this education and support, nurses must be knowledgeable about the prosthesis resources in the geographic area in which they practice. Optimally, nurses who make the referrals for fittings should know the fitter(s) and have visited the site where the fitting will occur. This helps nurses to provide guidance to patients prior to the fitting. When the healthcare provider knows the fitter, there is improved collaboration and more continuity of care.

Women need to realize that the decision to use a prosthesis or have reconstructive surgery is a personal one (Resnick & Belcher, 2002). There is not necessarily a right or wrong answer for any one woman. Women need to feel supported in their decision. Research suggests that women who explore their options carefully prior to surgery, are well educated about all options, and feel they have a major role in all aspects of the decision-making process tend to be more satisfied with whatever choice they make for breast restoration (Reaby, 2000). Nurses need to reassure women and support them in whatever decision they make in order to promote and improve their quality of life.

Unlike in the past, women who will need a full or partial-breast prosthesis now have many different options available. Nurses need to be aware of the many options that exist and encourage women that a good fit is possible. Although a prosthesis will never completely replace what was lost with surgery, a well-fitted prosthesis can make an enormous difference in how a woman ultimately adjusts to the diagnosis of cancer and the changes in her body image. A well-fitted prosthesis also will help to prevent long-term complications, including shoulder drop. Positive adjustment to these changes in body image ultimately improves the long-term quality of life for women diagnosed with breast cancer.

For some women weighing the decision of whether to use prosthesis or undergo reconstruction, it may be helpful to speak with women who have made the choice, are satisfied with the choice, and will not provide medical advice. Having contacts who have had positive experiences with both reconstruction and prostheses may be helpful.

One area in which oncology nurses can have a large impact is in assessment and referral for women who underwent surgery many years ago. Optimally, women should see prosthetic fitters approximately every two years. Changes in weight due to therapy, hormonal manipulation, or aging often necessitate a change in the prosthesis. Many women do not realize that the prosthesis will not last a lifetime and that insurance often will cover replacement costs. Nurses who see women during their follow-up should inquire about the fit of the prosthesis and when patients last saw a fitter for evaluation. Nurses then can encourage women to follow up with the fitter and can make referrals as needed. In addition to ensuring that the woman is wearing a well-fitted prosthesis, this assessment also communicates the nurse's continued care and concern about the survivor's overall well-being.

References

American Cancer Society. (2006). *Reach to recovery.* Retrieved September 6, 2006, from http://www.cancer.org/docroot/ESN/content/ESN_3_1x_Reach_to_Recovery_5.asp

Cohen, M.Z., Kahn, D.L., & Steeves, R.H. (1998). Beyond body image: The experience of breast cancer. *Oncology Nursing Forum, 25,* 835–841.

Reaby, L. (1998). Breast restoration decision making: Enhancing the process. *Cancer Nursing, 21,* 196–204.

Reaby, L. (2000). Women's perceptions regarding the advantages and disadvantages of postmastectomy breast restoration options. *International Journal of Cosmetic Surgery and Aesthetic Dermatology, 2,* 133–140.

Rees, C., & Bath, P.A. (2000). The information needs and source preferences of women with breast cancer and their family members: A review of the literature published between 1988 and 1998. *Journal of Advanced Nursing, 31,* 833–841.

Resnick, B., & Belcher, A.E. (2002). Breast reconstruction. Options, answers, and support for patients making a difficult personal decision. *American Journal of Nursing, 102*(4), 26–33.

Roberts, S., Livingston, P., White, V., & Gibbs, A. (2003). External breast prosthesis use: Experiences and views of women with breast cancer, breast care nurses, and prosthesis fitters. *Cancer Nursing, 26,* 179–186.

Wang, X., Cosby, L.G., Harris, M., & Liu, T. (1999). Major concerns and needs of breast cancer patients. *Cancer Nursing, 22,* 157–163.

CHAPTER 7

Systemic Treatment

Susan G. Yackzan, RN, MSN, AOCN®

Introduction

Breast cancer continues to be a diagnosis of significant proportion. In recent years, positive trends have developed that bear noting. Although the incidence of invasive breast cancer has continued to increase, the rate of this increase has slowed (Jemal et al., 2007; Wood, Muss, Solin, & Olopade, 2005). In addition, beginning in the 1990s, age-adjusted mortality rates have declined (Early Breast Cancer Trialists' Collaborative Group [EBCTCG], 2005; Jemal et al.). Early detection is an often-cited reason for both trends. Another important factor in the decline of mortality rates may be the use of adjuvant, aggressive, and multimodality treatment regimens.

Extensive surgical treatments such as radical mastectomies were based on the premise that breast cancer metastasized in a predictable manner—spreading locally, then regionally through and past the lymph nodes, and then systemically. Regional lymph nodes were thought of as barriers in this progression. Current understanding of breast cancer biology recognizes that breast cancer can be a systemic disease at diagnosis. Lymph nodes are now understood to be predictors of systemic disease rather than barriers (Kardinal & Cole, 2001). This understanding has allowed for phenomenal shifts in breast cancer treatment. Predictors of systemic disease can be assessed. Based on these predictors or characteristics, breast-conservation treatments may be an option, or adjuvant and aggressive combined-modality treatments may be offered. In addition, recent years have seen the advent of new endocrine therapies and targeted treatments for breast cancer.

Endocrine Therapy

Estrogen and progesterone are both steroid regulators of the endocrine system (Dickson, Pestell, & Lippman, 2005). Between puberty and menopause, estrogen is produced primarily in the ovaries. Estrogen also may be produced from adrenal androgens. Androgens are converted into estrogen by the enzyme aromatase, which exists throughout the body in adipose, muscle, brain, liver, breast, and even breast-cancer tissues (Chapman & Moore, 2005; Harwood, 2004). In postmenopausal women, the conversion of androgens is the primary source of estrogen, and the major site of this production is the subcutaneous fat (Smith & Dowsett, 2003).

Estrogen receptors (ERs) and progesterone receptors (PRs) are present in many body tissues. In normal breast tissue, estrogen and progesterone work together to direct cellular activities (Dickson et al., 2005). This cellular activity is brought about by the presence of nuclear receptor binding and subsequent intracellular signaling. In breast cancer, estrogen is the primary regulator of cellular activity and growth. The ER/PR status of tumors is important both as a prognostic variable and for the prescription of endocrine treatments (Dickson et al.).

Endocrine therapy involves the manipulation of hormone production, receptor binding, and cell signaling (see Table 7-1). This manipulation can be permanent, as with surgical oophorectomy, or temporary, as with medications such as tamoxifen. Breast cancers may exhibit resistance to endocrine therapy. Mechanisms of resistance are not well understood. Absent or weakly positive receptor status and human epidermal growth factor receptor 2 (HER2) overexpression may be predictors of resistance to endocrine therapy (Kardinal & Cole, 2001). Table 7-2 lists current endocrine therapies for breast cancer. Overall, the side effects of endocrine therapies are generally well tolerated. Side effects vary with the agent and may include hot flashes, vaginal discharge and dryness, skeletal effects including osteoporosis, arthralgias, sexuality and fertility changes, tumor flare, gastrointestinal disturbances, cognitive effects, and thromboembolic events. Endometrial changes have been noted, particularly with selective estrogen receptor modulators (SERMs).

Withdrawal responses sometimes occur in patients after discontinuation of endocrine therapies. These responses may include tumor regression or periods of disease stability. This effect may be employed as a treatment strategy sometimes described as a "drug holiday." Patients on endocrine therapies

Table 7-1. Endocrine Therapy Mechanism of Action in Breast Cancer

Category	Mechanism of Action
Selective estrogen receptor modulator	Estrogen receptor antagonist
Aromatase inhibitor	Blocks estrogen production by aromatization
Estrogen receptor downregulator	Targets and degrades estrogen receptors
Estrogen hormonal therapy	Endogenous estrogen antagonist Full mechanism of action unknown
Androgen hormonal therapy	Competes with estradiol for the estrogen receptor Blocks pituitary gonadotropin secretion
Progestin hormonal therapy	Full mechanism of action unknown
Luteinizing hormone-releasing hormone agonist	Decreases gonadotropin release
Ovarian ablation	Blocks estrogen production

who have positive responses and prolonged periods of disease stability are more likely to experience a withdrawal response (Wood et al., 2005).

Selective Estrogen Receptor Modulators

SERMs include tamoxifen, toremifene, and raloxifene. Tamoxifen has been the agent of choice for endocrine therapy of ER-positive breast cancer for a number of years. A 2005 review by the EBCTCG summarized the benefit of five years of adjuvant tamoxifen for ER-positive disease as a reduction in the annual breast cancer death rate by 31%. Tamoxifen has proven activity as a chemopreventive agent in the high-risk setting, as a treatment for both early and advanced invasive breast cancer, and in the metastatic setting (Chapman & Moore, 2005; Forbes, 2003; Wilkes & Barton-Burke, 2005). For ER-positive disease, five years of tamoxifen therapy is significantly more effective than one to two years for both recurrence and mortality rates (EBCTCG). In the ER-positive setting, a tamoxifen carryover effect has been described whereby the reduction of mortality benefit from tamoxifen continues beyond five years. This benefit at 15 years appears to be more than twice as large as the benefit at five years (EBCTCG; Forbes). Newer medications, such as aromatase inhibitors (AIs) and other SERMs, continue to be tested against and with tamoxifen.

Both tamoxifen and toremifene have breast cancer indications. They share similar efficacy patterns, and cross-resistance may exist between the two (Gerken, 2004; Wood et al.,

2005). Raloxifene is indicated for the prevention of osteoporosis and currently has no breast cancer indication. Several clinical trials are studying raloxifene in both the preventive and treatment setting.

SERMs have both antagonist and agonist effects. In breast tissue, SERMs work as antagonists, reversibly binding with ERs and directly competing with estrogen. In other tissues, SERMs stimulate estrogen-like effects. These effects may be both beneficial and potentially harmful. Beneficial effects include protection against osteoporosis and positive effects on lipid levels. Potentially harmful agonist effects include endometrial changes and endometrial cancer. Five years of tamoxifen treatment in postmenopausal women carries a 1% risk of endometrial cancer (Wood et al., 2005). The agonist activity of SERMs has been postulated as the reason for the acquired resistance that may develop with these agents (Mouridsen & Robert, 2005).

Aromatase Inhibitors

AIs block the production of estrogen from androgenic sources, resulting in decreased estrogen levels in tumors (Lake & Hudis, 2002). AIs exert their action by blocking the enzyme aromatase. AIs do not inhibit estrogen production by the ovaries. In premenopausal women, the usefulness of AIs is thought to be limited because the normal hypothalamus/pituitary feedback loop would stimulate the ovaries to produce estrogen in the presence of decreased estrogen levels (Smith & Dowsett, 2003). Unlike SERMs, AIs have no agonist activity. Patients with HER2-positive tumors may derive greater benefit from AIs than SERMs. Both de novo and acquired AI resistances have been noted (Osborne & Schiff, 2005; Wood et al., 2005).

Previously, medications in this category were defined as first-, second-, or third-generation AIs based on chronology of clinical release (Goss & Strasser, 2001; Smith & Dowsett, 2003). Aminoglutethimide, a first-generation AI, lacked specificity for estrogen deprivation and reduced levels of glucocorticoids and mineralocorticoids, resulting in significant toxicities. Newer, selective AIs are sometimes described as third-generation. They also may be classified as either steroidal/irreversible or nonsteroidal/reversible. Three of these agents are commercially available in the United States. Anastrozole and letrozole are nonsteroidal/reversible AIs, and exemestane is a steroidal/irreversible AI. A lack of cross-resistance may exist between those two groups, allowing for potential clinical benefit with crossover (Lake & Hudis, 2002).

In the postmenopausal receptor-positive setting, AIs are now considered to be an effective if not first-line endocrine option (Osborne & Schiff, 2005). Five years of anastrozole (Arimidex®, AstraZeneca Pharmaceuticals, Wilmington, DE) versus tamoxifen treatment was compared in the large-scale Arimidex or Tamoxifen Alone or in Combination trial. Data

	Table 7-2. Endocrine Therapy for Breast Cancer			
Category	Endocrine Therapy	Dose	Route of Administration	Possible Side Effects
Selective estrogen receptor modulators	Tamoxifen citrate (Nolvadex®, AstraZeneca Pharmaceuticals, Wilmington, DE)	20–40 mg daily (most common dose is 20 mg daily either as a once-a-day dose or 10 mg bid)	po	Hot flashes, flare reaction, vaginal bleeding, vaginal discharge, menstrual irregularities, endometrial changes, nausea, vomiting, anorexia, visual changes
	Toremifene citrate (Fareston®, GTx, Inc., Memphis, TN)	60 mg daily	po	Hot flashes, flare reaction, vaginal bleeding, vaginal discharge, menstrual irregularities, nausea, vomiting, anorexia, headache, dizziness, fatigue, visual changes
	Raloxifene hydrochloride* (Evista®, Eli Lilly and Co., Indianapolis, IN)	60 mg daily	po	Hot flashes, thromboembolic events, nausea, vomiting, dyspepsia, headache, flu-like syndrome, depression, insomnia, arthralgias, myalgias, leg cramps, arthritis
Aromatase inhibitors	Anastrozole (Arimidex®, AstraZeneca Pharmaceuticals)	1 mg daily	po	Hot flashes, vaginal dryness, thrombophlebitis, headache, weakness, nausea, vomiting, diarrhea, asthenia, dizziness
	Letrozole (Femara®, Novartis Pharmaceuticals Corp., East Hanover, NJ)	2.5 mg daily	po	Nausea, hot flashes, musculoskeletal pain, arthralgias, headache, fatigue, hot flashes, vomiting, anorexia, diarrhea, dizziness
	Exemestane (Aromasin®, Pfizer Inc., New York, NY)	25 mg daily	po	Nausea, fatigue, hot flashes, sweating, depression, insomnia, arthralgias, musculoskeletal pain
Estrogen receptor down-regulator	Fulvestrant (Faslodex®, AstraZeneca Pharmaceuticals)	250 mg monthly	IM	Hot flashes, asthenia, injection site pain and inflammation, musculoskeletal pain, nausea, dyspepsia, anorexia, vomiting, constipation, diarrhea, anemia, pharyngitis, dyspnea, headache
Estrogen hormonal therapy	Diethylstilbestrol	15 mg daily or 5 mg tid	po	Thromboembolic events, hypercalcemia, sodium and water retention, cardiotoxicity, nausea, vomiting, breast tenderness and engorgement, uterine prolapse, urinary incontinence
	Ethinyl estradiol	0.5–1 mg tid	po	Thromboembolic events, hypercalcemia, sodium and water retention, cardiotoxicity, nausea, vomiting, breast tenderness and engorgement, uterine prolapse, urinary incontinence
Androgen hormonal therapy	Fluoxymesterone (Halotestin®, Pfizer Inc.)	10–40 mg daily (divided doses)	po	Sodium and water retention, fertility and sexuality changes, hypercalcemia, erythropoiesis, alopecia, acne
Progestin hormonal therapy	Megestrol acetate (Megace®, Bristol-Myers Squibb Co., New York, NY)	40 mg qid	po	Thromboembolic events, nausea, vomiting, tumor flare, vaginal discharge, vaginal bleeding, carpal tunnel syndrome, hot flashes, sodium and water retention, hypercalcemia
	Medroxyprogesterone acetate* (Provera®, Pfizer Inc.)	400–500 mg daily	po	Fluid retention, thromboembolic events, menstrual irregularities, nausea, headache, insomnia, fatigue, edema

(Continued on next page)

Table 7-2. Endocrine Therapy for Breast Cancer *(Continued)*				
Category	Endocrine Therapy	Dose	Route of Administration	Possible Side Effects
Luteinizing hormone-releasing hormone agonists	Goserelin acetate (Zoladex®, AstraZeneca Pharmaceuticals)	3.6 mg every four weeks; 10.8 mg every 12 weeks	SC	Hot flashes, fertility and sexuality changes, cardiovascular changes, anxiety, depression, headache, nausea, vomiting, anorexia, rash, acne, fatigue, insomnia, depression, lethargy, tumor flare
	Leuprolide acetate* (Lupron® Depot, TAP Pharmaceuticals Inc., Lake Forest, IL)	3.75 mg every four weeks; 11.25 mg every three months	IM	Hot flashes, fertility and sexuality changes, cardiovascular changes, tumor flare, edema, depression, anorexia, nausea, vomiting, increased cholesterol and triglyceride concentration

*Not currently approved for use in breast cancer

Note. Based on information from Fischer et al., 2003; Gerken, 2004; Harwood, 2004; Kardinal & Cole, 2001; Wilkes & Barton-Burke, 2005; Wood et al., 2005.

continue to mature but have demonstrated improvements in breast cancer–related events (locoregional recurrence, distant metastases, or contralateral breast cancer) in the anastrozole group and no significant difference in disease-free survival between the groups (Wood et al., 2005). The trial also included a treatment arm of combination anastrozole and tamoxifen, which showed no additional benefit over tamoxifen alone (Osborne & Schiff; Ranger, 2005). Differences in the toxicity profiles of anastrozole and tamoxifen were reported. The anastrozole group showed a decreased incidence of endometrial cancer, vaginal bleeding and discharge, thrombotic events, and hot flashes as compared to the tamoxifen group. The anastrozole group experienced more musculoskeletal events, including fractures (Ranger; Wood et al.). Furthermore, memory and cognition areas of the brain have estrogen receptors. Because of the lack of estrogen agonist activity of AIs as compared with tamoxifen, an adverse effect on these functions has been suggested (Ranger).

The choice of AI treatment and course duration are under active investigation. Three main areas of investigation are the use of AIs in the early adjuvant setting, as early sequential adjuvant therapy, and as extended adjuvant therapy. Early adjuvant use involves the replacement of tamoxifen with AIs for five years of treatment following surgery. Early sequential adjuvant therapy involves sequencing of tamoxifen and AIs in the first five years after surgery. Extended adjuvant therapy involves the use of AIs after five years of postsurgery tamoxifen (Mouridsen & Robert, 2005).

Selective Estrogen Receptor Downregulators

Fulvestrant is the first agent available for clinical use that selectively destroys ERs. Like tamoxifen, it binds to ERs and blocks the action of estrogen. Unlike tamoxifen, however, the antiestrogen activity is not reversible. Fulvestrant causes a downregulation of the ER by degrading the receptors. Fulvestrant has no partial agonist activity and is indicated as second-line treatment in postmenopausal women with metastatic breast cancer (Versea & Rosenzweig, 2003). The drug is given as an intramuscular injection every month and generally is well tolerated (Hancock, 2003). Also, it lacks cross-resistance with tamoxifen and has a unique mechanism of action. Both qualities make fulvestrant a valuable option for breast cancer treatment (Howell et al., 2005).

Estrogens, Progestins, and Androgens

Estrogens, progestins, androgens, and adrenal corticosteroids have all been used in the treatment of breast cancer. Estrogens were the primary endocrine treatment for postmenopausal women with metastatic breast cancer before the advent of tamoxifen. Agents such as diethylstilbestrol, ethinyl estradiol, and conjugated estrogens have been used. The exact mechanism of action of these therapies is unknown. Suggestions have included activity as antagonists or pure agonists to endogenous estrogen or as apoptosis-inducing agents (Kardinal & Cole, 2001; Lake & Hudis, 2002; Osborne & Schiff, 2005).

Androgens act by competing with estradiol for the ER and by blocking pituitary gonadotropin secretion. Virilization side effects of these agents are significant and may include frontal baldness, acne, hirsutism, changes in libido, and fluid retention (Chapman & Moore, 2005; Kardinal & Cole, 2001).

Progestins include the agents megestrol acetate and medroxyprogesterone acetate. Progestins have been useful in the advanced, hormonally responsive breast cancer setting. The mechanism of action is not fully understood but may include inhibition of ER binding and androgen aromatization (Chapman & Moore, 2005; Kardinal & Cole, 2001).

Luteinizing Hormone-Releasing Hormone Agonists

Luteinizing hormone-releasing hormone (LHRH) agonists work at the level of the pituitary to decrease gonadotropin release. The use of these agents results in medical ovarian ablation. Trials in metastatic breast cancer have met with some success. Combinations of LHRH agonists and tamoxifen, in particular, appear to be superior to LHRH agonists alone (Kardinal & Cole, 2001; Wood et al., 2005). Agents in this class include goserelin acetate and leuprolide acetate.

Ovarian Ablation

Surgical ovarian ablation as a breast cancer treatment was first described in the literature in 1896 (Beatson). Other methods of ovarian ablation include radiation and drug-induced suppression. In the metastatic setting, ovarian ablation has been combined with other endocrine therapies. The combination of LHRH agonists with tamoxifen has previously been described. Ovarian ablation in combination with AIs also has been studied (Wood et al., 2005).

Chemotherapy

Chemotherapy regimens are employed as treatment for locoregional, locally advanced, and metastatic breast cancer. In the late 1960s, an 88% response rate was reported for the regimen CMFVP (cyclophosphamide, methotrexate, 5-fluorouracil [5-FU], vincristine, and prednisone) for hormone-resistant breast cancer. A plethora of chemotherapy clinical trials have followed. All major classes of chemotherapeutic agents have activity against breast cancer (Kardinal & Cole, 2001). Common combination regimens are listed in Table 7-3 and often include anthracyclines, alkylating agents, plant alkaloids, and antimetabolites. In addition, based on tumor characteristics, hormonal and targeted therapies also may be part of combination regimens. Toxicities are regimen-related and may include alopecia, fatigue, mucositis, myelosuppression, cardiac toxicity, neurotoxicity, nausea, vomiting, diarrhea, skin and nail changes, menopausal symptoms, and fertility and sexuality changes.

Patient education is an essential component of informed consent for treatment and includes information about medications, potential side effects, and plans for symptom management. Regimen-specific patient education includes information about planned medications, doses, and schedules. Potential side effects of each medication should be discussed and written information provided before therapy begins. Healthcare professionals should reinforce this same information throughout treatment. Patient education also should include information about the use of baseline assessments such as multiple-gated acquisition (MUGA) scans and blood tests, pretreatment interventions such as antiemetics, monitoring for side effects, and management options should side effects occur. Significant self-care and motivation are required to complete planned doses on time for treatment regimens that can involve months of therapy with multiple drug combinations. The patient's active participation in preventing, monitoring, and reporting symptoms is essential and should be supported with continuing education.

Anthracyclines

Doxorubicin and epirubicin are the two most commonly used anthracyclines in breast cancer regimens. Epirubicin was widely used in Europe and in more recent years has gained approval for use in the United States. Toxicity with both agents is significant and includes myelosuppression, nausea, vomiting, mucositis, and alopecia. Both are vesicants, and special care must be taken with administration. Cardiac toxicity is a major concern and is most often a cumulative toxicity. The incidence of cardiac toxicity increases once cumulative doses of doxorubicin have exceeded 450 mg/m^2 and once doses of epirubicin have exceeded 900–1,000 mg/m^2 (Kardinal & Cole, 2001; Miller & Sledge, 2002; Wood et al., 2005). To rule out baseline cardiac abnormalities, pretreatment cardiac assessment should include review of the patient's medical history and a physical examination. In addition, tests such as an echocardiogram or MUGA scan provide essential cardiac function information. Continued and careful cardiac assessment throughout treatment may include both physical examinations and serial tests for cardiac function.

Liposomal doxorubicin has a longer half-life and better affinity for tumor tissue. Use in the metastatic setting is increasing. The side effect profile of liposomal doxorubicin is different from that of free doxorubicin. Liposomal doxorubicin causes fewer gastrointestinal side effects and less alopecia, myelosuppression, and cardiotoxicity but more mucositis, hypersensitivity reactions, and skin toxicities such as palmar-plantar erythrodysesthesia (Hamilton & Hortobagyi, 2005).

Taxanes

The taxanes paclitaxel and docetaxel both have activity against breast cancer. Paclitaxel has been used in both adjuvant and metastatic breast cancer regimens. Paclitaxel is currently a favored agent in many adjuvant regimens. Originally administered in three-week cycles, paclitaxel may have enhanced efficacy when given on a weekly schedule. Toxicities of paclitaxel include alopecia, nausea, vomiting, myelosuppression, hypersensitivity reactions, and neurotoxicities (Hamilton & Hortobagyi, 2005). A new delivery method for paclitaxel can be used to decrease administration time and side effects. Paclitaxel in this formulation is contained in a nanoparticle albumin-bound (nab) shell. Higher doses of nab-paclitaxel

Table 7-3. Combination Chemotherapy Regimens for Breast Cancer				
Chemotherapy Regimen	Interval	Dose (mg/m^2)	Route	Schedule
AC	q 21 days			
Doxorubicin		60	IV	Day 1
Cyclophosphamide		600	IV	Day 1
AC followed by paclitaxel (sequential)	q 21 days			
Doxorubicin		60	IV	Day 1
Cyclophosphamide		600	IV	Day 1
then				
Paclitaxel		175	IV	Day 1
AC followed by docetaxel (sequential)	q 21 days			
Doxorubicin		60	IV	Day 1
Cyclophosphamide		600	IV	Day 1
then				
Docetaxel		100	IV	Day 1
AT	q 21 days			
Doxorubicin		50	IV	Day 1
Paclitaxel		220	IV	Day 2
ATC (sequential)	q 14 days			
Doxorubicin		60	IV	Day 1
then				
Paclitaxel		175	IV	Day 1
then				
Cyclophosphamide		600	IV	Day 1
A to CMF	q 21 days			
Doxorubicin		75	IV	Day 1
then				
Cyclophosphamide		600	IV	Day 1
Methotrexate		40	IV	Day 1
5-fluorouracil		600	IV	Day 1

(Continued on next page)

Table 7-3. Combination Chemotherapy Regimens for Breast Cancer *(Continued)*

Chemotherapy Regimen	Interval	Dose (mg/m^2)	Route	Schedule
CAF	q 28 days			
Cyclophosphamide		100	po	Daily, days 1–14
Doxorubicin		25	IV	Day 1, day 8
5-fluorouracil		500	IV	Day 1, day 8
or				
CAF	q 21 days			
Cyclophosphamide		500	IV	Day 1
Doxorubicin		50	IV	Day 1
5-fluorouracil		500	IV	Day 1
CEF	q 21 days			
Cyclophosphamide		500	IV	Day 1
Epirubicin		100	IV	Day 1
5-fluorouracil		500	IV	Day 1
CMF (oral)	q 28 days			
Cyclophosphamide		100	po	Daily, days 1–14
Methotrexate		40	IV	Day 1, day 8
5-fluorouracil		600	IV	Day 1, day 8
CMF (IV)	q 21 days			
Cyclophosphamide		600	IV	Day 1
Methotrexate		40	IV	Day 1
5-fluorouracil		600	IV	Day 1
or	q 28 days			
Cyclophosphamide		600	IV	Day 1, day 8
Methotrexate		40	IV	Day 1, day 8
5-fluorouracil		600	IV	Day 1, day 8
CNF	q 21 days			
Cyclophosphamide		600	IV	Day 1
Mitoxantrone		12	IV	Day 1
5-fluorouracil		600	IV	Day 1

(Continued on next page)

Table 7-3. Combination Chemotherapy Regimens for Breast Cancer *(Continued)*				
Chemotherapy Regimen	Interval	Dose (mg/m²)	Route	Schedule
FEC	q 21 days			
5-fluorouracil		500	IV	Day 1, day 8
Epirubicin		60	IV	Day 1, day 8
Cyclophosphamide		75	po	Daily, days 1–14
HEC	q 21 days			
Epirubicin		100	IV	Day 1
Cyclophosphamide		830	IV	Day 1
NA	q 21 days			
Vinorelbine		25	IV	Day 1, day 8
Doxorubicin		50	IV	Day 1
TAC	q 21 days			
Docetaxel		75	IV	Day 1
Doxorubicin		50	IV	Day 1
Cyclophosphamide		500	IV	Day 1
Dose Dense (sequential; given with hematopoietic growth factor)	q 14 days			
Doxorubicin		60	IV	Day 1
Cyclophosphamide		600	IV	Day 1
then				
Paclitaxel		175	IV	Day 1

Note. Based on information from Wilkes & Barton-Burke, 2005; Wood et al., 2005.

can be given over shorter administration times and without extensive premedication regimens.

Docetaxel is now a first-line treatment choice in the metastatic setting. Side effects include myelosuppression, alopecia, neurotoxicity, and fluid retention. Medication with oral dexamethasone is required to alleviate the fluid retention syndrome associated with this agent (Kardinal & Cole, 2001).

Antimetabolites

The antimetabolite 5-FU has a long-standing history as a part of several combination regimens for breast cancer. Both short IV administration and continuous-infusion 5-FU have been used. Capecitabine is an oral fluoropyrimidine prodrug of 5-FU. Capecitabine requires three enzymatic steps for activation. The third step involves thymidine phosphorylase, which is typically found in greater quantities in malignant tissue, thus producing greater quantities of 5-FU in malignant versus normal tissues. Side effects of both 5-FU and capecitabine include diarrhea, stomatitis, nausea, vomiting, myelosuppression, and hand-foot syndromes (Miller & Sledge, 2002). Methotrexate is another antimetabolite chemotherapy agent with a long history as a treatment for breast cancer. Methotrexate is part of the CMF (cyclophosphamide, methotrexate, 5-FU) regimen.

Alkylating Agents

Both cisplatin and carboplatin function as alkylating agents. As a breast cancer treatment, cisplatin has shown activity in chemotherapy-naïve patients but minimal activity in previously treated patients. Carboplatin is less effective against breast cancer but has fewer toxicities than cisplatin and is easier to administer. Both agents have been used in the metastatic setting and in high-dose chemotherapy regimens for breast cancer.

Other Chemotherapies

Mitoxantrone is structurally related to doxorubicin. Trials comparing mitoxantrone and doxorubicin in patients with metastatic disease have demonstrated similar response rates. The side effect profile of mitoxantrone is milder, with less nausea, vomiting, and alopecia than doxorubicin. Myelosuppression is the dose-limiting toxicity of this agent. Mitoxantrone can cause cardiac toxicity.

The chemotherapy agent gemcitabine has proven single-agent activity of 25%–40% for both chemotherapy-naïve and previously treated patients. As a single agent, the activity of gemcitabine has not been overwhelming, but its unique mechanism of action and side effect profile make it attractive for combination chemotherapy regimens. Gemcitabine is generally well tolerated. Nausea, myelosuppression, and fatigue are side effects of gemcitabine (Miller & Sledge, 2002).

Vinorelbine is a semisynthetic vinca alkaloid with activity in the metastatic setting. As a second-line therapy, it is capable of showing activity in previously treated patients (Miller & Sledge, 2002). It is well tolerated as a single agent with toxicities including myelosuppression, gastrointestinal toxicities, and peripheral neuropathy.

Targeted Agents

Trastuzumab is a humanized monoclonal antibody for the HER2/*neu* or c-*erb*-b2 transmembrane receptor. Binding of epidermal growth factor with the HER2/*neu* receptor initiates intracellular signaling. Tumor tissue can be assessed for HER2 overexpression by either fluorescence in situ hybridization or immunohistochemistry techniques. In the HER2-positive metastatic setting, trastuzumab can be used as either a single agent or as part of combination regimens. Synergy may exist between trastuzumab and several chemotherapy agents, including cisplatin, thiotepa, docetaxel, and etoposide (Gralow, 2005). Recent data regarding the efficacy of trastuzumab in the adjuvant setting have been reported (see the "Adjuvant Therapy" section for discussion). Trastuzumab is well tolerated but may result in cardiac toxicity, especially in patients with prior or concurrent anthracycline administration or baseline cardiac disease (Wood et al., 2005).

Early-Stage Breast Cancers

Early-stage breast cancers are those in which disease is limited to the breast or locoregional lymph nodes. Early-stage breast cancers are defined by the ability to surgically remove all detectable disease. Current understanding of breast cancer biology acknowledges the possibility of micrometastatic disease with even these early-stage tumors. The use of systemic adjuvant therapy in this setting has resulted in significant positive outcomes for patients.

Adjuvant Therapy

Both single-agent and combination chemotherapy regimens in the adjuvant setting reduce recurrence rates. Combination chemotherapy regimens also reduce mortality rates and are superior to single-agent therapies, especially among younger women (EBCTCG, 2005). Approximately one-third of patients with early-stage disease have improved chances of cure with adjuvant hormonal and chemotherapy regimens (Wood et al., 2005).

The use of adjuvant therapy demands careful consideration of metastatic risk and the individualized risk/benefit ratio of treatments. Prognostic factors can be used to identify patients who are at increased risk for micrometastatic disease. Patients with negative lymph nodes and a tumor size smaller than 1 cm have a less than 10% chance of recurrence at 10 years. Deferral of adjuvant therapy may be a reasonable alternative for these patients (Chapman & Moore, 2005). Positive lymph nodes and larger tumor sizes are indicative of more advanced disease, and stronger consideration of adjuvant chemotherapy is imperative. Hormone receptor status of the primary tumor also is an important indicator. Additional prognostic factors may include lymphovascular invasion, HER2 overexpression, and measures of tumor differentiation and proliferation, including ploidy and S-phase fractions. Tools are available to assist both patients and healthcare providers with adjuvant therapy decision making. These aids exist in print, interactive video, and computer-based forms (Whelan & Loprinzi, 2005).

Interest is growing in the use of predictive molecular markers for decision making regarding adjuvant treatments (Duffy, 2005). Oncotype DX™ (Genomic Health, Inc., Redwood City, CA) is a tissue-based assay that reviews tumors for the expression of 21 genes. A risk score is calculated from the assay and may be used to assist with decision making regarding adjuvant therapy.

The mainstay of adjuvant chemotherapy regimens continues to be the anthracyclines, either doxorubicin or epirubicin. In the most recent EBCTCG (2005) review, a direct comparison showed six months of anthracycline-containing regimens to be significantly more effective than CMF-based regimens. This was particularly true in women younger than age 50 but also was true for women ages 50–69. Fewer women older than 70 have taken part in clinical trials and, therefore, this group is understudied. CMF-based regimens are still effective and may be the regimen of choice in certain settings, such as with patients at increased risk for cardiac toxicity. Anthracycline-containing regimens may be superior for HER2-positive tumors (Wood et al., 2005).

New combination regimens containing taxanes or trastuzumab have shown great promise. Trials incorporating a taxane into AC (doxorubicin and cyclophosphamide) regimens have resulted in improvements in disease-free and overall survival rates. The side effect profile of such regimens includes more pronounced neutropenia, fatigue, and neurotoxicity. An active area of research for early-stage node-negative patients involves comparison of anthracycline-based regimens with non-anthracycline-containing regimens that usually include a taxane. Elimination of anthracyclines would be optimal for patients at risk for cardiac toxicity (Hamilton & Hortobagyi, 2005).

Studies using trastuzumab in adjuvant regimens for women with HER2-positive tumors with node-positive or high-risk node-negative disease recently have been reported. Results of the National Surgical Adjuvant Breast and Bowel Project B-31 trial and the North Central Cancer Treatment Group N9831 trial were jointly reported (Romond et al., 2005). Both studies compared sequential AC-paclitaxel regimens with sequential AC-paclitaxel plus trastuzumab. The addition of trastuzumab significantly improved disease-free and overall survival rates. However, it also created an additional risk of cardiac toxicity, so careful cardiac monitoring was necessary. The reported incidence of class III or IV congestive heart failure or death from cardiac causes was 4.1% in the B-31 trial and 2.9% in the N9831 trial (Romond et al.). The European Herceptin® (Genentech, Inc., South San Francisco, CA) Adjuvant (HERA) trial also studied the use of trastuzumab for early-stage HER2-positive patients. Approximately one-third of the patients in the HERA trial were node negative. Results are not yet mature, but the addition of trastuzumab resulted in better relapse-free and overall survival (Sledge, 2005).

Neoadjuvant Chemotherapy

Traditionally, adjuvant chemotherapy is delivered during the postoperative period. Preoperative or neoadjuvant chemotherapy also may be used. To date, most studies of neoadjuvant chemotherapy have been anthracycline-based. Benefits may include higher rates of breast conservation, the ability to clinically assess response to treatment, and the ability to refine prognosis based on the amount of residual disease after therapy (Hamilton & Hortobagyi, 2005).

Dose and Schedule

Delivering the planned chemotherapy dose on time is optimal, as is avoiding dose reductions whenever possible (Hamilton & Hortobagyi, 2005). This is described as dose intensity and is measured as the amount of drug delivered per unit of time. Higher dose intensity can be achieved by either dose escalation or dose density (Citron, 2004). Careful assess-

ment, anticipation of the need for hematopoietic support, and significant patient education regarding side effect monitoring are essential to achieving maximal dose intensity.

Dose escalation involves the use of increased doses of chemotherapy per cycle. This strategy has been employed in the use of high-dose chemotherapy and stem cell support as a breast cancer treatment. Throughout the 1990s, this method of treatment was rapidly accepted in the absence of randomized clinical trials. To date, however, high-dose chemotherapy for breast cancer has demonstrated only modest improvements in overall survival. These improvements have emerged in the face of significant morbidity and expense (Miller & Sledge, 2002). Several randomized trials currently are ongoing.

Dose-dense strategies use shorter times between chemotherapy cycles. This allows the total dose to be compressed into a shorter period of time. The standard cycle time of every 21 days is shortened to every 14 days and sometimes every 7 days with this approach. Hematopoietic growth factor support is essential. In the adjuvant setting, dose-dense regimens have demonstrated better outcomes in disease-free and overall survival rates (Citron, 2004; Hamilton & Hortobagyi, 2005; Wood et al., 2005).

Sequential dosing of chemotherapy also has been an area of study. Traditional combination chemotherapy regimens for breast cancer involved the administration of several agents on the same day of each cycle. The concept of sequential dosing is an attempt to achieve maximum dose intensity for each chemotherapy agent. With this strategy, one agent or a combination of agents is given repeatedly before another is started, either alone or in combination with other agents.

Locally Advanced and Inflammatory Breast Cancers

Locally advanced breast cancers carry a high risk of metastasis. In the United States, tumors in this group account for only 2%–5% of all breast cancers (Wood et al., 2005), but in developing countries and in ethnic groups with screening and early detection challenges, locally advanced disease represents a larger proportion of breast cancer cases. Breast cancers in this category are a heterogenous group including large or unresectable primary tumors, cancers with fixed or matted axillary nodes, cancers with positive supraclavicular nodes, and inflammatory carcinomas. Staging systems have changed over time, but these tumors generally fall into the stage III category of the American Joint Committee on Cancer staging system (Chapman & Moore, 2005; Kardinal & Cole, 2001).

Local therapies alone have not provided favorable long-term disease-free or overall survival rates for locally advanced breast cancers. Combined modality approaches including surgery, systemic treatment, and radiation therapy represent the current standard of care. Neoadjuvant chemotherapy is a favored approach in many settings, and most regimens contain doxorubicin or epirubicin. As in the adjuvant breast cancer setting, taxanes also may show efficacy in this setting (Wood et al., 2005). Hormonal therapy may be useful in receptor-positive disease, and trastuzumab for HER2-positive tumors. The benefits of neoadjuvant treatment include the ability to downstage tumors for breast-conservation options, the ability to decrease tumor size for a more cosmetically appealing lumpectomy, and the ability to assess for response to chemotherapy. Radiation therapy may be employed in the postoperative setting and for inoperable tumors.

Inflammatory breast cancer (IBC) is the most aggressive type of breast cancer. Clinical characteristics mimic the signs of infection and include redness, warmth, edema (peau d'orange), breast enlargement, and tenderness. The onset of symptoms usually is quite rapid. IBC can present as lobular, ductal, or any other type of breast cancer. Presence of cancer cells in the dermal lymphatics is indicative of IBC, although a diagnosis can be made on clinical presentation alone. A mass may or may not be palpable, and axillary nodes often are positive at the time of presentation (Cole & Kardinal, 2002; Cristofanilli, Buzdar, & Hortobagyi, 2003; Giordano & Hortobagyi, 2003; Moore, 2005).

In cases of IBC, local therapy alone results in consistently poor outcomes with no long-term survivors. Evidence-based treatment is not easily discernible, and few large-scale trials have been undertaken. IBCs account for a very small portion of breast cancer cases, and the aggressive nature of the disease makes travel and referral for a clinical trial more difficult. Multimodality treatment, beginning with induction chemotherapy, is the standard of care. As in the adjuvant setting, anthracycline-based regimens make up most combination chemotherapy regimens, and interest has turned to the addition of taxanes. In a trial at the University of Texas M.D. Anderson Cancer Center, 178 patients with IBC were treated with combination chemotherapy. Patients were randomized to five different treatment arms. No significant differences in disease-free or overall survival rates were noted among the groups, although the regimen containing paclitaxel showed a marginal improvement. The median duration of survival was 37 months. Disease-free survival rates at 5, 10, and 15 years were 32%, 28%, and 28%, respectively. Response to induction chemotherapy is a very important predictor of survival (Cristofanilli et al., 2003; Giordano & Hortobagyi, 2003). HER2 overexpression frequently is present in cases of IBC. Adding trastuzumab to the chemotherapy regimen in those cases should be considered (Moore, 2005).

Metastatic Breast Cancer

Approximately 40,460 women are expected to die of breast cancer in 2007, accounting for 15% of all female deaths from cancer (Jemal et al., 2007). The vast majority of these deaths are the result of metastatic disease. The median survival time after discovery of metastatic breast cancer is two to three years, yet the advent of more successful treatments has allowed 10% of patients with metastatic breast cancer to achieve survival of 10 years of more (Wood et al., 2005).

Initial sites of recurrence usually are bone metastases or local sites involving lymph nodes or the chest wall. A longer disease-free interval, a single site of metastasis, prior positive response to systemic chemotherapy, hormone receptor positivity, and lack of significant visceral or central nervous system metastasis are favorable metastatic findings. Bone metastases are more likely with ER-/PR-positive tumors, whereas visceral metastases are more likely with ER-/PR-negative tumors (Wood et al., 2005). The major goals of treatment in this setting are to maintain quality of life, offer palliation, and control the disease. Symptom control is of the utmost importance. Depending on the course of metastatic progression, symptom control may focus on pain control, organ toxicity effects from prior treatment, hypercalcemia, dyspnea, and management of depression and anxiety, along with many other issues.

Treatment choices for metastatic disease depend on patient condition, response to previous therapies, time interval from prior treatments, and characteristics of the tumor. Systemic treatments include both endocrine therapies and chemotherapies.

Endocrine Therapies for Metastatic Breast Cancer

Endocrine therapies for metastatic disease include all agents discussed previously in this chapter. Tumors previously positive for ER and/or PR receptors may lose this receptor status upon recurrence. Tissue should be tested for receptor status at the time of recurrence whenever possible (Chapman & Moore, 2005).

For many years, tamoxifen has been the first-line treatment choice for metastatic breast cancer. For postmenopausal women with metastatic disease, recent data have demonstrated favorable results for anastrozole, exemestane, and letrozole when compared to tamoxifen. AIs are now accepted as first-line treatment in this setting. Clinical trials comparing fulvestrant with both anastrozole and tamoxifen have been completed. No significant difference in time to progression (TTP) or overall survival was seen in comparisons of fulvestrant and anastrozole. In comparison with tamoxifen, fulvestrant showed similar TTP and overall survival, but greater clinical benefit occurred with tamoxifen (Gralow, 2005). In summary, tamoxifen, fulvestrant, or AIs may all be used in the metastatic setting. Crossover among the agents may be beneficial. After progression on these therapies, the use of estrogens, progestins, and androgens may be considered (Wood et al., 2005).

For premenopausal metastatic breast cancer, tamoxifen and ovarian ablation have shown similar efficacy in clinical trials. Ovarian ablation induces menopause, and AIs may then be used. Androgens and progestins also may be considered (Wood et al., 2005).

Chemotherapy for Metastatic Breast Cancer

Chemotherapy for metastatic disease must take into consideration the potential benefits and toxicities of the therapy. Single-agent, sequential, and combination chemotherapy may be prescribed. Single-agent chemotherapy is effective as both first- and second-line treatment. Agents include doxorubicin (including liposomal doxorubicin), epirubicin, paclitaxel, docetaxel, capecitabine, gemcitabine, and vinorelbine. Response rates for initial therapy range from 20%–68% depending on the agent. Greatest activity usually is found with the anthracyclines and taxanes (Gralow, 2005). Median TTP is approximately six months, and response rates decrease by about half when these agents are used as second- or third-line treatments (Wood et al., 2005). Previous exposure to taxanes or anthracyclines in adjuvant regimens may decrease response to those agents in the metastatic setting. Exposure to chemotherapy within the previous 12 months suggests the need to use different chemotherapies (Gralow).

When compared with single-agent therapy, combination regimens result in higher response rates and longer TTP but no survival advantage. Toxicities are increased with combination regimens. The effects that changing a combination regimen to a sequential administration plan has on response, TTP, and survival are of great interest. Administration of sequential chemotherapy results in less toxicity (Gralow, 2005; Hamilton & Hortobagyi, 2005).

Breast Cancer in Select Populations

Special consideration should be given in regard to use of systemic therapy in select populations. Clinical presentation and tumor characteristics may influence selection of treatments.

Male Breast Cancer

Breast cancer in males is an uncommon occurrence, accounting for less than 1% of all breast cancers. All histologic subtypes have been noted in male breast cancer, but the majority have been invasive ductal carcinomas. In situ cancers and IBCs also have been described. Disease most often presents as a subareolar mass (Winchester, 2002). Male breast cancers more often are hormone receptor positive and present more frequently in the locally advanced stage as compared with female breast cancers. Because of the rare occurrence of the disease, no large-scale randomized trials have been undertaken.

Systemic treatment recommendations have been derived from the treatment of female breast cancer. Hormonal therapy with tamoxifen has been a standard approach in receptor-positive disease. Orchiectomy may be used as a hormone-ablating procedure in males. Estrogens, progestins, androgens, and LHRH agonists all have reported activity in male breast cancer (Kardinal & Cole, 2001).

Breast Cancer During Pregnancy

Breast cancer during pregnancy may be referred to as gestational breast cancer or pregnancy-associated breast cancer (PABC). The annual estimated occurrence is 30,000 women worldwide, or 10% of breast cancers diagnosed in premenopausal women (Ahrendt, 2002; Saunders, Hickey, & Ives, 2004). PABC is more likely to present at an advanced stage at diagnosis. This presumably occurs because of a delay in diagnosis that may be related to several factors, including difficult assessment of breasts because of changes associated with pregnancy, low index of suspicion on the part of primary care providers, and reluctance to obtain breast imaging studies during pregnancy. Mammography with appropriate shielding is considered to be safe during pregnancy.

Systemic therapy is not given in the first trimester because of the risk of fetal harm. Antimetabolite agents such as 5-FU and methotrexate in particular are avoided. Chemotherapy can be given during the second and third trimesters. Chemotherapy is scheduled to stop two to three weeks before planned delivery or at 35 weeks of gestation before spontaneous delivery. Stopping chemotherapy at these times is important to avoid maternal myelosuppression at the time of delivery. Stopping chemotherapy before delivery also is important because the neonate's liver and kidneys may not be able to metabolize and excrete the chemotherapeutic agents (Ahrendt, 2002; Saunders et al., 2004).

Breast Cancer in African American Women

Ethnic disparities in breast cancer incidence and survival have been noted. Despite a lower incidence of breast cancer in African American women, this population experiences higher mortality rates than do Caucasian women with breast cancer. A trend toward later-stage disease at presentation has been noted in African American women, which may be attributed to screening and prevention challenges. The possibility of different breast cancer biology in this population also exists. A larger percentage of African American women have premenopausal breast cancer as compared to Caucasian women. As would be expected in premenopausal presentation, ER-negative status also is more prevalent in these tumors. Higher nuclear grade and S-phase fraction also have been noted (Chapman & Moore, 2005; Hershman et al., 2005).

Breast Cancer in Older Adults

Great strides have been made in the research of breast cancer treatment, but few clinical trials have included women older than 65. A recently published study from Giordano, Hortobagyi, Kau, Theriault, and Bondy (2005) reviewed the care of 1,568 patients ages 55 years and older at a single institution. Treatments for that population were compared to institutional guidelines. The results of the study showed that older women were less likely to receive standard treatment for surgical therapy, postlumpectomy radiation, adjuvant chemotherapy, and adjuvant hormonal therapy.

Breast cancers in older women generally exhibit more favorable and less aggressive features. They are more likely to be hormone receptor positive, HER2 negative, and node negative (Kimmick & Muss, 2004; Wood et al., 2005). Older women may present with locally advanced disease, especially if screening and detection practices have ceased or become infrequent. Screening mammography should continue in any woman with a life expectancy of four years or more (Kimmick & Muss).

In addition, comorbidities may be more pronounced in older adults. Other illnesses may be life threatening. Systemic therapy choices must include consideration of disease status, life expectancy, and comorbidities.

In early-stage disease, adjuvant treatment with chemotherapy and/or hormonal therapy may be considered. Treatment regimens not containing anthracycline often are used to minimize the potential for cardiac toxicity. Mitoxantrone, liposomal doxorubicin, and taxanes also have been attractive alternatives. Trastuzumab for HER2 overexpression has been used in this population. In locally advanced or metastatic disease, the same considerations regarding chemotherapy should be made. Primary hormonal therapy alone may be the best choice in cases when surgery is not an option or when life expectancy is limited. Several endocrine therapies have a history of use in this setting (Mano et al., 2005).

New Agents and Future Directions

Insight into the biology of breast cancer has formed the basis of breast-conservation and adjuvant therapies, which have been very successful. Better understanding of breast cancer biology will further assist with treatment decisions. Study of predictive molecular markers in a tumor may assist in treatment decision making by stratifying patients with early-stage breast cancer into groups of those for whom adjuvant therapy will be of benefit and those for whom little benefit might be expected. Study of tumors also may assist with therapy choice by defining susceptibilities to chemotherapeutic and hormonal agents.

The availability of systemic agents for breast cancer treatment continues to advance as new agents are discovered, researched, and incorporated into clinical practice. New agents of interest in treatment include angiogenesis inhibitors, targeted agents for the epidermal growth factor receptors, and farnesyl transferase inhibitors. Cyclooxygenase pathway inhibitors and statins also may prove useful as breast cancer therapies (Wood et al., 2005). As with many cancers, immunologic treatments continue to be of interest. Breast cancer antigens such as HER2 and breast cancer–specific mucin may serve as targets for vaccines or other immune therapies (Sabel & Nehs, 2005).

The manner in which systemic therapies are administered has changed over the history of systemic breast cancer treatments. Trials with new combinations of therapies continue. Sequencing of systemic therapies with each other and with surgery and radiation therapy continues to be studied. All systemic therapies cause untoward effects. Alleviation of toxicities and palliation of symptoms must continue to be an important endeavor in both research and clinical practice. Education needs should be anticipated and answered as patients and healthcare providers continue to navigate the many treatment options, which involve complex decision making and risk-benefit analyses from patients.

Conclusion

Significant progress has been made in the systemic treatment of breast cancer in recent years. However, much work remains to be done. More than 180,000 new cases of breast cancer are expected to be diagnosed in 2007, accounting for 26% of all cancers diagnosed in women (Jemal et al., 2007). Even small gains in response, survival, and palliation will have a significant impact on a disease that affects so many.

References

Ahrendt, G.M. (2002). Pregnancy and breast cancer. In W.L. Donegan & J.S. Spratt (Eds.), *Cancer of the breast* (5th ed., pp. 909–915). Philadelphia: Saunders.

Beatson, G.T. (1896). On the treatment of inoperable cases of carcinoma of the mamma: Suggestions for a new method of treatment with illustrative cases. *Lancet, 2,* 104–107, 162–165.

Chapman, D.D., & Moore, S. (2005). Breast cancer. In C.H. Yarbro, M.H. Frogge, & M. Goodman (Eds.), *Cancer nursing: Principles and practice* (6th ed., pp. 1022–1088). Sudbury, MA: Jones and Bartlett.

Citron, M.L. (2004). Dose density in adjuvant chemotherapy for breast cancer. *Cancer Investigation, 22,* 555–568.

Cole, J., & Kardinal, C.G. (2002). Locally advanced and inflammatory breast cancer. In W.L. Donegan & J.S. Spratt (Eds.), *Cancer of the breast* (5th ed., pp. 579–595). Philadelphia: Saunders.

Cristofanilli, M., Buzdar, A.U., & Hortobagyi, G.N. (2003). Update on the management of inflammatory breast cancer. *Oncologist, 8,* 141–148.

Dickson, R.B., Pestell, R.G., & Lippman, M.E. (2005). Molecular biology of breast cancer. In V.T. DeVita, Jr., S. Hellman, & S.A. Rosenberg (Eds.), *Cancer: Principles and practice of oncology* (7th ed., pp. 1399–1414). Philadelphia: Lippincott Williams & Wilkins.

Duffy, M.J. (2005). Predictive markers in breast and other cancers: A review. *Clinical Chemistry, 51,* 494–503.

Early Breast Cancer Trialists' Collaborative Group. (2005). Effects of chemotherapy and hormonal therapy for early breast cancer on recurrence and 15-year survival: An overview of the randomised trials. *Lancet, 365,* 1687–1717.

Fischer, D.S., Knobf, M.T., Durivage, H.J., & Beaulieu, N.J. (2003). *The cancer chemotherapy handbook* (6th ed.). Philadelphia: Mosby.

Forbes, J.F. (2003). Breast cancer. In C. Williams (Ed.), *Evidence-based oncology* (pp. 428–464). London: BMJ Publishing Group.

Gerken, P. (2004). Toremifene citrate (Fareston). *Clinical Journal of Oncology Nursing, 8,* 529–530.

Giordano, S.H., & Hortobagyi, G.N. (2003). Inflammatory breast cancer: Clinical progress and the main problems that must be addressed. *Breast Cancer Research, 5,* 284–288.

Giordano, S.H., Hortobagyi, G.N., Kau, S.C., Theriault, R.L., & Bondy, M.L. (2005). Breast cancer treatment guidelines in older women. *Journal of Clinical Oncology, 23,* 783–791.

Goss, P.E., & Strasser, K. (2001). Aromatase inhibitors in the treatment and prevention of breast cancer. *Journal of Clinical Oncology, 19,* 881–894.

Gralow, J.R. (2005). Optimizing the treatment of metastatic breast cancer. *Breast Cancer Research and Treatment, 89*(Suppl. 1), S9–S15.

Hamilton, A., & Hortobagyi, G. (2005). Chemotherapy: What progress in the last 5 years? *Journal of Clinical Oncology, 23,* 1760–1775.

Hancock, C.M. (2003). Fulvestrant antiestrogen for treatment of breast cancer. *Clinical Journal of Oncology Nursing, 7,* 201–202.

Harwood, K.V. (2004). Advances in endocrine therapy for breast cancer: Considering efficacy, safety, and quality of life. *Clinical Journal of Oncology Nursing, 8,* 629–635.

Hershman, D., McBride, R., Jacobson, J.S., Lamerato, L., Roberts, K., Grann, V.R., et al. (2005). Racial disparities in treatment and survival among women with early-stage breast cancer. *Journal of Clinical Oncology, 23,* 6639–6646.

Howell, A., Pippen, J., Elledge, R.M., Mauriac, L., Vergote, I., Jones, S.E., et al. (2005). Fulvestrant versus anastrozole for the treatment of advanced breast carcinoma: A prospectively planned combined survival analysis of two multicenter trials. *Cancer, 104,* 236–239.

Jemal, A., Siegel, R., Ward, E., Murray, T., Xu, J., & Thun, M.J. (2007). Cancer statistics, 2007. *CA: A Cancer Journal for Clinicians, 57,* 43–66.

Kardinal, C.G., & Cole, J.T. (2001). Chemotherapy of breast cancer. In M.C. Perry (Ed.), *The chemotherapy source book* (3rd ed., pp. 647–689). Philadelphia: Lippincott Williams & Wilkins.

Kimmick, G., & Muss, H.B. (2004). Breast cancer in older patients. *Seminars in Oncology, 31,* 234–248.

Lake, D.E., & Hudis, C. (2002). Aromatase inhibitors in breast cancer: An update. *Cancer Control, 9,* 490–498.

Mano, M., Fraser, G., McIlroy, P., Stirling, L., MacKay, H., Ritchie, D., et al. (2005). Locally advanced breast cancer in octogenarian women. *Breast Cancer Research and Treatment, 89,* 81–90.

Miller, K.D., & Sledge, G.W. (2002). Chemotherapy for early and advanced breast cancer. In W.L. Donegan & J.S. Spratt (Eds.), *Cancer of the breast* (5th ed., pp. 659–687). Philadelphia: Saunders.

Moore, S. (2005). Inflammatory breast cancer. *Oncology Nursing Forum, 32,* 907–911.

Mouridsen, H.T., & Robert, N.J. (2005). The role of aromatase inhibitors as adjuvant therapy for early breast cancer in postmenopausal women. *European Journal of Cancer, 41,* 1678–1689.

Osborne, C.K., & Schiff, R. (2005). Aromatase inhibitors: Future directions. *Journal of Steroid Biochemistry and Molecular Biology, 95,* 183–187.

Ranger, G.S. (2005). Current concepts in the endocrine therapy of breast cancer: Tamoxifen and aromatase inhibitors. *Journal of Clinical Pharmacy and Therapeutics, 30,* 313–317.

Romond, E.H., Perez, E.A., Bryant, J., Suman, V.J., Geyer, C.E., Davidson, N.E., et al. (2005). Trastuzumab plus adjuvant chemotherapy for operable HER2-positive breast cancer. *New England Journal of Medicine, 353,* 1673–1684.

Sabel, M.S., & Nehs, M.A. (2005). Immunologic approaches to breast cancer treatment. *Surgical Oncology Clinics of North America, 14,* 1–31.

Saunders, C., Hickey, M., & Ives, A. (2004). Breast cancer during pregnancy. *International Journal of Fertility and Women's Medicine, 49,* 203–207.

Sledge, G.W., Jr. (2005). New developments in adjuvant therapy for breast cancer. *Clinical Advances in Hematology and Oncology, 3,* 688–690.

Smith, I.E., & Dowsett, M. (2003). Aromatase inhibitors in breast cancer. *New England Journal of Medicine, 348,* 2431–2442.

Versea, L., & Rosenzweig, M. (2003). Hormonal therapy for breast cancer: Focus on fulvestrant. *Clinical Journal of Oncology Nursing, 7,* 307–311.

Whelan, T.J., & Loprinzi, C. (2005). Physician/patient decision aids for adjuvant therapy. *Journal of Clinical Oncology, 23,* 1627–1630.

Wilkes, G.M., & Barton-Burke, M. (2005). *2005 oncology nursing drug handbook.* Sudbury, MA: Jones and Bartlett.

Winchester, D.J. (2002). Male breast cancer. In W.L. Donegan & J.S. Spratt (Eds.), *Cancer of the breast* (5th ed., pp. 951–958). Philadelphia: Saunders.

Wood, W.C., Muss, H.B., Solin, L.J., & Olopade, O.I. (2005). Malignant tumors of the breast. In V.T. DeVita, Jr., S. Hellman, & S.A. Rosenberg (Eds.), *Cancer: Principles and practice of oncology* (7th ed., pp. 1415–1477). Philadelphia: Lippincott Williams & Wilkins.

CHAPTER 8

Symptom Management in Breast Cancer

Carole H. Martz, RN, MS, AOCN®, and Katina Kirby, MS, OTR/L, CLT-LANA

Introduction

Survivors of breast cancer number in the millions as a result of strides made in early detection and improved multimodal therapy. Yet, the potential to cure or prolong the lives of women has not come without a price for those women experiencing side effects. These side effects can range from minor to life altering. Some can contribute to a decrease in quality of life (QOL) and psychological well-being. This chapter will review the most common side effects of breast cancer treatment along with symptom management strategies.

Surgical Complications

The most common long-term side effects from breast cancer surgery are pain and numbness, limited shoulder and arm range of motion (ROM), and lymphedema (LE) (Baron, Fey, Borgen, & Van Zee, 2004; Bosompra, Ashikaga, O'Brien, Nelson, & Skelly, 2002; Karki, Simonen, Malkia, & Selfe, 2005; Schrenk, Rieger, Shamiyeh, & Wayand, 1999; Swenson et al., 2002). The incidence of these side effects varies by the length of follow-up, measurement techniques used, and patient- and treatment-related factors (Kakuda, Stuntz, Trivedi, Klein, & Vargas, 1999; Kuehn et al., 2000; McCredie et al., 2001). The severity of these symptoms can range from mild to severe and can affect QOL many years later (Dow, Ferrell, Leigh, Ly, & Gulasekaram, 1996; Rietman et al., 2003).

Recent studies comparing the frequency of side effects from axillary lymph node dissection (ALND) to sentinel lymph node biopsy (SLN) indicate a trend to more favorable outcomes with the latter procedure (Schrenk et al., 1999; Sener et al., 2001; Swenson et al., 2002). Most of the studies comparing ALND to SLN have been of small sample size and without significant long-term follow-up. Retrospective and prospective studies currently are available for review, many of which are based on patient self-reports of symptoms.

Surgery-Related Pain and Limitation of Movement

In a review by Rietman et al. (2003), the incidence of post-surgery pain was noted to range from 12% to 51%. The type of breast pain experienced has been described as tightness in the breast scar and axilla, tenderness at the incision(s), and nerve entrapment symptoms (burning and stabbing) sometimes referred to as postmastectomy pain syndrome (Baron et al., 2004; Bosompra et al., 2002; Karki et al., 2005; Lierman, 1998; Stevens, Dibble, & Miaskowski, 1995; Swenson et al., 2002). Patients in the Bosompra et al. study who underwent modified radical mastectomy were more likely to complain of problems with scar tightness than patients undergoing breast-conserving surgery. Baron et al. (2004) found that tenderness at the incision site(s) was the most common symptom at baseline for patients who had SLN and persisted in more than 40% of the women at two years. Breast cancer survivors also used the terms *twinges* and *soreness* to describe their symptoms. In patients undergoing ALND, more patients complained of tightness, numbness, and pain at baseline, and tightness, numbness, pulling, and tingling at 24 months. Numbness was the most distressing symptom in the ALND group at baseline and at 24 months.

Stiffness was the only sensation that was significant in patients who had both a total mastectomy and SLN in the Baron et al. (2004) study, and it likely had some impact on shoulder and arm ROM. The biggest drop in the level of distress for all pain-related symptoms was between baseline and three months after surgery. In this study, 56% of patients undergoing mastectomy were found to experience phantom breast sensations at least one time during the 24-month evaluation period. Overall, the level of severity and distress for this symptom was low. The incidence of phantom breast sensations was 26% in a study by Kroner, Knudsen, Lundby, and Hvid (1992). Rowland et al. (2000) found that women undergoing mastectomy with or without reconstruction had more physical symptoms, particularly discomfort at the surgical site, than women undergoing breast conservation. Symptoms described included pins and needles (26% incidence in mastectomy-alone patients) and numbness occurring in 52% of patients undergoing reconstruction. Most studies find that although women report a high prevalence of numbness following surgery, it does not affect their daily lives and activities after the first year. Most breast cancer survivors learn to adjust to the surgical complications. Shoulder and arm ROM difficulties at one year following surgery range from 1.5% to 23% and are more commonly seen in women undergoing ALND, mastectomy, and radiation therapy (Deutsch & Flickinger, 2001; Duff et al., 2001; Kakuda et al., 1999; Karki et al., 2005; Keramopoulos, Tsionou, Minaretzis, Michalas, & Aravantinos, 1993; Sugden, Rezvani, Harrison, & Hughes, 1998; Swenson et al., 2002). Most ROM limitations improved during follow-up (Knopf & Sun, 2005).

Altered sensations result from injury or resection of specific nerves in the operative field. The intercostobrachial cutaneous nerve innervates the axilla and medial upper arm. This nerve is directly in the path of surgeons as they perform ALND and often is sacrificed to gain wider access to the axillary lymph nodes during SLN. Even when preserved, it can be injured. A recent literature search by Kim et al. (2005) looked at SLN technique and the risk of increased postoperative sensory changes. A lower rate of changes occurred when lymphoscintigraphy (LS) was used to assist in localization of the sentinel lymph node(s) compared to when LS was not used. Numbness was more frequent when blue dye or an intraoperative handheld probe without LS or skin markings was used, suggesting that a change in surgical technique could affect the development of postmastectomy pain.

Injury to motor nerves is a very rare occurrence in the hands of a skilled surgeon. The brachial plexus may be injured as a result of hyperabduction of the arm on the operating room table. Women who receive radiation therapy to the brachial plexus region also can develop chronic pain in the ipsilateral arm (Gutman, Kersz, Barzilai, Haddad, & Reiss, 1990).

Nonpharmacologic measures for treating mild pain include resting the arm on a pillow, limiting movement, applying heat (may be contraindicated in patients at risk for LE), or icing the painful area, taking care to protect the skin from thermal injury. The use of over-the-counter nonsteroidal anti-inflammatory drugs (NSAIDs), acetaminophen, and prescription cyclooxygenase-2 inhibitors may be helpful for pain. Distraction also may help.

Katz et al. (2005) found that more severe acute postoperative pain increased the risk of chronic pain following breast cancer surgery. Postsurgical complications such as the development of a seroma, hematoma, or infection have been shown to increase the risk of developing chronic pain (Tasmuth, von Smitten, Hietanen, Katja, & Kalso, 1995). Most chronic pain syndromes associated with surgery are related to dysesthesias. The treatment depends on the severity of the symptom and its impact on the patient's QOL. Both pharmacologic and non-

pharmacologic strategies have been employed. Randomized clinical trials have looked at topical capsaicin and EMLA® (eutectic mixture of local anesthetics [lidocaine and prilocaine], AstraZeneca Pharmaceuticals, Wilmington, DE) application for the prevention of postmastectomy pain at varying dosages and administration times. All achieved a good to excellent response, with the main side effect of the medications being a burning sensation (Fassoulaki, Sarantopoulos, Melemeni, & Hogan, 2000; Watson & Evans, 1992). Other pharmaceutical options include NSAIDs, tricyclic antidepressants, and anticonvulsants. Kalso, Tasmuth, and Neuvonen (1996) found that amitriptyline 50 mg significantly relieved neuropathic pain in the arm and around the breast scar. However, the drug's side effects affected patients' willingness to take the drug. Venlafaxine (Effexor®, Wyeth Pharmaceuticals, Philadelphia, PA) also has been shown to be effective in the management of neuropathic pain associated with breast surgery. Reuben, Makari-Judson, and Lurie (2004) examined the effect of venlafaxine starting the night before partial or radical mastectomy and two weeks after with surgeries that included ALND. A significant decrease occurred in the incidence of chest wall, arm, and axillary pain at follow-up six months after surgery. Fassoulaki, Triga, Melemeni, and Sarantopoulos (2005) evaluated the effect of multimodal analgesia on acute and chronic pain after breast cancer surgery using gabapentin (Neurontin®, Pfizer Inc., New York, NY), EMLA, and ropivacaine in the wound, each of which reduced acute and chronic pain compared to controls. If these measures do not control the pain, a weak opioid such as codeine or hydrocodone should be added, followed by a more potent narcotic, or referral to a pain clinic for consideration of nerve blocks (National Comprehensive Cancer Network [NCCN], 2005a).

Restrictions in shoulder and arm movement can persist for up to two years after surgery in both SLN and ALND groups. Radiation therapy can contribute to scarring, adding additional restrictions. Now that more patients are receiving adjuvant chemotherapy and trastuzumab (Herceptin®, Genentech, Inc., South San Francisco, CA), the start of radiation treatments may be delayed following surgery. Patients should be advised that ROM limitations might recur during radiation therapy. All patients undergoing axillary surgery should be advised about the possibility of ROM limitations and should be provided with exercises to decrease long-term restrictions (Isaksson & Feuk, 2000). Postoperative physical therapy can help to restore motion and strength (Gutman et al., 1990). Timing of postoperative exercises is controversial, with randomized clinical trials showing mixed results. Some researchers suggest delaying exercises until one week after surgery in order to reduce seroma formation (Petrek et al., 1990; Schultz, Barholm, & Grondal, 1997; Shamley, Barker, Simonite, & Beardshaw, 2005). Patients who exhibit limited ROM for four to six weeks postoperatively will benefit from referral to a physical medicine specialist (McAnaw & Harris, 2002). Figures 8-1 through 8-3 show examples of exercises for after

Figure 8-1. Exercises in Lying Position

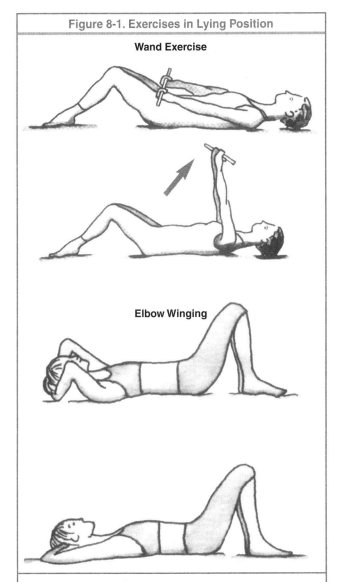

Wand Exercise

Elbow Winging

Figure 8-2. Exercises in Sitting Position

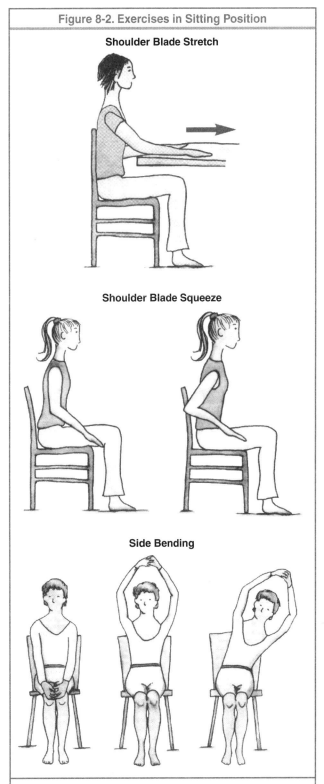

Shoulder Blade Stretch

Shoulder Blade Squeeze

Side Bending

breast surgery. Patients should perform these exercises following a warm shower and should do the exercises until they feel a slow stretch. Patients should hold the stretch for a count of five and repeat the set five to seven times. The entire routine is to be repeated twice a day until normal flexibility and strength are regained (American Cancer Society, 2001). Patients must be advised that the stretch may cause some discomfort. The use of pain medication 30–45 minutes prior to beginning these exercises can limit the degree of discomfort.

Identification of people with preexisting mobility difficulties or significant early postoperative ROM problems

Figure 8-3. Exercises in Standing Position

Chest Wall Stretch

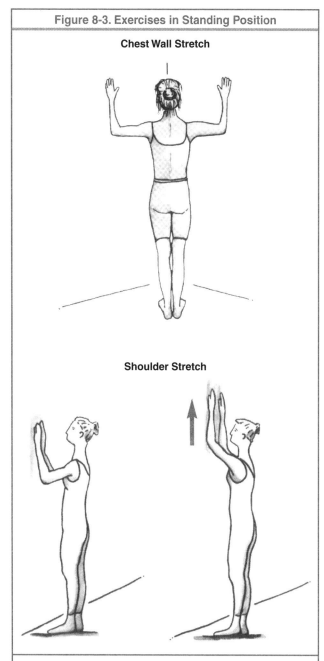

Shoulder Stretch

Note. From *Exercises After Breast Surgery,* by the American Cancer Society, 2006. Retrieved July 17, 2006, from http://www. cancer.org/docroot/CRI/content/CRI_2_6x_Exercises_After_ Breast_Surgery.asp?sitearea=. Copyright 2006 by the American Cancer Society, Inc., from www.cancer.org. All rights reserved. Reprinted with permission.

of symptoms (Reedijk, Boerner, Ghazarian, & McCready, 2005). Exercise programs are aimed at preventing joint ROM limitation, LE, and postural alterations. Box, Reul-Hirche, Bullock-Saxton, and Furnival (2002) found that LE after ALND was decreased with the use of a monitoring, counseling, and early physiotherapy intervention.

Side effects from surgical treatment are varied. Patients and their families must be aware of the expected side effects (mild discomfort, tightness, numbness) and which side effects will require intervention (limited ROM, pain that disrupts daily activities). This information should be discussed during preoperative teaching and reviewed during postoperative education. Additional teaching should be done during follow-up examinations to alleviate concerns when symptoms develop (Johnson, Rice, Fuller, & Endress, 1978).

Lymphedema

Over the past few years, a noticeable increase has occurred in the awareness of the effects of LE on individuals after breast cancer surgery. LE is a well-known complication of ALND that often is downplayed in the era of conservative breast surgeries (Simon & Cody, 1992). Limited research has been done on LE. The majority of material published on the topic focuses on case studies, small or limited research studies, and textbooks from Germany, Austria, and Australia. LE is defined as "the protein-rich edema that occurs when the lymph load (volume) exceeds lymph transport capacity in any body segment. As more and more protein and other macromolecules accumulate in the interstitial spaces, colloid osmotic pressure rises and edema worsens" (Lerner, 2000, p. 1227). LE has two types: primary and secondary. Primary LE is caused by a failure in the lymphatic system itself, and secondary LE is caused by a known insult to the lymphatic system, such as removal of lymph nodes or radiation therapy for the treatment of cancer (Browse, Burnard, & Mortimer, 2003; Casley-Smith & Casley-Smith, 1997). See Figure 8-4 for an example of a patient experiencing LE following breast surgery.

Ipsilateral upper extremity LE may occur at any point after treatment. Stanton, Levik, and Mortimer (1996) suggest that the percentage of women who develop LE following full ALND varies from 8% to 63%. Two recent studies reported an LE rate of 3%–3.5% in women after SLN in the first two years following surgery (Sener et al., 2001; Swenson et al., 2002). Sener et al. determined that ipsilateral upper extremity LE was more common when tumors were located in the upper outer quadrant of the breast, regardless of the type of surgery. No follow-up studies have been reported on this cohort of patients.

The two main functions of the lymphatic system are drainage and transport (Foldi, Foldi, & Kubic, 2003; Weissleder & Schuchhardt, 2001). The lymphatics carry "proteins and large particulate matter away from the tissue spaces, neither

should lead to earlier intervention. A rarely reported axillary web syndrome, also termed *banding* or *cording,* can result in pain along a cord leading from the axilla to the elbow (and occasionally extending to the wrist) with associated limitation in ROM. This syndrome can develop in the immediate postoperative period or months later. Therapy can result in relief

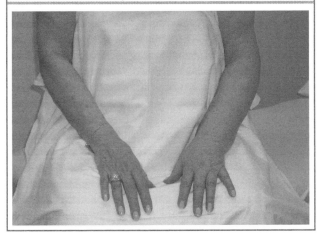

Figure 8-4. Secondary Lymphedema Following Mastectomy With Axillary Dissection

of which can be removed by absorption directly into the blood capillaries" (Guyton, 1997, p. 170). The lymphatic system relies on active/passive muscle contractions, arterial pulsation, respiration, and lymphangion contractions to transport fluid (Foldi et al.). A Starling's law equilibrium is responsible for the creation of lymph fluid (Casley-Smith & Casley-Smith, 1997; Foldi et al.; Simon & Cody, 1992). As Simon and Cody explained, "Under normal physiologic conditions, tissue fluid is in balance with outflow from the arterial side of the capillary bed, inflow on the venous side, and lymph drainage removing excess fluids and protein" (p. 545). In essence, when homeostasis becomes disrupted, LE may occur as a result of a "mechanical failure" in the lymph.

LE can be measured circumferentially (through the use of a tape measure), volumetrically (by water displacement or calculated through circumference measures), or by weight. However, no agreed-upon quantitative definition currently is available for LE following breast cancer surgery (Browse et al., 2003; Stanton et al., 1996). As a result, no universally accepted measure exists that would articulate at what level of increase in circumference or at what increase in volume a diagnosis of LE is warranted. Most physicians use a range scale and rely on patient symptoms to make a diagnosis. Symptoms may include fullness, tightness, loss of mobility, and/or heaviness (Kelly, 2002). These symptoms and sensations may be experienced in any at-risk area "surrounding and distal to the lymph vessel disruption" (Kelly, p. 32). Areas at risk include the ipsilateral upper extremity, chest wall (including but not limited to the breast), and upper back quadrant. Assessment for LE should include all of these areas. The International Society of Lymphology (2003) developed consensus guidelines with a new staging schema for LE (see Table 8-1).

Once LE is suspected, the patient should be evaluated by an experienced physician and LE therapist. If LE is identified, a treatment protocol including complete decongestive therapy

(also known as complex physical therapy or complete decongestive physiotherapy) can be developed. Treatment should consist of skin care, manual lymphatic drainage (sometimes called manual lymphatic treatment), compression bandaging, compression garments, and possibly a compression pump (Casley-Smith & Casley-Smith, 1997; Foldi et al., 2003).

In addition, the skin should be screened for incidental lesions and breaks in skin integrity (Cheville & Gergich, 2004). Lymphedematous tissue may crack and provide an entry for bacteria (Okhuma, 1990). A study performed by Simon and Cody (1992) demonstrated that cellulitis was more likely to occur in the first year after surgery in women who underwent lumpectomy with radiation, and women who underwent more radical surgical procedures, generally without radiation, had cellulitis after a longer time frame. Individuals with repeated cellulitis may require prophylactic antibiotic therapy (Feldman, 2005).

Manual lymphatic drainage "is a massage technique that stimulates lymph vessels to contract more frequently and to channel lymphatic fluid towards adjacent, functioning lymph systems" (Ko, Lerner, Klose, & Cosimi, 1998, p. 454). Specific gentle movements begin on the contralateral quadrant of the body, working from proximal to distal yet always directing the fluid proximally (Browse et al., 2001).

Compression bandaging consists of many layers (i.e., protective stockinet, padding, and elastic bandage) (Browse et al., 2001; Casley-Smith & Casley-Smith, 1997; Foldi et al., 2003). The bandages used are low elastic that have a low resting pressure and high working pressure placed in a gradient manner (more pressure distally than proximally) (Casley-Smith & Casley-Smith). An example of LE bandaging can be seen in Figure 8-5.

Table 8-1. International Society of Lymphology Lymphedema Staging	
Lymphedema Stage	**Definition**
Stage 0	Latent or subclinical condition where swelling is not evident despite impaired lymph transport
Stage 1	Early accumulation of fluid relatively high in protein content, which subsides with limb elevation (pitting may occur)
Stage 2	May or may not pit as tissue fibrosis supervenes
Stage 3	Lymphostatic elephantiasis where pitting is absent and trophic skin changes such as acanthosis, fat deposits, and warty overgrowths develop

Note. Based on information from International Society of Lymphology, 2003.

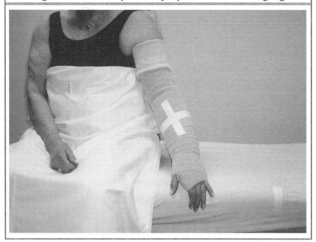

Figure 8-5. Example of Lymphedema Bandaging

A patient with LE should wear a compression bandage throughout therapy until measures have stabilized. The individual's circumferential and volumetric measurements should steadily decrease, and then remain fairly constant. At this point, the individual should be fitted for a compression garment. Afterward, the individual will use the compression bandage as a source of reduction and the compression garment as a form of maintenance. Patients are instructed to wear the garment continuously during the day and remove the garment at night (Casley-Smith & Casley-Smith, 1997). Garments should be checked every six months for proper fit (Weissleder & Schuchhardt, 2001). It is important to note that use of an Ace® (Becton, Dickinson and Co., Franklin Lakes, NJ) wrap bandage is contraindicated. Studies by Ko et al. (1998) and Boris, Weindorf, and Lasinski (1997) showed that patients demonstrated a significantly increased rate of maintenance and decreased LE because of the use of complete decongestive therapy.

The use of compression pumps for LE therapy remains controversial (Casley-Smith, Casley-Smith, Lasinski, & Boris, 1996). Studies evaluating the use of compression pumps in lower extremity LE have shown worsening of symptoms. However, the use of compression pumps may be applicable for "the patient who cannot or will not tolerate LE bandaging, for the patient with minimal fibrotic changes to subcutaneous tissues, and the patient who cannot come for daily treatment" (Kelly, 2002, p. 103). No official indications for pump therapy exist.

Complete decongestive therapy should be administered by a therapist (i.e., an occupational therapist, physical therapist, or RN with special training) who specializes in LE. The Lymphology Association of North America (2005) has developed a national certifying examination for competency standards in LE therapy. Lymphologists, physicians who specialize in the treatment of LE, are not numerous in the United States. As a result, the physician referring the patient for treatment is frequently the primary care physician or oncologist, thus making the skill level of the therapist critical.

No medications currently are available to treat LE. Researchers in Australia studied benzopyrenes for LE reduction. However, this drug's use may have caused acute liver toxicity and therefore was never approved by the U.S. Food and Drug Administration (Kalinowski, 2004). Currently, the National Institutes of Health has two clinical trials studying the treatment of LE. A randomized, double-blind, placebo-controlled trial through the National Center for Complementary and Alternative Medicine (NCCAM) is evaluating the use of Pycnogenol® (Horphag Research LTD, Guernsey, United Kingdom) for the treatment of LE of the arm in breast cancer survivors (2003c). NCCAM (2003b) also is conducting a randomized, single-blind study of massage therapy for breast cancer treatment–related swelling of the arms. Surgical procedures have never shown a durable response and have required the use of compression bandages and sleeves to effect any longstanding change (Servelle, 1987).

It is important to educate women about the risk of LE and how to potentially decrease the risk of developing it. The literature does not report a direct correlation between education and either a reduction in LE development or a delay in onset. Anecdotal case reports have driven the development of most of the guidelines for risk reduction. It is assumed that risk is decreased if an individual avoids triggers that can further "decrease the transport capacity of the lymph vessels and/or unnecessarily increase the lymphatic fluid and protein load of the lymphatic system of the affected region" (Kelly, 2002, p. 33). The National Lymphedema Network (NLN) Medical Advisory Committee (2005b) has published a concise list of triggers in *Lymphedema Risk Reduction Practices.* Triggers include trauma to the skin, infection, sunburn, weight gain, intense upper body activities, limb constriction, ill-fitting compression garments, and temperature extremes (e.g., saunas, hot tubs). A complete copy of this position statement is available at the NLN Web site (www.lymphnet.org/pdfDocs/nlnriskreduction.pdf). Table 8-2 describes LE triggers, pathophysiology, and risk-reduction strategies.

A review of the literature demonstrates that exercise is important for an individual with or at risk for LE. Exercise produces muscle contraction, which is believed to increase pressure in the interstitium, increase uptake of initial lymphatics, promote muscle strengthening, and mobilize the joints (Browse et al., 2003; Casley-Smith & Casley-Smith, 1997; Foldi et al., 2003; Kelly, 2002; NLN Medical Advisory Committee, 2005a). Discussions have arisen as to whether the kind of exercise one engages in decreases or increases the risk of developing LE. Researchers have conducted studies to determine whether isometric exercise, exercises following drainage pathways, or simply any exercise that an individual performs has a higher impact over another in preventing or prolonging the onset of LE. No strong conclusions have been reached. The NLN position statement on exercise suggests that

Table 8-2. Lymphedema Triggers, Pathophysiology, and Risk-Reduction Examples		
Triggers	**Pathophysiologic Basis**	**Risk Reduction**
Cuts/scrapes to at-risk area	Bacteria may enter through cracks, causing a cellulitic infection (Cheville & Gergich, 2004; Kelly, 2002; Okhuma, 1990; Simon & Cody, 1992).	Wear gloves while washing dishes or gardening. Keep skin pliable and well lubricated. Avoid needle punctures on area at risk.
Constriction	Constriction may slow or stop lymphatic flow (Kelly, 2002).	Avoid wearing tight-fitting clothing (e.g., bra straps/bands). Avoid taking blood pressure readings on arm at risk.
Exercise	More lymph fluid may be produced secondary to (a) increased pulse leading to increased arterial blood flow and (b) overuse syndrome (National Lymphedema Network [NLN] Medical Advisory Committee, 2005a).	Wear a form of compression while exercising, and monitor for signs of edema.
Air travel	Pressure may decrease in cabin, changing interstitial pressures in the body (NLN Medical Advisory Committee, 2004).	Wear a form of compression while traveling. (External pressure may decrease potential of fluid accumulation in tissue.)

a person with or at risk for LE wear compression bandages or garments while exercising (NLN Medical Advisory Committee, 2005a). Also, weight training or resistive exercises may pose a greater risk. Currently, no studies are available to help practitioners in advising patients as to weight-lifting limits, nor is there a formula to decide how much an individual may lift. According to the NLN Medical Advisory Committee (2005a), "The introduction of weights should be gradual with the individual's response monitored in order to avoid injury, overuse, and exacerbation of lymphedema" (p. 2).

Research has shown that some symptoms may be predictors of breast cancer LE (Armer, Radina, Porock, & Culbertson, 2003). These prodromal symptoms include heaviness, swelling, and numbness. Early identification of patients experiencing these symptoms may enable healthcare professionals to target women to refer for early LE evaluation, review precautions, and establish criteria for the use of compression garments.

The NLN Medical Advisory Committee (2004) recommends that people with LE wear a compression garment or compression bandages while traveling by air. Patients are advised to don the compression garment or bandage prior to the flight and remove it once the final destination is reached. People at risk for LE must make a decision about sleeve use with the guidance of their physician. The rationale for compression during airplane travel is that changes in cabin pressure can impact the interstitial pressures in the limb, causing increased swelling (NLN Medical Advisory Committee, 2004). External pressure (i.e., compression) on the limb may decrease the potential of fluid accumulation in the tissue. The lack of activity (i.e., walking) while on an airplane lends itself to edema development because of less muscle pumping to propel the fluid. Therefore, people with or at risk for LE are encouraged to ambulate and/or perform

frequent, simple upper extremity ROM exercises while on an airplane (NLN Medical Advisory Committee, 2004). Additionally, patients need to keep in mind that traveling usually involves carrying or pulling luggage—recognized triggers for LE development. Although no research is documented, considerations should be given as to what precautions should be taken based on the length and mode (i.e., car, train, or bus) of travel.

The risk of infection is another consideration with LE. As explained by Simon and Cody (1992), "Lymphatic impairment favors development of infection due to impaired host response, and the stagnated lymph fluid provides an ideal medium for bacterial growth" (p. 546). *Cellulitis, erysipelas,* and *dermatolymphangioadenitis* are terms often used synonymously for a lymphatic infection (Foldi et al., 2003). Most breast and arm infections are caused by *Staphylococcus aureus,* penicillin-sensitive *Streptococcus,* or fungus (Chikly, 2001). Symptoms include, but are not limited to, redness, warmth, fever, chills, generalized malaise, pain, and edema (Browse et al., 2003; Casley-Smith & Casley-Smith, 1997). Treatment of infection consists of rest, elevation of the affected limb, and oral or IV antibiotics. In some cases, prophylactic antibiotics are prescribed for patients with recurrent infections (Browse et al.). Complete decongestive therapy can decrease the incidence of infection in women who currently have LE (Browse et al.; Casley-Smith & Casley-Smith; Foldi et al.).

Although LE is not life threatening, it does pose a substantial threat to QOL for breast cancer survivors. It can affect relationships with family and friends, ability to perform activities of daily living, and one's body image and self-esteem (Armer et al., 2003). The current literature (or lack thereof) demonstrates the need for research to better understand the true incidence and prevalence of LE, whether preventive interventions are valid, and whether less-invasive lymph node staging will result in long-term decreases in LE. Moreover, a quantification system with universally accepted data is needed.

Radiation Skin Changes

The majority of patients with breast cancer receiving radiation therapy will develop skin toxicity. Skin damage is caused by the effect of radiation on the rapidly dividing cells of the basal layer of the epidermis and the dermis (Williams et al., 1996). Sekine et al. (2000) suggested that sweat gland damage also might play a role. The intensity of side effects depends on the fractionation, total dose, anatomic area, radiation type, and patient characteristics (Perera, Chisela, Stitt, Engel, & Venkatesan, 2005; Poti et al., 2004; Turesson, Nyman, Holmberg, & Oden, 1996). Treatment delays may be required for severe reactions. Acute skin reactions occur during radiation treatment and for as long as six months after therapy. Modern radiotherapy causes less skin toxicity and fewer late complications. However, new radiation techniques treating smaller volumes of tissue with different doses and fractionations recently have gained favor (Baglan et al., 2003; Balfour & Goa, 1997), and long-term data regarding side effects are lacking.

The most commonly identified acute skin changes are erythema, increased pigmentation, pruritus, dry desquamation (peeling), and moist desquamation. Other symptoms include breast heaviness, mild discomfort, and shooting pains. The degree of skin toxicity is variable and is related to concurrent chemotherapy, concurrent tamoxifen use, larger breast size, smoking history, boost or bolus skin fields, treatment of the chest wall, and African American ancestry (Deutsch & Flickinger, 2003; Heggie et al., 2002; Okumura et al., 2003; Wells et al., 2004). Supraclavicular fields can result in skin reactions on the woman's upper back. Transient erythema can occur with the first treatment. More intense erythema and hyperpigmentation generally occur after two to three weeks of treatment (Blackmar, 1997; Knopf & Sun, 2005). Destruction of the basal layer of the skin can result in dry desquamation. Higher doses of radiation can cause moist desquamation characterized by a bright erythema, clear serous exudate, and pain, which usually occurs toward the end of the treatment course. Skin folds within the treatment field (axilla and inframammary crease) are at greater risk for developing skin toxicity because of the movement of skin on skin, warmth, and moisture buildup (Blackmar).

The most commonly cited radiation-related breast symptoms reported in a prospective longitudinal study by Knopf and Sun (2005) were skin changes in 36%–100% of patients, sensation changes in 28%–79%, and breast swelling in 11%–28%. Severity ratings were mild to moderate but higher by the end of the treatment, with gradual improvement over the following three months. One hundred percent of the patients

developed skin changes by week 5 or 6, and the ratings of symptom severity were higher in the final three weeks of treatment yet still rated as mild. Skin irritation was described as red, itchy, and sensitive. However, the sensation of heaviness persisted over the next three months. Studies by Wengstrom, Haggmark, Strander, and Forsberg (2000) and Munro and Potter (1996) have reported similar findings. Study sample sizes were small, thus limiting generalization.

Skin care recommendations vary and are based on individual practice patterns rather than empirically based in many radiation departments. A review of radiation skin care studies from 1967–2001 found that few studies showed improvement in symptoms (Wickline, 2004). Several randomized clinical trials involving patients with breast cancer found trends favoring the use of sucralfate (Maiche, Isokangas, & Grohn, 1994) and mometasone furoate (Bostrom, Lindman, Swartling, Berne, & Bergh, 2001) in preventing radiation skin effects. Aloe vera was found to have a protective effect when higher doses of radiation were used (Olsen et al., 2001). Tegaderm® (3M Health Care, St. Paul, MN) and Vigilon® (C.R. Bard, Inc., Murray Hill, NJ) wound dressings and Biafine® (OrthoNeutrogena, Los Angeles, CA) topical emulsion were found to promote patient comfort (Fisher et al., 2000; Shell, Stanutz, & Grimm, 1986; Strunk & Maher, 1993).

More recently, Heggie et al. (2002) showed that an aqueous cream was useful in reducing dry desquamation and pain. Graham et al. (2004) found that Cavilon™ No Sting Barrier Film (3M Health Care) reduced pruritus and the duration and frequency of moist desquamation in women undergoing chest wall radiation. Miko Enomoto et al. (2005) showed that the use of RayGel™ (ITI Wellness, Green Bay, WI), a combination of glutathione and anthocyanins, promoted patient comfort and protection compared with standard skin care therapies. Table 8-3 lists commonly recommended self-care strategies to promote skin integrity during radiation therapy.

Breast edema, mild hyperpigmentation, fibrosis, and telangiectasia are some of the late side effects that are seen following breast irradiation (Perera et al., 2005; Poti et al., 2004). Acute skin reactions predict the incidence of skin pigmentation and telangiectasia. They are related to boost doses and higher skin doses seen with some newer therapies (Perera et al.; Romestaing et al., 1997). Edema and fibrosis incidence peak at one year after treatment and may resolve in some patients. Severe fibrosis, seen in a small number of patients, is related to older age, clinical tumor size, use of chemotherapy, and high boost dose and may result in patient dissatisfaction with cosmetic outcome (Borger et al., 1994; Taylor et al., 1995). Breast edema is more commonly seen in women with ALND. Breast erythema in an edematous breast following radiation must be viewed as a possible infection, and inflammatory breast cancer recurrence must be included in the differential diagnosis. However, a syndrome of lymphangitis or cellulitis of the breast has been recognized and was described previously. In addition, the phenomenon of

Table 8-3. Skin Care Instructions for Patients Undergoing Breast Irradiation	
Precautions	**Skin Care**
Avoid temperature extremes in the treatment field.	Do not use hot water bottles, hot soaks, heating pads, or ice packs in the area of treatment. Do not expose treatment field to cold wind or intense sunlight. Skin in the area will remain sun-sensitive for years to come. Do not take cold or hot baths or use a sauna. Lukewarm water is preferred.
Avoid trauma to the skin in the treatment field.	Do not scrub the skin. Pat skin dry. Use mild soap, and take care to avoid rubbing off any skin markings. Wear soft, loose, cotton clothing. Do not scratch or rub skin in the treatment area. Do not shave in the treatment area. Hair loss may be permanent.
Avoid application of topical agents to skin in the treatment field.	Do not apply powder, deodorant, perfume, or lotions to the treatment area. Cornstarch may be used to control itching. Use only radiation therapy–approved lotions or creams. Apply two hours prior to treatment.

Note. Based on information from National Cancer Institute, 2005.

radiation recall—namely, erythema of the skin in the treatment field—can occur with the administration of chemotherapy at a later time.

Patient education regarding expected side effects from breast irradiation can promote comfort, reduce severity of reactions, and allay anxiety. Reinforcement that acute skin reactions will heal is extremely important for patients experiencing moist desquamation. Long-term cosmetic changes are more difficult to predict and generally are not modifiable by the patient and type of skin care used. As radiation therapy techniques evolve, cutaneous and cosmetic outcomes may become more or less apparent. Patients should be aware of late changes that they should report to their healthcare provider, namely breast erythema, breast swelling, and changes noticed during self-exam. Prompt evaluation in most cases can alleviate patient concerns regarding recurrence of their breast cancer or enable timely treatment.

Chemotherapy-Induced Nausea and Vomiting

Despite medical advances in the treatment of chemotherapy-induced nausea and vomiting (CINV), nausea and emesis continue to be a major concern for women undergoing moderately and highly emetic chemotherapy for breast cancer. Fear of vomiting is the most concerning symptom for patients undergoing chemotherapy. CINV can lead to poor QOL, electrolyte imbalances, dehydration, poor nutrition, and diminished ability to work (Wickham, 2004).

The most commonly used drugs to treat breast cancer in the adjuvant setting are a combination of two or more of the following medications: cyclophosphamide (Cytoxan®, Bristol-Myers Squibb Co., Princeton, NJ), methotrexate (Rheumatrex®, Trexall™, Barr Laboratories, Pomona, NY),

5-fluorouracil, paclitaxel (Taxol®, Bristol-Myers Squibb Co.), docetaxel (Taxotere®, Sanofi-Aventis U.S., Bridgewater, NJ), doxorubicin (Adriamycin®, Bedford Laboratories, Bedford, OH), and epirubicin (Ellence®, Pfizer Inc.). Cyclophosphamide, methotrexate, 5-fluorouracil, and doxorubicin are considered moderately emetic at the doses commonly used. Moderately emetic chemotherapy is defined as chemotherapy that produces vomiting in 30%–60% of patients who do not receive effective nausea and vomiting treatment (NCCN, 2006). Doxorubicin or epirubicin in combination with cyclophosphamide is considered highly emetic, whereby at least 90% of patients will develop CINV without treatment (NCCN, 2006).

The causal mechanisms of nausea and vomiting are multifactorial. Patients frequently use the terms *queasiness, upset stomach,* and *throwing up* to describe their symptoms. CINV can be categorized as anticipatory, acute, delayed, or refractory (see Table 8-4). Each process seems to be caused by different mechanisms, as drugs designed to manage acute CINV are not as effective in managing the other types of CINV. The primary mediators of acute nausea and vomiting result from direct or indirect stimulation of the chemoreceptor trigger zone and vomiting center, or emetic zone. Olfactory, emotional, and peripheral stimuli from the gastrointestinal tract also can affect the development of nausea and trigger emesis. Key brain and gastrointestinal receptors involved in this process are serotonin ($5HT_3$), dopamine, and neurokinin (NK-1) (Bender et al., 2002; Gralla et al., 1999). Other conditions that can cause nausea in the breast cancer population include concurrent use of opiates or antibiotics, constipation, hypercalcemia, progressive disease, brain metastasis, hyperglycemia, hyponatremia, and renal or hepatic failure (Wickham, 2004).

Table 8-4. Definitions of Chemotherapy-Induced Nausea and Vomiting (CINV)	
Type of CINV	**Definition**
Anticipatory	Occurs day(s) before the administration of chemotherapy and is likely a conditioned response; more common in patients who had poorly controlled CINV. Nausea is more common than vomiting.
Acute	Occurs within the first minutes to first 24 hours after drug administration; peak incidence of vomiting at 5–6 hours after dose
Delayed	Occurs 24 hours after chemotherapy, peaking at 48–72 hours after administration; can last as long as 6–7 days
Breakthrough	Emesis that is unresponsive to medication and may require the addition of less commonly used or higher-level antiemetics to control symptoms
Refractory	Emesis that occurs during subsequent treatment cycles having failed prophylactic and rescue medications

Note. Based on information from Eckert, 2001; National Comprehensive Cancer Network, 2006.

Patient-related risk factors for CINV include female gender, history of vomiting with prior exposure to chemotherapy, poor performance status, emetogenicity of the drugs, younger age, preexisting fatigue, low level of social functioning, low alcohol consumption, a history of anxiety, motion sickness, and nausea, and vomiting during pregnancy (Dibble, Israel, Nussey, Casey, & Luce, 2003; Goodman, 1997). A study by Roscoe et al. (2004) showed that patient expectation of nausea is a strong predictor of subsequent nausea but not emesis. However, this observation is not documented as a risk factor in antiemetic guidelines or taken into account when prescribing medications. An interesting finding by Dibble et al. (2003) was that women with a larger body mass index had worse CINV than their smaller counterparts. This may be associated with underdosing of antiemetics. African American women also seem to be at greater risk, suggesting genetic differences in drug metabolism.

Acute nausea and acute emesis in patients undergoing moderately emetic chemotherapy for breast cancer continued to be problematic in studies by Dibble, Casey, Nussey, Israel, and Luce (2004) and Grunberg et al. (2004). The prevalence of delayed nausea was high, as well. Since then, the addition of aprepitant (Emend®, Merck and Co., Inc., Whitehouse Station, NJ), an NK-1 receptor antagonist, to treatment guidelines has led to improvements in the management of both acute and delayed nausea and vomiting, but there is still room for improvement (Grunberg et al.; Herrstedt et al., 2005; Warr et al., 2005). Other commonly used and frequently effective 5HT$_3$ antagonists include ondansetron (Zofran®, GlaxoSmithKline, Research Triangle Park, NC), granisetron (Kytril®, Roche Laboratories Inc., Nutley, NJ), and dolasetron (Anzemet®, Sanofi-Aventis U.S.).

A consensus panel developed and recently revised a decision tree to assist clinicians in CINV management, which is available online at www.nccn.org/professionals/physician_gls/PDF/antiemesis.pdf (NCCN, 2006) (see Figure 8-6). Most chemotherapy protocols for breast cancer use highly and moderately emetic drugs given in combination. Practitioners must be cognizant that the risk for emesis with these protocols extends for at least four days and should prescribe antiemetics accordingly. If nausea or vomiting occurs after the first cycle of chemotherapy, a change in antiemetic protocol is recommended. For breakthrough nausea, a change in 5HT$_3$ receptor antagonist is suggested, with the addition of one of the following medications: prochlorperazine (Compazine®, GlaxoSmithKline), metoclopramide (Reglan®, Wyeth Pharmaceuticals) with or without diphenhydramine (Benadryl®, Pfizer Inc.), lorazepam, haloperidol (Haldol®, Ortho-McNeil Pharmaceutical, Inc., Raritan, NJ), dronabinol (Marinol®, Solvay Pharmaceuticals, Inc., Marietta, GA), dexamethasone (Decadron®, Merck and Co., Inc.), promethazine (Phenergan®, Wyeth Pharmaceuticals), or olanzapine (Zyprexa®, Eli Lilly and Co., Indianapolis, IN). For patients who develop indigestion during treatment, the addition of antacids (H$_2$ blockers and proton pump inhibitors) can be beneficial (NCCN, 2006).

According to experts, as many as 1 in 3 patients undergoing chemotherapy experiences anticipatory nausea, and 1 in 10 has anticipatory emesis. This is thought to be a conditioned response. Sensory stimuli associated with chemotherapy administration are the triggers. After repeated exposures, any associated stimuli can elicit the symptoms (King, 1997). The most significant risk factors for anticipatory emesis appear to be the occurrence, magnitude, and duration of CINV experienced. Treatment for patients who develop anticipatory emesis includes behavioral therapy such as relaxation, guided imagery, hypnosis, systematic desensitization, and music therapy. Antianxiety medications the night prior to the next chemotherapy cycle and on the morning of treatment may be useful. Antinausea medications also may be started prior to chemotherapy. Behavioral interventions can assist patients in gaining a sense of control over their symptoms, are easy to use, and can be self-administered. Additional nonpharmacologic interventions under study include acupuncture, foot massage, progressive muscle relaxation, acupressure, and music therapy. Eckert (2001) and Bender et al. (2002) provide a thorough overview of these techniques. Most of these interventions, however, are based on pilot studies with small sample sizes.

Figure 8-6. Decision Tree for the Treatment of Chemotherapy-Related Nausea and Vomiting (Levels 3–5)

NCCN® Practice Guidelines in Oncology – v.2.2006

Antiemesis

Guidelines Index
Antiemesis Table of Contents
MS, References

HIGH EMETIC RISK CHEMOTHERAPY - EMESIS PREVENTION[b,c,d]

HIGH[a] →

- Start before chemotherapy[b,c,d]
  - Aprepitant[e] 125 mg PO day 1, 80 mg PO daily days 2-3
  - Dexamethasone 12 mg PO or IV day 1, 8 mg PO or IV daily days 2-4
    and
  - 5-HT3 antagonist:[f]
    Ondansetron 16-24 mg PO or 8-12 mg (maximum 32 mg) IV day 1
    or
    Granisetron 2 mg PO or 1 mg PO bid or 0.01 mg/kg (maximum 1 mg) IV day 1
    or
    Dolasetron 100 mg PO or 1.8 mg/kg IV or 100 mg IV day 1
    or
    Palonosetron 0.25 mg IV day 1[e]
    and
  - ± Lorazepam 0.5-2 mg PO or IV or sublingual either every 4 or every 6 h days 1-4

→ See Breakthrough Treatment (AE-5)

See Principles of Emesis Control (AE-1)

[a]Data for post-cisplatin (> 50 mg/m^2) emesis prevention are category 1, others are category 2A.
[b]Antiemetic regimens should be chosen based on emetogenic potential of the chemotherapy regimen.
[c]Lowest fully efficacious dose.
[d]See Principles for Managing Multi-day Emetogenic Chemotherapy Regimens (AE-A).
[e]See New Antiemetic Agents for Treating Nausea and Vomiting (AE-B).
[f]Order of listed antiemetics does not reflect preference.

Note: All recommendations are category 2A unless otherwise indicated.
Clinical Trials: NCCN believes that the best management of any cancer patient is in a clinical trial. Participation in clinical trials is especially encouraged.

 AE-2

(Continued on next page)

Figure 8-6. Decision Tree for the Treatment of Chemotherapy-Related Nausea and Vomiting (Levels 3–5) *(Continued)*

NCCN® Practice Guidelines in Oncology – v.2.2006 | Antiemesis

MODERATE EMETIC RISK CHEMOTHERAPY - EMESIS PREVENTION[b,c,d]

Day 1

- Start before chemotherapy[b,c,d]
  ‣ Aprepitant 125 mg PO in select patients[e,h]
  ‣ Dexamethasone 12 mg PO or IV
  and
  ‣ 5-HT3 antagonist:[f]
    Palonosetron 0.25 mg IV[e] (category 1)
    or
    Ondansetron 16-24 mg PO or 8-12 mg (maximum 32 mg) IV (category 1)
    or
    Granisetron 1-2 mg PO or 1 mg PO bid (category 1) or 0.01 mg/kg (maximum 1 mg) IV
    or
    Dolasetron 100 mg PO or 1.8 mg/kg or 100 mg IV
  and
  ‣ ± Lorazepam 0.5-2 mg PO or IV or sublingual either every 4 or every 6 h

MODERATE[g] →

Days 2-4

- ‣ Aprepitant 80 mg PO days 2-3 if used on Day 1[e]
  and
  ‣ Dexamethasone 8 mg PO or IV daily
  ‣ ± Lorazepam 0.5-2 mg PO or IV or sublingual either every 4 or every 6 h
  or
  ‣ Dexamethasone 8 mg PO or IV daily or 4 mg PO or IV bid (preferred)
  or
  ‣ 5-HT3 antagonist:[f]
    Ondansetron 8 mg PO bid or 16 mg PO daily or 8 mg (maximum 32 mg) IV
    or
    Granisetron 1-2 mg PO daily or 1 mg PO bid or 0.01 mg/kg (maximum 1 mg) IV
    or
    Dolasetron 100 mg PO daily or 1.8 mg/kg IV or 100 mg IV
    or
    Metoclopramide 0.5 mg/kg PO or IV every 6 h or 20 mg PO 4 times daily ± Diphenhydramine 25-50 mg PO or IV either every 4 or every 6 h prn

→ See Breakthrough Treatment (AE-5)

---

[b]Antiemetic regimens should be chosen based on emetogenic potential of the chemotherapy regimen.
[c]Lowest fully efficacious dose.
[d]See Principles for Managing Multi-day Emetogenic Chemotherapy Regimens (AE-A).
[e]See New Antiemetic Agents for Treating Nausea and Vomiting (AE-B).
[f]Order of listed antiemetics does not reflect preference.

[g]Data for post-carboplatin ≥ 300 mg/m², cyclophosphamide ≥ 600-1000 mg/m², doxorubicin ≥ 50 mg/m² emesis prevention are category 1.
[h]Aprepitant should be added for patients receiving the combination of an anthracycline and cyclophosphamide and select patients receiving other chemotherapies of moderate emetic risk (for example, carboplatin, cisplatin, doxorubicin, epirubicin, ifosfamide, irinotecan or methotrexate).

Note: All recommendations are category 2A unless otherwise indicated.
Clinical Trials: NCCN believes that the best management of any cancer patient is in a clinical trial. Participation in clinical trials is especially encouraged.

AE-3

(Continued on next page)

Figure 8-6. Decision Tree for the Treatment of Chemotherapy-Related Nausea and Vomiting (Levels 3–5) *(Continued)*

NCCN Practice Guidelines in Oncology – v.2.2006

Antiemesis

Guidelines Index
Antiemesis Table of Contents
MS, References

BREAKTHROUGH TREATMENT FOR CHEMOTHERAPY INDUCED NAUSEA/VOMITING[c,d,i]

No nausea/emesis ⟶ No change in antiemetic regimen

Any nausea/emesis ⟶

- General principle of breakthrough treatment is to give an additional agent from a different drug class
  - ▸ Prochlorperazine 25 mg supp pr every 12 h or 10 mg PO or IV every 4 or every 6 h or 15 mg Spansule PO every 8 or every 12 h
    or
  - ▸ Metoclopramide 20-40 mg PO either every 4 or every 6 h or 1-2 mg/kg IV either every 3 or every 4 h ± Diphenhydramine 25-50 mg PO or IV either every 4 or every 6 h
    or
  - ▸ Lorazepam 0.5-2 mg PO either every 4 or every 6 h
    or
  - ▸ Ondansetron 16 mg PO or 8 mg IV daily
    or
  - ▸ Granisetron 1-2 mg PO daily or 1 mg PO bid or 0.01 mg/kg (maximum 1 mg) IV
    or
  - ▸ Dolasetron 100 mg PO daily or 1.8 mg/kg IV or 100 mg IV
    or
  - ▸ Haloperidol 1-2 mg PO q 4-6 h or 1-3 mg IV either every 4 or every 6 h
    or
  - ▸ Dronabinol 5-10 mg PO either every 3 or every 6 h
    or
  - ▸ Dexamethasone 12 mg PO or IV daily, if not previously given
    or
  - ▸ Olanzapine 2.5-5 mg PO bid prn (category 2B)[j]
    or
  - ▸ Promethazine 12.5-25 mg PO or IV every 4 h

RESPONSE TO BREAKTHROUGH ANTIEMETIC TREATMENT

SUBSEQUENT CYCLES

Nausea and emesis controlled ⟶ Continue breakthrough medications, on a schedule, not prn

Nausea and/or emesis uncontrolled ⟶ Consider changing antiemetic therapy to higher-level primary treatment

See Principles of Emesis Control (AE-1)

[c] Lowest fully efficacious dose.
[d] See Principles for Managing Multi-day Emetogenic Chemotherapy Regimens (AE-A).
[i] See Principles of Managing Breakthrough Treatment (AE-C).
[j] See blackbox warning/label indication regarding type II diabetes and hyperglycemia.

Note: All recommendations are category 2A unless otherwise indicated.
Clinical Trials: NCCN believes that the best management of any cancer patient is in a clinical trial. Participation in clinical trials is especially encouraged.

Version 2.2006, 04-25-06 © 2006 National Comprehensive Cancer Network, Inc. All rights reserved. These guidelines and this illustration may not be reproduced in any form without the express written permission of NCCN.

AE-5

As another intervention strategy to counteract nausea, patients often are encouraged to use dietary measures that they found helpful during pregnancy, illness, or stressful periods. Altering food preparation and freezing meals for later can help to avoid exposure to strong odors during cooking at times of heightened sensitivity. Other helpful hints include eating smaller, more frequent meals; keeping the mouth clean and moist; drinking a glass of wine with meals; eating cold or room-temperature foods, which give off fewer odors than hot foods; eating sour foods; eating crackers, breadsticks, and toast; sitting up while eating; and sucking on hard candies such as peppermints or lemon drops. Most clinicians recommend that patients avoid their favorite foods on the day of chemotherapy and during periods of potential nausea so that they do not develop food aversions. Other foods to avoid include fatty foods, which delay gastric emptying, and spicy, salty, and sweet foods (Wickham, 2004). Herbal teas such as peppermint, cinnamon, or chamomile may help to soothe dyspepsia as well as lessen nausea and vomiting (Deng, Cassileth, & Yeung, 2004). Currently, NCCAM (2003a) is conducting a randomized, double-blind, placebo-controlled study evaluating the use of ginger in controlling CINV.

In the present era of cost containment, the use of expensive antiemetics as first-line therapy has been slow to gain acceptance. Insurance coverage of outpatient oral medications remains variable, although this may change with the implementation of the Medicare drug benefit plan and the recent revision of the NCCN antiemetic guidelines. Letters of medical necessity may be needed to petition insurance carriers to authorize their use. Because of the profound impact of CINV on the quality of life of patients with breast cancer, research into more gender-effective antiemetics, complementary and behavioral adjunct measures, and the development of chemoprotective agents is essential. Patients should report new symptoms to their healthcare provider so that effective treatment can be utilized and planned for later treatments. Healthcare providers must be aware of the significant impact that unrecognized delayed CINV has on their patients and act proactively.

Cancer-Related Fatigue

Cancer-related fatigue (CRF) is the most distressing symptom experienced by patients with cancer, surpassing that of nausea and vomiting (Vogelzang et al., 1997). CRF occurs in 80%–100% of patients receiving chemotherapy (Jacobsen et al., 1999). Trends toward the use of regimens with higher doses and dose densities in patients receiving breast cancer chemotherapy may result in an increase in incidence. Fatigue also is a commonly reported and distressing side effect of radiation therapy (Knopf & Sun, 2005; Magnan & Mood, 2003; Munro & Potter, 1996). Furthermore, 30%–75% of cancer survivors report experiencing fatigue months to years after the end of treatment (Andrykowski, Curran, & Lightner, 1998; Bower et al., 2000; Broeckel, Jacobsen, Horton, Balducci, & Lyman, 1998; Gelinas & Fillion, 2004).

The definition of CRF is "a persistent subjective sense of tiredness related to cancer or its treatment that interferes with usual functioning" (NCCN, 2005b, p. 5). CRF is different from fatigue in healthy individuals and has been found to adversely affect the QOL of cancer survivors (Curt et al., 2000). The cause of CRF is multifactorial and has physical, psychological, and situational elements (Curt et al.). It has been associated with insomnia, sleep disturbances, hot flashes, and pain, suggesting a symptom cluster effect (Beck, Dudley, & Barsevick, 2005). For instance, a study by Beck et al. showed that relieving pain was an important strategy in improving sleep and reducing fatigue.

NCCN (2005b) published guidelines for the screening, assessment, and management of CRF. These guidelines are available free of charge through the American Cancer Society. The consensus is that all patients with cancer should be screened for CRF at their initial visit and at regular intervals thereafter. Although many sophisticated assessment tools exist, most clinicians assess fatigue by using a 0–10 scale or by allowing patients to categorize it as mild, moderate, or severe. If mild fatigue is identified at the initial visit, it should be monitored for increase in severity at follow-up visits. This also provides a teachable moment to educate patients about CRF and known patterns of fatigue development during and after treatment. This can help to prevent patients from assuming that increasing fatigue indicates disease progression. Self-care interventions that might be useful for women include practicing energy conservation, pacing activities, requesting help with household tasks, getting daily exercise, using distraction, taking short naps, eating balanced meals, and managing stress (Barsevick, Whitmer, Sweeney, & Nail, 2002; NCCN, 2003). Dietary counseling also may be useful if nutritional deficiencies are contributory.

Any patient experiencing moderate or severe fatigue should receive a more thorough evaluation. Clinical conditions that can contribute to CRF are pain, emotional distress, sleep disturbances, anemia, nutritional deficiencies, decreased physical activity levels, and comorbidities such as heart disease, hypothyroidism, and electrolyte imbalances. If fatigue remains unrelieved after implementing interventions directed at these conditions, other causes should be considered (Berger et al., 2003; Mock & Olsen, 2003; Nail, 2002).

The most common cause of CRF is anemia. It can occur as a result of bone marrow suppression from treatment, poor dietary intake, or disease progression. The symptoms of mild anemia can easily go unrecognized. However, symptoms of severe anemia, such as shortness of breath, weakness, tachycardia, and decreased exercise and activity tolerance, generally are easier to recognize.

Magnan and Mood (2003) found that women who experienced CRF while undergoing radiation therapy developed it during the second week of treatment, and it worsened by the fifth week and resolved within two weeks following the end of therapy. Earlier onset may occur because of preexisting treatment such as recent surgery or chemotherapy, lower hemoglobin levels, and symptom and mood distress. Most studies of radiation therapy for breast cancer have found a return to baseline level by three months after treatment (Greenberg, Sawicka, Eisenthal, & Ross, 1992; Irvine, Vincent, Graydon, Bubela, & Thompson, 1994).

Nonpharmacologic measures to treat CRF include education and coping strategies as previously described. Of all the coping strategies, exercise appears to be the most credible (Ahlberg, Ekman, Gaston-Johansson, & Mock, 2003; Stricker, Drake, Hoyer, & Mock, 2004). Mock et al. (2001) evaluated the effectiveness of a walking program in adult patients with breast cancer undergoing radiation treatment or chemotherapy and found that women experienced lower levels of fatigue, increased ability to perform daily tasks, less psychological distress, and greater QOL while participating in exercise intervention. This walking program was 20–30 minutes in length, occurred five to six times a week, and was moderately intensive, causing an increase in resting heart rate. It is important for patients to know how to balance rest and activity to prevent deconditioning.

The pharmacologic management of CRF includes medication to correct anemia in patients with a hemoglobin level lower than 11 g/dl. If the anemia is cancer therapy–related, epoetin alfa (Epogen®, Amgen Inc., Thousand Oaks, CA; Procrit®, Ortho Biotech, Bridgewater, NJ), darbepoetin alfa (Aranesp®, Amgen Inc.), or transfusion can be recommended depending on how rapidly a correction is needed. Several randomized clinical trials have shown a benefit in QOL and functional status with this drug therapy (Boccia et al., 2006; Cella, Dobrez, & Glaspy, 2003; Littlewood et al, 2001; Waltzman et al., 2005). A recent report of increased mortality and thrombotic events in patients with cancer treated with these drugs requires further investigation and caution (Bohlius et al., 2006). Other medications that may help to relieve fatigue include thyroid replacement hormone for women with hypothyroidism, iron supplementation for those experiencing iron deficiency anemia, and vitamin therapy, psychostimulants (i.e., modafinil, dextroamphetamine), corticosteroids, and antidepressants (Burks, 2001; Mock, 2001). A randomized clinical trial evaluating the use of coenzyme Q10 in relieving fatigue and depression in patients with breast cancer who are undergoing chemotherapy currently is enrolling patients (National Cancer Institute, 2004).

Persistent CRF at the completion of breast cancer treatment has a negative impact on patients' return to normal functioning. It is more common in women who have undergone chemotherapy and has been found to last for as long as two years following treatment (Andrykowski et al., 1998; Bower et al., 2000; Lindley, Vasa, Sawyer, & Winer, 1998). Gelinas and Fillion (2004) found that in a group of women who had completed radiation therapy 3–24 months prior, menopausal symptoms and pain, as well as stress, were related to persistent fatigue. Woo, Dibble, Piper, Keating, and Weiss (1998) reported that the younger the woman with breast cancer, the more likely she was to perceive cancer stressors in her life, and the more fatigued she was, the less likely she was to use active coping skills.

Clearly, the impact of CRF is significant for women whose roles in society are those of caretaker, wife, mother, coworker, and employer. Continued research into this side effect of treatment is imperative. Healthcare providers should focus on instituting prompt interventions when this side effect is noted. Early communication to both patients and their significant others that this problem may occur is essential to enable women to prepare for it and for their families to accept it as a known side effect. Too often, women are expected by their loved ones to get on with their lives following treatment and to assume the roles they had before cancer therapy. This can be a difficult expectation for women experiencing prolonged CRF.

Cognitive Dysfunction

The incidence of "chemo brain" or "chemo fog" in women who are undergoing breast cancer chemotherapy is variable, ranging from 16% to 50% (Tannock, Ahles, Ganz, & van Dam, 2004). Cognitive defects have been observed up to 10 years following treatment (Ahles et al., 2002). Cognitive dysfunction adversely affects patients' QOL and may reduce their ability to make the transition back into a "normal" life after treatment. Changes are subtle and cross a variety of cognitive domains, including verbal memory, nonverbal memory, information processing speed, multitasking, and visuospatial functioning (Bender, Paraska, Seirika, Ryan, & Berga, 2001). Of note, many women demonstrate impaired cognitive functioning before the initiation of adjuvant chemotherapy, thus making a baseline assessment imperative when studying cognitive dysfunction (Wefel, Lenzi, Theriault, Davis, & Meyers, 2004).

Causes of cancer treatment–related cognitive dysfunction have yet to be fully identified. It is hypothesized that direct injury to the cerebral gray and white matter occurs with chemotherapy, that microvascular injury may occur, and that immune-mediated inflammatory responses may predispose some patients to develop cognitive dysfunction (Saykin, Ahles, & McDonald, 2003; Tuxen & Werner, 1994). An additional risk factor may be a genetic predisposition caused by a variant of the *apolipoprotein E* gene, which has been associated with an increased risk of early

Alzheimer disease and preclinical cognitive decline (Ahles et al., 2003).

Comparison of the research studies documenting the incidence of cognitive dysfunction in patients with breast cancer has been limited because of differences in the assessment tools, definitions of dysfunction, types of chemotherapy agents used, menopausal status, and frequency of evaluation; the use of cross-sectional design; and the lack of baseline assessments in some studies. However, a review of studies on cognitive dysfunction in patients receiving chemotherapy showed a trend toward greater dysfunction when compared to controls (Phillips & Bernhard, 2003).

Several longitudinal studies have shown that the dose and type of chemotherapy may influence cognitive impairment, showing a worse effect in higher-dose protocols (van Dam et al., 1998) and in those regimens that include cyclophosphamide compared to doxorubin (Schagen et al., 2002). No data are available on the use of taxanes at this point (Rugo & Ahles, 2003). Concurrent medications such as steroids and analgesics during treatment may have an additive effect (Shilling, Jenkins, Morris, Deutsch, & Bloomfield, 2005). Wefel, Lenzi, Theriault, Buzdar, et al. (2004) found that women who had more invasive surgery, were menopausal, and had not previously used hormone replacement therapy appeared to be more likely to present with greater cognitive impairment. Age, IQ, and pretest levels of cognitive dysfunction must be taken into consideration. Normal age-related changes at the beginning of chemotherapy may cause older patients to have less capacity to overcome the cognitive effects of chemotherapy. Most studies have shown an associated increase in levels of fatigue and endocrine symptoms in patients experiencing cognitive dysfunction. Patients who indicated that they were experiencing cognitive problems were more likely to have emotional distress related to their symptoms than women who were found to have limitations noted on sequential evaluation only (Shilling et al.).

Because of the very detailed analysis of neurocognitive testing, depression and anxiety can be separated as causes of affective distress. The addition of tamoxifen to chemotherapy regimens showed a worsening of cognitive dysfunction in a study by Castellon et al. (2004). A longitudinal study of patients with anemia associated with chemotherapy administration showed increases in fatigue and cognitive dysfunction in control subjects. Those patients who received epoetin alfa prior to the beginning of chemotherapy and weekly thereafter were found to experience fewer changes in hemoglobin levels, improved energy levels, improved overall QOL, and less deterioration in cognitive function than controls (Shilling et al., 2005). However, no difference in cognitive function was noted among patients at six months after completion of chemotherapy. Epoetin alfa is believed to have neuroprotective effects (O'Shaughnessy et al., 2005; Shilling et al.). A study by Wefel Lenzi, Theriault, Buzdar, et al. (2004) found that 61% of patients with breast cancer experienced a change in attention, learning, and pro-

cessing speed, but at the end of one year, half of the patients had improved in function and most of the people affected had been able to return to work.

A study of raloxifene (Evista®, Eli Lilly and Co.) for osteoporosis prevention found a trend toward lower declines in verbal memory and attention in the women taking the medication as a secondary end point of a study in healthy women. This may hold promise for patients with breast cancer in the future (Yaffe et al., 2001). However, its use should be discouraged in women who have received hormonal therapy, specifically tamoxifen and aromatase inhibitors, as part of their treatment. In the QOL portion of the randomized trial comparing letrozole (Femara®, Novartis Pharmaceuticals Corp., East Hanover, NJ) to megestrol acetate (Megace®, Bristol-Myers Squibb Co.) in women with advanced breast cancer, patients taking letrozole experienced improvement in subjective cognitive function (Weinfurt, Wait, Boyko, & Schulman, 1998). Other medications that may have an impact on improving cognitive function or preventing cognitive decline include cholinesterase inhibitors and aminobutyric acid derivatives (Sherwin, 2000).

Interventions to assist patients in overcoming cognitive dysfunction continue to be explored. Barton and Loprinzi (2002) have outlined two interventional approaches for chemotherapy-induced cognitive changes that include behavioral and pharmacologic interventions. Ferguson and Ahles (2003) formulated an intervention that involved stress management techniques for long-term survivors of breast cancer who continued to experience dysfunction. Medications that are being explored to counteract this side effect include methylphenidate, herbs such as ginkgo biloba and ginseng, NSAIDs, and vitamins (Rugo & Ahles, 2003). Currently, the National Cancer Institute (2002) is sponsoring a randomized clinical trial evaluating the use of the drug EGb761 in the prevention of cognitive dysfunction in patients with breast cancer undergoing chemotherapy.

Self-care strategies that often are recommended to patients to improve memory include avoiding distraction, asking people to repeat information, practicing activities like crossword puzzles, writing down events in daily organizers, keeping a journal, posting reminders for themselves, managing stress, getting enough sleep, exercising regularly, maintaining routines, and using mnemonic devices (Mayo Foundation for Medical Education and Research, 2004). Researchers are studying brain function in patients at baseline and during chemotherapy to assess brain changes using magnetic resonance imaging and positron-emission tomography scanning (Saykin et al., 2003). Other research areas in cognitive dysfunction include the development of easier tools to assess and monitor decline and to identify patients at risk with the goal of discovering ways to prevent its development.

Healthcare providers must prepare patients with breast cancer for this potential side effect at the onset of therapy. Women and their families must be aware so that adjustments to their lives can be anticipated because of the effects on multiple domains. Special precautions may be needed for people with preexisting cognitive dysfunction.

Menopausal Effects of Breast Cancer Treatment

Management of estrogen deficiency states in breast cancer survivors is complicated by concerns related to the use of hormone replacement therapy to counteract the two most prevalent hormone-related side effects of adjuvant therapy—hot flashes and bone loss. Hot flashes are problematic in breast cancer survivors because many women are diagnosed around the time of natural menopause, and acute menopause may result from treatment. In addition, the expanding indications for the use of chemotherapy and increased use of antiestrogen agents have resulted in more breast cancer survivors being at risk for menopausal symptom development. Other risk factors found to have an impact on hot flashes in healthy women include smoking, higher body mass index, lack of exercise, African American ancestry, and lower socioeconomic status (Avis et al., 2001; Schwingl, Hulka, & Harlow, 1994; Whiteman et al., 2003).

Hot Flashes

Hot flashes have been defined as sudden episodes of flushing, sweating, and a sensation of heat often preceded or followed by chills (Kronenberg, 1990) and are estimated to occur in 65% of breast cancer survivors (Carpenter et al., 1998; Couzi, Helzlsouer, & Fetting, 1995). The physiology of hot flashes (or flushes) is associated with reduced hormone levels that are believed to affect the thermoregulatory system of the body, resulting in the sensation of heat (Stearns & Hayes, 2002). Hot flashes have become recognized as a frequent, severe, and bothersome side effect among survivors (Carpenter, Johnson, Wagner, & Andrykowski, 2005). Women who discontinue hormone replacement therapy at the time of diagnosis are more likely to experience hot flashes if they had them in the past or were having them at the time of discontinuation of therapy (Hammar et al., 1999). The effects of chemotherapy on the ovaries vary depending on age, dose, and type of chemotherapy or hormonal therapy. Younger women are better able to tolerate higher doses of chemotherapy and are less likely to undergo permanent menopause (Bines, Oleske, & Cobleigh, 1996). However, younger premenopausal women have more hot flashes during endocrine therapy than older postmenopausal women. As many as 4% of breast cancer survivors discontinue tamoxifen prior to the five-year recommended interval because of the intolerance of hot flashes (Morales et al., 2004).

Carpenter et al. (2002) compared healthy controls to breast cancer survivors and found that survivors experienced greater hot flash severity and bother and had more daily hot flashes with a longer duration of symptoms compared to healthy controls. Emotional factors were more commonly noted in breast cancer survivors, and hot flashes caused greater interference with daily activities and QOL—affecting sleep, concentration, mood, and sexuality. They found that when comparing healthy women to breast cancer survivors, the menopause experience for breast cancer survivors was significantly different than the natural menopause experience. The most common self-care behaviors used by breast cancer survivors were fanning, removing clothing, and moving to a cooler environment. In addition, exercise, vitamin therapy, and diet were used to ameliorate symptoms, although these interventions lack empirical evidence supporting their use.

Interventions to manage hot flashes can be categorized as pharmacologic and nonpharmacologic. Treatment should match the severity of the symptoms reported by the patient. Mild to moderate hot flashes that do not seem to interfere with sleep patterns or the ability to work can be managed with behavioral and nonprescription methods. Vitamin E 400–800 IU was tested in a randomized, placebo-controlled clinical trial and was found to decrease hot flash frequency and severity by 30% without toxicity (Barton et al., 1998). In addition, the use of measures to keep cool may be useful, such as dressing in cotton layers, using fans, or drinking cold drinks. Avoidance of potential triggers such as alcohol and spicy foods also may be helpful. Stress management using paced respiration and relaxation techniques also has been shown to be beneficial (Carpenter et al., 2002).

For women with moderate to severe hot flashes that have a greater impact on their QOL, stronger or additional interventions may be necessary. Several selective serotonin and norepinephrine reuptake inhibitors and antidepressant medications have been tested in clinical trials and found to be effective in reducing hot flashes in breast cancer survivors. They include venlafaxine (Effexor XR®, Wyeth Pharmaceuticals), paroxetine (Paxil®, GlaxoSmithKline) and fluoxetine (Prozac®, Eli Lilly and Co.), citalopram (Celexa®, Forest Pharmaceuticals, Inc., St. Louis, MO), and gabapentin (Neurontin) (Boekhout, Beijnen, & Schellens, 2006; Carpenter, 2005; Loprinzi et al., 2000; Loprinzi, Barton, et al., 2002; Loprinzi, Sloan, et al., 2002; Stearns & Loprinzi, 2003; Stearns et al., 2005). Transdermal clonidine (Catapres®, Boehringer Ingelheim Pharmaceuticals, Inc., Ridgefield, CT) also has been shown to moderately reduce hot flashes compared to placebo (Goldberg et al., 1994). Doses may need to be titrated. Side effects can be problematic and decrease compliance.

For those women whose hot flashes continue to alter QOL or for those who are unable to tolerate the side effects of medications used to control symptoms, hormone replacement therapy can be considered. It is essential that breast cancer survivors be provided with an adequate explanation of the possible risks and benefits, as there is a potential for increased risk of breast cancer recurrence (von Schoultz & Rutqvist, 2005). Hormonal medications that have been found to be useful include traditional hormone replacement therapy, megestrol acetate, and medroxyprogesterone acetate (known as MPA) (Bertelli et al., 2002; Pritchard, 2001).

Complementary products that have undergone clinical trial evaluation and were found not to be better than placebo include soy, red clover, dong quai, evening primrose oil, kava kava, and Chinese herbs (Kronenberg & Fugh-Berman, 2002). Pilot studies on behavioral interventions such as paced respiration, relaxation techniques, exercise, and acupuncture have been encouraging (Ganz et al., 2000; Wyon, Wijma, Nedstrand, & Hammar, 2004). Currently the NCCAM (2004a, 2004b, 2005) is studying hypnosis, hydrotherapy, and acupuncture in the treatment of menopausal symptoms in breast cancer survivors.

Osteoporosis

Patients with breast cancer are at increased risk for cancer treatment–induced bone loss (CTIBL) as a result of hypogonadism from treatment and antiestrogen medication side effects (Pfeilschifter & Diel, 2000). According to Viale and Yamamoto (2003), "Osteoporosis is characterized by low bone mass and deterioration of bone, leading to bone weakness and an increased susceptibility to fractures" (p. 393). Bone undergoes a continual process of loss and formation throughout a woman's life. Women who go through natural menopause experience a sharp decrease in bone mass within five years after the end of menses, with gradual loss thereafter. Unless the bone formation rate increases, osteopenia and, eventually, osteoporosis will develop.

Risk factors for the development of osteoporosis in healthy women are categorized as modifiable and nonmodifiable. Nonmodifiable risks include female gender, age, Caucasian or Asian ancestry, small body frame, and family history of osteoporosis. Modifiable risks include cigarette smoking, low calcium and vitamin D intake, sedentary lifestyle, alcohol intake, and low body weight. These risk factors should be taken into consideration to determine additive risk in women undergoing cancer treatment. It is important to note that the incidence of osteoporosis in women in the United States has increased in the past decade, placing more women at risk at the time of their breast cancer development (Kuehn, 2005).

CTIBL can begin one year after chemotherapy and continues for the next two to five years in women with permanent menopause. It can be accelerated with the use of aromatase inhibitors such as anastrozole (Arimidex®, AstraZeneca Pharmaceuticals) (Gnant et al., 2002) and letrozole (Femara) in postmenopausal women, and fulvestrant (Faslodex®, AstraZeneca Pharmaceuticals) or tamoxifen (Nolvadex®, AstraZeneca Pharmaceuticals) in premenopausal women (Powles, Hickish, Kanis, Tidy, & Ashley, 1996). In a study

by Sverrisdottir, Fornander, Jacobsson, von Schoultz, and Rutqvist (2004), two years of ovarian ablation with goserelin (Zoladex®, AstraZeneca Pharmaceuticals) therapy caused a significant reduction in bone mineral density (BMD), but a partial recovery occurred after cessation of treatment. Ovarian insufficiency generally develops within one year of therapy in 63%–96% of premenopausal women with breast cancer who receive cyclophosphamide, methotrexate, 5-fluorouracil, or doxorubicin. The risk of ovarian injury is related to the age of the patient at the time of treatment, the cumulative dose of the drug administered, and the duration of treatment (Pfeilschifter & Diel, 2000). The incidence of fractures caused by CTIBL has not been reported. However, a trial comparing anastrozole to tamoxifen indicated that the anastrozole group was more likely to experience bone loss, and the incidence of fracture was 5.9% in the anastrozole group compared to 3.7% in the tamoxifen group (Baum et al., 2003). Studies of other aromatase inhibitors show a trend toward increased bone loss.

The World Health Organization has established criteria for categorizing bone density. Measurement of the density by dual x-ray absorptiometry scan is considered the gold standard. Results are reported as T scores that represent the number of standard deviations between an individual's BMD and the mean value for a group of young adults of the same sex (Cummings et al., 1993). Women with T scores above –1 are considered to have normal bone density with minimal risk of hip fracture. Women with T scores of –1 to –2.5 have osteopenia and are at 2.6–7 times greater risk of hip fracture than normal controls. Women with T scores less than –2.5 are considered to have osteoporosis and are at 7–11 times greater risk of having a hip fracture. Women with T scores less than –2.5 who have already experienced one or more fractures are considered to have severe osteoporosis and are at 11 times or greater risk of sustaining a hip fracture (Cummings et al.). Optimal timing of BMD testing for CTIBL has not been established. A thorough review of the patient's history including duration of menses, current dietary and activity lifestyles, vertebral deformities, height loss, abdominal protrusion, and paraspinal muscle pain may help to identify preexisting vertebral fractures caused by osteoporosis (Pfeilschifter & Diel, 2000). Serum chemistries assessing for kidney or liver disease and parathyroid hormone, thyroid-stimulating hormone, vitamin D, serum calcium, phosphorus, and alkaline phosphatase levels may help in the evaluation (Pfeilschifter & Diel). Although cancer therapies cause the biggest increase in osteoporosis risk in breast cancer survivors, patients also should be instructed about the importance of smoking cessation, moderate alcohol consumption, and the importance of regular weight-bearing exercise. Resistance and weight-bearing exercises and a daily intake of 1,200–1,500 mg of calcium and 600–800 IU of vitamin D should be recommended (Hillner et al., 2003).

According to the American Society of Clinical Oncology (ASCO) bone health guidelines for breast cancer survivors, women should be stratified into low- and high-risk groups depending on the presence of risk factors (Hilner et al., 2003). Breast cancer survivors who are considered high risk are women age 65 and older, postmenopausal women receiving aromatase inhibitors, premenopausal women with premature menopause, and women age 60–64 with general osteoporosis risk factors. These individuals are advised to undergo baseline hip and spine BMD testing and be counseled about lifestyle and dietary changes (Hillner et al.). It is recommended that patients with a T score of –2.5 or lower be treated with oral or IV bisphosphonates such as alendronate (Fosamax®, Merck and Co., Inc.), risedronate (Actonel®, Proctor and Gamble Pharmaceuticals, Cincinnati, OH), or zoledronic acid (Zometa®, Novartis Pharmaceuticals Corp.). Raloxifene is considered an option, except in women who have received tamoxifen in the past or who are currently receiving an aromatase inhibitor. Annual BMD screening is recommended in follow-up. ASCO recommends that low-risk patients not undergo bone density screening until age 65 but should have assessment of risk factors done annually with ongoing counseling on diet and lifestyle changes (Hilner et al.). Other clinicians have disagreed with this position and instead recommend baseline BMD screening with repeat measurements performed every three to five years (Twiss et al., 2001).

Tamoxifen is modestly effective in preventing bone loss in postmenopausal women. Currently, clinical trials are evaluating the use of IV bisphosphonates for the prevention of osteoporosis in women with a history of breast cancer. Although patients do not experience gastrointestinal symptoms from the IV drugs, these drugs are expensive to administer (must be given in the clinic by an RN) and require close monitoring of serum creatinine and blood counts. However, a study by Reid et al. (2002) showed that a single yearly infusion of zoledronic acid (Zometa) significantly increased BMD in healthy postmenopausal women with osteoporosis. The Z-FAST randomized, open-label study preliminary results also show promise in the use of zoledronic acid in preventing bone loss in women randomized to an early intervention plan while undergoing treatment with letrozole (Brufsky et al., 2005). Intranasal calcitonin (Miacalcin®, Novartis Pharmaceuticals Corp.) has not been well studied in breast cancer survivors but can be a reasonable option for women who cannot tolerate the gastrointestinal side effects of oral medications. Teriparatide (Forteo®, Eli Lilly and Co.) and ibandronate sodium (Boniva®, GlaxoSmithKline) have not been tested in breast cancer survivors and should be used only after patients discuss it with their healthcare provider.

Research on nonpharmacologic interventions for CTIBL has been quite varied. Waltman et al. (2003) tested a 12-month multicomponent intervention for preventing osteoporosis in 21 postmenopausal women who had completed breast cancer treatment (excluding tamoxifen). The intervention used a home-based strength and weight training exercise program combined with alendronate, vitamin D, and calcium, along with education about osteoporosis. Each of the breast cancer survivors had improvements in function, and 3 in 21 women who had measurable bone loss at baseline had normal BMD after the intervention. This pilot study shows that a combination of strategies along with education can assist breast cancer survivors in taking a proactive approach to health. See Table 8-5 for a listing of common pharmacologic treatments for osteoporosis in breast cancer survivors.

Management of CTIBL is likely to become a significant health issue in the next few years as the benefits of adjuvant therapy are better defined. Patients must be educated about the bone effects of treatment and should be encouraged to make lifestyle changes to promote bone health. Healthcare professionals must be proactive in doing follow-up BMD studies to identify worsening bone health and take prompt corrective measures. Research into better tolerated and less expensive treatments is needed. For patients who are refractive to oral osteoporosis medications, serious consideration should be given to the use of IV bisphosphonate drug therapy.

Conclusion

Symptom distress can adversely alter the experience of women diagnosed with breast cancer. Close review of the most commonly experienced side effects from treatment show clear but complex interrelationships. Although most women with early-stage breast cancer do not experience severe side effects, even minor symptoms can serve as a constant reminder of their cancer diagnosis. Healthcare providers must ensure that women are well informed about potential side effects. Doing so will help to lessen patients' anxiety, avoid misconceptions, and reduce their fear of recurrence. Promotion of self-care strategies helps to empower women to take back control of their lives. Research into improved surgical techniques; kinder, gentler chemotherapy and hormonal therapy regimens; and more targeted symptom management strategies, taking into consideration genetic and gender differences, is needed to further improve women's QOL. Long-term follow-up of survivors after treatment for breast cancer is critical to enable prompt identification of post-treatment problems, to educate women about potential side effects and strategies to manage them, and to share medical updates. Education regarding cancer treatment side effects should be provided to all healthcare professionals involved the care of these patients, including nurses, primary care practitioners, and specialists. As these issues become a healthcare priority, the emotional and physical well-being of millions of women who are breast cancer survivors will be enhanced.

Table 8-5. Pharmacologic Interventions for Osteoporosis Prevention and Cancer Treatment–Induced Bone Loss

Drug	Dosage	Special Considerations and Side Effects
Calcium citrate	1,200 mg–1,500 mg daily in divided doses of 500 mg	Avoid taking with iron supplements and caffeine. Drink with 8 oz of water. Can cause constipation, bloating, and gas
Calcium carbonate	Same as above	Same as with calcium citrate Concern with use in patients with renal insufficiency
Vitamin D	400–800 IU	Can also be gained by daily sun exposure
Calcitonin nasal spray (Miacalcin®)	200 units intranasally (one nostril per day)	Rhinitis and, rarely, epistaxis
Alendronate (Fosamax®)	10 mg po daily or 70 mg po weekly	Must stay upright for 30 minutes after taking medication; take on empty stomach. Drink with 8 oz of water. Can cause upper gastrointestinal irritation, myalgias, and arthralgias
Risedronate (Actonel®)	5 mg po daily or 35 mg po weekly	Same as with alendronate
Raloxifene (Evista®)	60 mg po daily	Not recommended for use after tamoxifen therapy or with aromatase inhibitors Can cause hot flashes, leg cramps, and, rarely, deep vein thrombosis
Tamoxifen (Nolvadex®)	10 mg po bid or 20 mg po daily	Should not be used with raloxifene or aromatase inhibitors Can cause hot flashes, weight gain, cataract formation, deep vein thrombosis, and endometrial cancer Has been found to promote bone loss in premenopausal women
Zoledronic acid (Zometa®)	4 mg IV once or twice annually, given over 15 minutes	Check creatinine clearance before each dose. Ensure adequate hydration. Avoid in people with history of aspirin-sensitive asthma. Osteonecrosis of the jaw has occurred following dental procedures in people with prior or concurrent chemotherapy and dexamethasone therapy. Can cause flu-like symptoms, nausea, vomiting, fever, flushing, and loss of appetite

Note. Based on information from Brufsky et al., 2005; Gnant et al., 2002; Hillner et al., 2003; Maxwell & Viale, 2005; Viale & Yamamoto, 2003.

References

Ahlberg, K., Ekman, T., Gaston-Johansson, F., & Mock, V. (2003). Evaluation and management of cancer-related fatigue: A review. *Lancet, 362,* 640–650.

Ahles, T.A., Saykin, A.J., Furstenberg, C.T., Cole, B., Mott, L.A., Skalla, K., et al. (2002). Neuropsychologic impact of standard-dose systemic chemotherapy in long-term survivors of breast cancer and lymphoma. *Journal of Clinical Oncology, 20,* 485–493.

Ahles, T.A., Saykin, A.J., Noll, W.W., Furstenberg, C.T., Guerin, S., Cole, B., et al. (2003). The relationship of APOE genotype to neuropsychological performance in long-term cancer survivors treated with standard dose chemotherapy. *Psycho-Oncology, 12,* 612–619.

American Cancer Society. (2001). *Exercises after breast surgery* (No. 4668, pp. 4–12). Atlanta, GA: Author.

Andrykowski, M.A., Curran, S.L., & Lightner, R. (1998). Off-treatment fatigue in breast cancer survivors: A controlled comparison. *Journal of Behavioral Medicine, 21,* 1–18.

Armer, J., Radina, M., Porock, D., & Culbertson, S. (2003). Predicting breast cancer-related lymphedema using self-reported symptoms. *Nursing Research, 52,* 370–379.

Avis, N.E., Stellato, R., Crawford, S., Bromberger, J., Ganz, P., Cain, V., et al. (2001). Is there a menopausal syndrome? Menopausal status and symptoms across racial/ethnic groups. *Society of Scientific Medicine, 52,* 345–356.

Baglan, K.L., Sharpe, M.B., Jaffray, D., Frazier, R.C., Fayad, J., Kestin, L.L., et al. (2003). Accelerated partial breast irradiation using 3D conformal radiation therapy (3D-CRT). *International Journal of Radiation Oncology, Biology, Physics, 55,* 302–311.

Balfour, J.A., & Goa, K.L. (1997). Dolasetron: A review of its pharmacology and therapeutic potential in the management of nausea and vomiting induced by chemotherapy, radiotherapy or surgery. *Drugs, 54,* 273–298.

Baron, R.H., Fey, J.V., Borgen, P.I., & Van Zee, K.J. (2004). Eighteen sensations after breast cancer surgery: A two year comparison of sentinel lymph node biopsy and axillary lymph node dissection. *Oncology Nursing Forum, 31,* 691–698.

Barsevick, A., Whitmer, K., Sweeney, C.A., & Nail, L.M. (2002). A pilot study examining conservation for cancer treatment-related fatigue. *Cancer Nursing, 25,* 333–341.

Barton, D., & Loprinzi, C. (2002). Novel approaches to preventing chemotherapy-induced cognitive dysfunction in breast cancer: The art of the possible. *Clinical Breast Cancer, 3*(Suppl. 3), S121–S127.

Barton, D.L., Loprinzi, C.L., Quella, S.K., Sloan, J.A., Veeder, M.H., Egner, J.R., et al. (1998). Prospective evaluation of vitamin E for hot flashes in breast cancer survivors. *Journal of Clinical Oncology, 16,* 495–500.

Baum, M., Budzar, A., Cuzick, J., Forbes, J., Houghton, J., Howell, A., et al. (2003). Anastrozole alone or in combination with tamoxifen versus tamoxifen alone for adjuvant treatment of postmenopausal women with early-stage breast cancer: Results of the ATAC (Arimidex, Tamoxifen Alone, or in Combination) trial efficacy and safety update analyses. *Cancer, 98,* 1802–1810.

Beck, S.L., Dudley, W.N., & Barsevick, A. (2005). Pain, sleep disturbance, and fatigue in patients with cancer: Using a mediation model to test a symptom cluster [Online exclusive]. *Oncology Nursing Forum, 32,* E48–E55.

Bender, C.M., McDaniel, R.W., Murphy-Ende, K., Pickett, M., Rittenberg, C.N., Rogers, M.P., et al. (2002). Chemotherapy-induced nausea and vomiting. *Clinical Journal of Oncology Nursing, 6,* 94–102.

Bender, C.M., Paraska, K.K., Seirika, S.M., Ryan, C.M., & Berga, S.L. (2001). Cognitive function and reproductive hormones in adjuvant therapy for breast cancer: A critical review. *Journal of Pain and Symptom Management, 21,* 407–424.

Berger, A.M., Von Essen, S., Kuhn, B.R., Piper, B.F., Farr, L., Agrawal, S., et al. (2003). Adherence, sleep, and fatigue outcomes after adjuvant breast cancer chemotherapy: Results of a feasibility intervention study. *Oncology Nursing Forum, 30,* 513–522.

Bertelli, G., Venturini, M., Del Mastro, L., Bergaglio, M., Sismondi, P., Biglia, N., et al. (2002). Intramuscular depot medroxyprogesterone versus oral megestrol for the control of postmenopausal hot flashes in breast cancer patients: A randomized study. *Annals of Oncology, 13,* 883–888.

Bines, J., Oleske, D.M., & Cobleigh, M.A. (1996). Ovarian function in premenopausal women treated with adjuvant chemotherapy for breast cancer. *Journal of Clinical Oncology, 14,* 1718–1729.

Blackmar, A. (1997). Radiation-induced skin alterations. *MedSurg Nursing, 6,* 172–175.

Boccia, R., Malik, I.A., Raja, V., Kahanic, L., Liu, R., Lillie, T., et al. (2006). Darbepoetin alfa administered every three weeks is effective for the treatment of chemotherapy-induced anemia. *Oncologist, 11,* 409–417.

Boekhout, A.H., Beijnen, J.H., & Schellens, J.H.M. (2006). Symptoms and treatment in cancer therapy-induced early menopause. *Oncologist, 11,* 641–654.

Bohlius, J., Wilson, J., Seidenfeld, J., Piper, M., Schwarzer, G., Sandercock, J., et al. (2006). Recombinant human erythropoietins and cancer patients: Updated meta-analysis of 57 studies including 9353 patients. *Journal of the National Cancer Institute, 98,* 708–714.

Borger, J.H., Kemperman, H., Smitt, H.S., Hart, A., van Dongen, J., Lebesque, J., et al. (1994). Dose and volume effects on fibrosis after breast conservation. *International Journal of Radiation Oncology, Biology, Physics, 30,* 1073–1081.

Boris, M., Weindorf, S., & Lasinski, B. (1997). Persistence of lymphedema reduction after complex therapy. *Oncology, 11,* 99–109.

Bosompra, K., Ashikaga, T., O'Brien, P.J., Nelson, L., & Skelly, J. (2002). Swelling, numbness, pain, and their relationship to arm function among breast cancer survivors: A disablement process model perspective. *Breast Journal, 8,* 338–348.

Bostrom, A., Lindman, H., Swartling, C., Berne, B., & Bergh, J. (2001). Potent corticosteroid cream (mometasone furoate) significantly reduces acute radiation dermatitis: Results from a double-blind, randomized study. *Radiotherapy and Oncology, 59,* 257–265.

Bower, J.E., Ganz, P.A., Desmond, K.A., Rowland, J.H., Meyerowitz, B.E., & Belin, T.R. (2000). Fatigue in breast cancer survivors: Occurrence, correlates, and impact on quality of life. *Journal of Clinical Oncology, 18,* 743–753.

Box, R.C., Reul-Hirche, H.M., Bullock-Saxton, J.E., & Furnival, C.M. (2002). Shoulder movement after breast cancer surgery: Results of a randomized controlled study of postoperative physiotherapy. *Breast Cancer Research and Treatment, 75,* 35–50.

Broeckel, J.A., Jacobsen, P.B., Horton, J., Balducci, L., & Lyman, G.H. (1998). Characteristics and correlates of fatigue after adjuvant chemotherapy for breast cancer. *Journal of Clinical Oncology, 16,* 1689–1696.

Browse, N., Burnard, K.G., & Mortimer, P.S. (2003). *Diseases of the lymphatics.* London: Arnold.

Brufsky, A., Harker, J.T., Beck, R., Carroll, E., Tan-Chiu, C., Seidler, L., et al. (2005). Zoledronic acid (ZA) effectively inhibits cancer treatment-induced bone loss (CTIBL) in postmenopausal women (PMW) with early breast cancer (BCa) receiving adjuvant letrozole (Let): 12 mos BMD results of the Z-FAST trial. *Journal of Clinical Oncology, 23*(Suppl. 16), 533.

Burks, T.F. (2001). New agents for the treatment of cancer-related fatigue. *Cancer, 92*(Suppl. 6), 1714–1718.

Carpenter, J.S. (2005). State of the science: Hot flashes and cancer, part 2: Management and future directions. *Oncology Nursing Forum, 32,* 969–978.

Carpenter, J.S., Andrykowski, M.A., Cordova, M., Cunningham, L., Studts, J., McGrath, P., et al. (1998). Hot flashes in postmenopausal women treated for breast carcinoma: Prevalence, severity, correlates, management, and relation to quality of life. *Cancer, 82,* 1682–1691.

Carpenter, J.S., Johnson, D.H., Wagner, L.J., & Andrykowski, M.A. (2002). Hot flashes and related outcomes in breast cancer survivors and matched comparison women [Online exclusive]. *Oncology Nursing Forum, 29,* E16–E25.

Casley-Smith, J.R., & Casley-Smith, J.R. (1997). *Modern treatment of lymphoedema* (5th ed.). Adelaide, Australia: Lymphedema Association of Australia.

Casley-Smith, J.R., Casley-Smith, J.R., Lasinski, B., & Boris, M. (1996). The dangers of pumps in lymphoedema therapy. *Lymphology, 29,* 232–234.

Castellon, S.A., Ganz, P.A., Bower, J.E., Peterson, L., Abraham, L., & Greendale, G.A. (2004). Neurocognitive performance in breast cancer survivors exposed to adjuvant chemotherapy and tamoxifen. *Journal of Clinical and Experimental Neuropsychology, 26,* 955–969.

Cella, D., Dobrez, D., & Glaspy, J. (2003). Control of cancer-related anemia with erythropoietin agents: A review of evidence for improved clinical outcomes. *Annals of Oncology, 14,* 511–519.

Cheville, A., & Gergich, N. (2004). Lymphedema: Implications for wound care. In P.J. Sheffield, A.P.S. Smith, & C. Fife (Eds.), *Wound care practice* (pp. 285–303). Flagstaff, AZ: Best Publishing Co.

Chikly, B. (2001). *Silent waves: The theory and practice of lymph drainage therapy: With applications for lymphedema, chronic pain, and inflammation.* Scottsdale, AZ: I.H.H. Publishing.

Couzi, R.J., Helzlsouer, K.J., & Fetting, J.H. (1995). Prevalence of menopausal symptoms among women with a history of breast cancer and attitudes toward estrogen replacement therapy. *Journal of Clinical Oncology, 13,* 2737–2744.

Cummings, S.S., Black, D.M., Nevitt, M.C., Browner, W., Cauley, J., Enstrud, K., et al. (1993). Bone density of various sites for prediction of hip fracture. The Study of Osteoporotic Fracture Research Group. *Lancet, 341,* 72–75.

Curt, G.A., Breitbart, W., Cella, D., Groopman, J.E., Horning, S.J., Itri, L.M., et al. (2000). Impact of cancer-related fatigue on the lives of patients: New findings from the Fatigue Coalition. *Oncologist, 5,* 353–360.

Deng, G., Cassileth, B.R., & Yeung, K.S. (2004). Complementary therapies for cancer-related symptoms. *Journal of Supportive Oncology, 2,* 419–429.

Deutsch, M., & Flickinger, J.C. (2001). Shoulder and arm problems after radiotherapy for primary breast cancer. *American Journal of Clinical Oncology, 24,* 172–176.

Deutsch, M., & Flickinger, J.C. (2003). Patient characteristics and treatment factors affecting cosmesis following lumpectomy and breast irradiation. *American Journal of Clinical Oncology, 26,* 350–353.

Dibble, S.L., Casey, K., Nussey, B.A., Israel, J., & Luce, J. (2004). Chemotherapy-induced vomiting in women treated for breast cancer [Online exclusive]. *Oncology Nursing Forum, 31,* E1–E8.

Dibble, S.L., Israel, J., Nussey, B., Casey, K., & Luce, J. (2003). Delayed chemotherapy-induced nausea in women treated for breast cancer [Online exclusive]. *Oncology Nursing Forum, 30,* E40–E47.

Dow, K.H., Ferrell, B.R., Leigh, S., Ly, J., & Gulasekaram, P. (1996). An evaluation of the quality of life among long-term survivors of breast cancer. *Breast Cancer Research and Treatment, 39,* 261–273.

Duff, M., Hill, A., McGreal, G., Walsh, S., McDermott, E.W., & Higgins, N. (2001). Prospective evaluation of the morbidity of axillary clearance for breast cancer. *British Journal of Surgery, 88,* 114–117.

Eckert, R.M. (2001). Understanding anticipatory nausea. *Oncology Nursing Forum, 28,* 1553–1558.

Fassoulaki, A., Sarantopoulos, C., Melameni, A., & Hogan, Q. (2000). EMLA reduces acute and chronic pain after breast surgery for cancer. *Regional Anesthesia and Pain Management, 25,* 350–355.

Fassoulaki, A., Triga, A., Melemeni, A., & Sarantopoulos, C. (2005). Multimodal analgesia with gabapentin and local anesthetics prevents acute and chronic pain after breast surgery for cancer. *Anesthesia and Analgesia, 101,* 1427–1432.

Feldman, J. (2005). The challenge of infection in lymphedema. *LymphLink, 17*(4), 1–2, 27.

Ferguson, R.J., & Ahles, T.A. (2003). Low neuropsychologic performance among adult cancer survivors treated with chemotherapy. *Current Neurology and Neuroscience Reports, 3,* 215–222.

Fisher, J., Scott, C., Stevens, R., Marconi, B., Champion, L., Freedman, G., et al. (2000). Randomized phase III study comparing best supportive care to Biafine as a prophylactic agent for radiation-induced skin toxicity for women undergoing breast irradiation: Radiation Therapy Oncology Group (RTOG) 97-13. *International Journal of Radiation Oncology, Biology, Physics, 48,* 1307–1310.

Foldi, M., Foldi, E., & Kubic, S. (Eds.). (2003). *Text of lymphology.* Munich, Germany: Urban and Fischer.

Ganz, P.A., Greendale, G.A., Petersen, L., Zibecchi, L., Kahn, B., & Belin, T.R. (2000). Managing menopausal symptoms in breast cancer survivors: Result of a randomized controlled trial. *Journal of the National Cancer Institute, 92,* 1054–1065.

Gelinas, C., & Fillion, L. (2004). Factors related to persistent fatigue following completion of breast cancer treatment. *Oncology Nursing Forum, 31,* 269–278.

Gnant, M., Hausmaninger, H., Samonigg, H., Mlineritsch, B., Taucher, S., Luschin-Ebengreuth, G., et al. (2002). Changes in bone mineral density caused by anastrozole or tamoxifen in combination with goserelin (± zoledronate) as adjuvant treatment for hormone receptor-positive premenopausal breast cancer: Results of a randomized multicenter trial [Abstract]. *Breast Cancer Research and Treatment, 76*(Suppl. 1), S31.

Goldberg, R.M., Loprinzi, C.L., O'Fallon, J.R., Veeder, M.H., Miser, S.W., Mailliard, J.A., et al. (1994). Transdermal clonidine for ameliorating tamoxifen-induced hot flashes. *Journal of Clinical Oncology, 12,* 155–158.

Goodman, M. (1997). Risk factors and antiemetic management of chemotherapy-induced nausea and vomiting. *Oncology Nursing Forum, 24*(Suppl. 7), 20–32.

Graham, P., Browne, L., Capp, A., Fox, C., Graham, J., Hollis, J., et al. (2004). Randomized, paired comparison of No-Sting Barrier Film versus sorbolene cream (10% glycerine) skin care during postmastectomy irradiation. *International Journal of Radiation Oncology, Biology, Physics, 58,* 241–246.

Gralla, R.J., Osoba, D., Kris, M.G., Kirkbride, P., Hesketh, P.J., Chinnery, L.W., et al. (1999). Recommendations for the use of antiemetics: Evidence-based, clinical practice guidelines. American Society of Clinical Oncology. *Journal of Clinical Oncology, 17,* 2971–2994.

Greenberg, D.B., Sawicka, J., Eisenthal, S., & Ross, D. (1992). Fatigue syndrome due to localized radiation. *Journal of Pain and Symptom Management, 7,* 38–45.

Grunberg, S.M., Deuson, R.R., Mavros, P., Geling, O., Hansen, M., Cruciani, G., et al. (2004). Incidence of chemotherapy-induced nausea and emesis after modern antiemetics: Perception versus reality. *Cancer, 100,* 2261–2268.

Gutman, M., Kersz, T., Barzilai, T., Haddad, M., & Reiss, R. (1990). Achievements of physical therapy in patients after modified radical mastectomy compared with quadrantectomy, axillary dissection, and radiation for carcinoma of the breast. *Archives of Surgery, 125,* 389–391.

Guyton, A.C. (1997). The microcirculation and the lymphatic system: Capillary fluid exchange, interstitial fluid dynamics and lymph flow. In A.C. Guyton & J.E. Hall (Eds.), *Human physiology and mechanism of disease* (6th ed., pp. 162–174). Philadelphia: Saunders.

Hammar, M., Ekblad, S., Lonnberg, B., Berg, G., Lindgren, R., & Wyon, Y. (1999). Postmenopausal women without previous or current vasomotor symptoms do not flush after abruptly abandoning estrogen replacement therapy. *Maturitas, 31,* 117–122.

Heggie, S., Bryant, G.P., Tripcony, L., Keller, J., Rose, P., Glendenning, M., et al. (2002). A phase III study on the efficacy of topical aloe vera gel on irradiated breast tissue. *Cancer Nursing, 25,* 442–451.

Herrstedt, J., Muss, H.B., Warr, D.G., Hesketh, P.J., Eisenberg, P.D., Raftopoulos, H., et al. (2005). Efficacy and tolerability of aprepitant for the prevention of chemotherapy-induced nausea and emesis over multiple cycles of moderately emetogenic chemotherapy. *Cancer, 104,* 1548–1555.

Hillner, B.E., Ingle, J.N., Chlebowski, R.T., Gralow, J., Yee, G.C., Janjan, N.A., et al. (2003). American Society of Clinical Oncology 2003 update on the role of bisphosphonates and bone health issues in women with breast cancer. *Journal of Clinical Oncology, 21,* 4042–4057.

International Society of Lymphology. (2003). The diagnosis and treatment of peripheral lymphedema. Consensus document of the International Society of Lymphology. *Lymphology, 36,* 84–91.

Irvine, D., Vincent, L., Graydon, J.E., Bubela, N., & Thompson, L. (1994). The prevalence and correlates of fatigue in patients receiving treatment with chemotherapy and radiotherapy. *Cancer Nursing, 17,* 367–378.

Isaksson, G., & Feuk, B. (2000). Morbidity from axillary treatment in breast cancer—a follow-up study in a district hospital. *Acta Oncologica, 39,* 335–336.

Jacobsen, P.B., Hann, D.M., Azzarello, L.M., Horton, J., Balducci, L., & Lyman, G.H. (1999). Fatigue in women receiving adjuvant chemotherapy for breast cancer: Characteristics, course and correlates. *Journal of Pain and Symptom Management, 18,* 233–242.

Johnson, J.E., Rice, V.H., Fuller, S.S., & Endress, M.P. (1978). Sensory information, instruction in a coping strategy, and recovery from surgery. *Research in Nursing and Health, 1,* 4–17.

Kakuda, J., Stuntz, M., Trivedi, V., Klein, S., & Vargas, H. (1999). Objective assessment of axillary morbidity in breast cancer treatment. *American Surgeon, 65,* 995–998.

Kalinowski, B. (2004). Lymphedema. In C.H. Yarbro, M.H. Frogge, & M. Goodman (Eds.), *Cancer symptom management* (3rd ed., pp. 461–472). Sudbury, MA: Jones and Bartlett.

Kalso, E., Tasmuth, T., & Neuvonen, P.J. (1996). Amitriptyline effectively relieves neuropathic pain following treatment of breast cancer. *Pain, 64,* 293–302.

Karki, A., Simonen, R., Malkia, E., & Selfe, J. (2005). Impairments, activity limitations and participation restrictions 6 and 12 months after breast cancer operation. *Journal of Rehabilitation Medicine, 37,* 180–188.

Katz, J., Poleshuck, E.L., Andrus, C.H., Hogan, L.A., Jung, B.F., Kulick, D.I., et al. (2005). Risk factors for acute pain and its persistence following breast cancer surgery. *Pain, 119*(1–3), 16–25.

Kelly, D.G. (2002). *A primer on lymphedema.* Upper Saddle River, NJ: Prentice Hall.

Keramopoulos, A., Tsionou, C., Minaretzis, D., Michalas, S., & Aravantinos, D. (1993). Arm morbidity following treatment of breast cancer with total axillary dissection: A multivariated approach. *Oncology, 50,* 445–449.

Kim, S.C., Kim, D.W., Moadel, R.M., Kim, C.K., Chatterjee, S., Shafir, M.K., et al. (2005). Using the intraoperative hand held probe without lymphoscintigraphy or using only dye correlates with higher sensory morbidity following sentinel lymph node biopsy in breast cancer: A review of the literature [Electronic version]. *World Journal of Surgical Oncology, 3,* 64.

King, C.R. (1997). Nonpharmacologic management of chemotherapy-induced nausea and vomiting. *Oncology Nursing Forum, 24*(Suppl. 7), 41–48.

Knopf, M.T., & Sun, Y. (2005). A longitudinal study of symptoms and self-care activities in women treated with primary radiotherapy for breast cancer. *Cancer Nursing, 28,* 210–218.

Ko, D.S.C., Lerner, R., Klose, G., & Cosimi, A.B. (1998). Effective treatment of lymphedema of the extremities. *Archives of Surgery, 133,* 452–458.

Kronenberg, F. (1990). Hot flashes: Epidemiology and physiology. *Annals of the New York Academy of Sciences, 592,* 52–86.

Kronenberg, F., & Fugh-Berman, A. (2002). Complementary and alternative medicine for menopausal symptoms: A review of randomized, controlled trials. *Annals of Internal Medicine, 137,* 805–813.

Kroner, K., Knudsen, U.B., Lundby, L., & Hvid, H. (1992). Long-term phantom breast syndrome after mastectomy. *Clinical Journal of Pain, 8,* 346–350.

Kuehn, B.M. (2005). Better osteoporosis management a priority: Impact predicted to soar with aging population. *JAMA, 293,* 2453–2458.

Kuehn, T., Klauss, W., Darsow, M., Regele, S., Flock, F., Maiterth, C., et al. (2000). Long-term morbidity following axillary dissection in breast cancer patients—clinical assessment, significance for life quality and the impact of demographic, oncologic and therapeutic factors. *Breast Cancer Research and Treatment, 64,* 275–286.

Lerner, R. (2000). Chronic lymphedema. In J.B. Chang, E. Olsen, P. Kailash, & B. Sumpio (Eds.), *Textbook of angiology* (pp. 1227–1236). New York: Springer.

Lierman, L.M. (1988). Phantom breast experiences after mastectomy. *Oncology Nursing Forum, 15,* 41–44.

Lindley, C., Vasa, S., Sawyer, W.T., & Winer, E.P. (1998). Quality of life and preferences for treatment following systemic adjuvant therapy for early-stage breast cancer. *Journal of Clinical Oncology, 16,* 1380–1387.

Littlewood, T.J., Bajetta, E., Nortier, J.W.R., Vercammen, E., Rapoport, B., & Epoetin Alfa Study Group. (2001). Effects of epoetin alfa on hematologic parameters and quality of life in cancer patients receiving nonplatinum chemotherapy. *Journal of Clinical Oncology, 19,* 2865–2874.

Loprinzi, C.L., Barton, D.L., Sloan, J.A., Zahasky, K.M., Smith, D.A., Pruthi, S., et al. (2002). Pilot evaluation of gabapentin for treating hot flashes. *Mayo Clinic Proceedings, 77,* 1159–1163.

Loprinzi, C.L., Kugler, J.W., Sloan, J.A., Mailliard, J.A., La Vasseur, B., Barton, D.L., et al. (2000). Venlafaxine in management of hot flashes in survivors of breast cancer: A randomized controlled trial. *Lancet, 356,* 2059–2063.

Loprinzi, C.L., Sloan, J.A., Perez, E.A., Quella, S.K., Stella, P.J., Mailliard, J.A., et al. (2002). Phase III evaluation of fluoxetine for treatment of hot flashes. *Journal of Clinical Oncology, 20,* 1578–1583.

Lymphology Association of North America. (2005). *Certification makes a difference.* Wilmette, IL: Author.

Magnan, M.A., & Mood, D.W. (2003). The effects of health state, hemoglobin, global symptom distress, mood disturbance, and treatment site on fatigue onset, duration, and distress in patients receiving radiation therapy [Online exclusive]. *Oncology Nursing Forum, 30,* E33–E39.

Maiche, A., Isokangas, O., & Grohn, P. (1994). Skin protection by sucralfate cream during electron beam therapy. *Acta Oncologica, 33,* 201–203.

Maxwell, C., & Viale, P.H. (2005). Cancer treatment-induced bone loss in patients with breast or prostate cancer. *Oncology Nursing Forum, 32,* 589–601.

Mayo Foundation for Medical Education and Research. (2004, October 15). *Chemobrain: When cancer treatment disrupts your thinking and memory skills.* Retrieved December 8, 2005, from http://www.mayoclinic.com/health/cancer-treatment/CA00044

McAnaw, M.B., & Harris, K.W. (2002). The role of physical therapy in the rehabilitation of patients with mastectomy and breast reconstruction. *Breast Disease, 16,* 163–174.

McCredie, M., Diter, G., Porter, L., Maskiell, J., Giles, G., Phillips, K.A., et al. (2001). Prevalence of self-reported arm mobility following treatment for breast cancer in the Australian Breast Cancer Family Study. *Breast, 10,* 515–522.

Miko Enomoto, T., Johnson, T., Peterson, N., Homer, L., Walts, D., & Johnson, N. (2005). Combination glutathione and anthocyanins as an alternative for skin care during external-beam radiation. *American Journal of Surgery, 189,* 627–630.

Mock, V. (2001). Fatigue management: Evidence and guidelines for practice. *Cancer, 92*(Suppl. 6), 1699–1707.

Mock, V., & Olsen, M. (2003). Current management of fatigue and anemia in patients with cancer. *Seminars in Oncology Nursing, 19*(4 Suppl. 2), 36–41.

Mock, V., Pickett, M., Ropka, M.E., Muscari Lin, E., Stewart, K.J., Rhodes, V.A., et al. (2001). Fatigue and quality of life outcomes of exercise during cancer treatment. *Cancer Practice, 9,* 119–127.

Morales, L., Neven, P., Timmerman, D., Christiaens, M.R., Vergote, I., Van Limbergen, E., et al. (2004). Acute effects of tamoxifen and third-generation aromatase inhibitors on menopausal symptoms of breast cancer patients. *Anti-Cancer Drugs, 15,* 753–760.

Munro, A.J., & Potter, S. (1996). A quantitative approach to the distress caused by symptoms in patients treated with radical radiotherapy. *British Journal of Cancer, 74,* 640–647.

Nail, L. (2002). Fatigue in patients with cancer. *Oncology Nursing Forum, 29,* 537–545.

National Cancer Institute. (2002, October). *EGb761 in maintaining mental clarity in women receiving chemotherapy for newly diagnosed breast cancer.* Retrieved February 25, 2006, from http://www.clinicaltrials.gov/ct/show/NCT00046891

National Cancer Institute. (2004, November). *Coenzyme Q10 in relieving treatment-related fatigue in women with breast cancer.* Retrieved February 25, 2006, from http://clinicaltrials.gov/ct/show/NCT00096356

National Cancer Institute. (2005, December). *Radiation therapy and you: A guide to self-help during cancer treatment.* Retrieved December 5, 2005, from http://www.cancer.gov/cancertopics/radiation-therapy-and-you/page5

National Center for Complementary and Alternative Medicine. (2003a, November). *Ginger control of chemotherapy induced nausea and vomiting.* Retrieved December 6, 2005, from http://clinicaltrials.gov/show/NCT00065221

National Center for Complementary and Alternative Medicine. (2003b, January). *Massage therapy for breast cancer treatment-related swelling of the arms.* Retrieved December 6. 2005, from http://www.clinicaltrials.gov/show/NCT00058851

National Center for Complementary and Alternative Medicine. (2003c, August). *Pycnogenol for the treatment of lymphedema of the arm in breast cancer survivors.* Retrieved December 6, 2005, from http://clinicaltrials.gov/show/NCT00064857

National Center for Complementary and Alternative Medicine. (2004a, April). *Acupuncture for the treatment of hot flashes in breast cancer patients.* Retrieved December 6, 2005, from http://clinicaltrials.gov/show/NCT00081965

National Center for Complementary and Alternative Medicine. (2004b, April). *Hypnosis for hot flashes in breast cancer survivors.* Retrieved December 6, 2005, from http://clinicaltrials.gov/show/NCT00094133

National Center for Complementary and Alternative Medicine. (2005, November). *Hydrotherapy against menopausal symptoms in breast cancer survivors.* Retrieved February 25, 2006, from http://clinicaltrials.gov/ct/show/NCT00243607

National Comprehensive Cancer Network. (2005a, August). *Cancer pain treatment guidelines for patients, version II.* Atlanta, GA: American Cancer Society and Author. Retrieved August 18, 2006, from http://www.NCCN.org/patients/patient_gls/_english/pdf/NCCN%20Pain%20guidelines.pdf

National Comprehensive Cancer Network. (2005b, November). *Cancer-related fatigue and anemia treatment guidelines for patients, version III.* Atlanta, GA: American Cancer Society and Author. Retrieved August 18, 2006, from http://www.nccn.org/patients/patient_gls/_english/pdf/NCCN%20Fatigue%20guidelines.pdf

National Comprehensive Cancer Network. (2006). *NCCN clinical practice guidelines in oncology: Antiemesis, version 2.2006.* Jenkintown, PA: Author. Retrieved August 18, 2006, from http://www.nccn.org/professionals/physician_gls/PDF/antiemesis.pdf

National Lymphedema Network Medical Advisory Committee. (2004). *Position statement of the National Lymphedema Network topic: Air travel.* Retrieved September 20, 2005, from http://www.lymphnet.org/pdfDocs/nlnairtravel.pdf

National Lymphedema Network Medical Advisory Committee. (2005a). *Position statement of the National Lymphedema Network topic: Exercise.* Retrieved September 20, 2005, from http://www.lymphnet.org/pdfDocs/nlnexercise.pdf

National Lymphedema Network Medical Advisory Committee. (2005b, July). *Position statement of the National Lymphedema Network topic: Lymphedema risk reduction practices.* Retrieved October 2, 2005, from http://www.lymphnet.org/pdfDocs/nlnriskreduction.pdf

Okhuma, M. (1990). Cellulitis seen in lymphoedema. In M. Mishi, S. Uchino, & S. Yabukis (Eds.), *Progress in lymphology XII. Excerpto medica, International Congress Series 887* (pp. 401–402). Amsterdam, Netherlands: Elsevier.

Okumura, S., Mitsumori, M., Kokubo, M., Yamauchi, C., Kawamura, S., Oya, N., et al. (2003). Late skin and subcutaneous soft tissue changes after 10-Gy boost for breast conserving therapy. *Breast Cancer, 10,* 129–133.

Olsen, D., Raub, W., Bradley, C., Johnson, M., Macias, J., Love, V., et al. (2001). The effect of aloe vera gel/mild soap versus mild soap alone in preventing skin reactions in patients undergoing radiation therapy. *Oncology Nursing Forum, 28,* 543–547.

O'Shaughnessy, J.A., Vukelja, S.J., Holmes, F.A., Savin, M., Jones, M., Royall, D., et al. (2005). Feasibility of quantifying the effects of epoetin alfa therapy on cognitive function in women with breast cancer undergoing adjuvant or neoadjuvant chemotherapy. *Clinical Breast Cancer, 5,* 439–446.

Perera, F., Chisela, F., Stitt, L., Engel, J., & Venkatesan, V. (2005). TLD skin dose measurements and acute and late effects after lumpectomy and high-dose rate brachytherapy only for early breast cancer. *International Journal of Radiation Oncology, Biology, Physics, 62,* 1283–1290.

Petrek, J.A., Peters, M.M., Nori, S., Knauer, C., Kinne, D.W., & Rogatko, A. (1990). Axillary lymphadenectomy. A prospective, randomized trial of 13 factors influencing drainage, including early or delayed arm mobilization. *Archives of Surgery, 125,* 378–382.

Pfeilschifter, J., & Diel, I.J. (2000). Osteoporosis due to cancer treatment: Pathogenesis and management. *Journal of Clinical Oncology, 18,* 1570–1593.

Phillips, K., & Bernhard, J. (2003). Adjuvant breast cancer treatment and cognitive function: Current knowledge and research directions. *Journal of the National Cancer Institute, 95,* 190–197.

Poti, A., Nemeskeri, C., Fekeshazy, A., Safrany, G., Bajzik, G., Nagy, Z.P., et al. (2004). Partial breast irradiation with interstitial 60 CO brachytherapy results in frequent grade 3 or 4 toxicity. Evidence based on a 12-year follow-up of 70 patients. *International Journal of Radiation Oncology, Biology, Physics, 58,* 1022–1033.

Powles, T.J., Hickish, T., Kanis, J.A., Tidy, A., & Ashley, S. (1996). Effect of tamoxifen on bone mineral density measured by dual-energy x-ray absorptiometry in healthy premenopausal and postmenopausal women. *Journal of Clinical Oncology, 14,* 78–84.

Pritchard, K.I. (2001). Hormone replacement in women with a history of breast cancer. *Oncologist, 6,* 353–362.

Reedijk, M., Boerner, S., Ghazarian, D., & McCready, D. (2006). A case of axillary web syndrome with subcutaneous nodules following axillary surgery. *Breast,* 411–413.

Reid, I.R., Brown, J.P., Burckhardt, P., Horowitz, Z., Richardson, P., Trechsel, U., et al. (2002). IV zoledronic acid in postmenopausal women with low bone mineral density. *New England Journal of Medicine, 346,* 653–661.

Reuben, S.S., Makari-Judson, G., & Lurie, S.D. (2004). Evaluation of efficacy of the perioperative administration of venlafaxine XR in the prevention of postmastectomy pain syndrome. *Journal of Pain and Symptom Management, 27,* 133–139.

Rietman, J.S., Dijkstra, P.U., Hoekstra, H.J., Eisman, W.H., Szabo, B.G., Groothoff, J.W., et al. (2003). Late morbidity after treatment of breast cancer in relation to daily activities and quality of life: A systematic review. *European Journal of Surgical Oncology, 29,* 229–238.

Romestaing, P., Lehingue, Y., Carrie, C., Coquard, R., Montbarbon, X., Ardiet, J.M., et al. (1997). Role of a 10-Gy boost in the conservative treatment of early breast cancer: Results of a randomized clinical trial in Lyon, France. *Journal of Clinical Oncology, 15,* 963–968.

Roscoe, J.A., Bushunow, P., Morrow, G.R., Hickok, J.T., Kuebler, P.J., Jacobs, A., et al. (2004). Patient expectation is strong predictor of severe nausea after chemotherapy. *Cancer, 101,* 2701–2708.

Rowland, J.H., Desmond, K.A., Meyerowitz, B.E., Belin, T.R., Wyatt, G.E., & Ganz, P.A. (2000). Role of breast reconstructive surgery in physical and emotional outcomes among breast cancer survivors. *Journal of the National Cancer Institute, 92,* 1422–1429.

Rugo, H.S., & Ahles, T. (2003). The impact of adjuvant therapy for breast cancer on cognitive function: Current evidence and directions for research. *Seminars in Oncology, 30,* 749–762.

Saykin, A.J., Ahles, T.A., & McDonald, B.C. (2003). Mechanisms of chemotherapy-induced cognitive disorders: Neuropsychological, pathophysiological, and neuroimaging perspectives. *Seminars in Clinical Neuropsychiatry, 8,* 201–216.

Schagen, S.B., Muller, M.J., Boogerd, W., Rosenbrand, R.M., van Rhijn, D., Rodenhuis, S., et al. (2002). Late effects of adjuvant chemotherapy on cognitive function: A follow-up study in breast cancer patients. *Annals of Oncology, 13,* 1387–1397.

Schrenk, P., Rieger, R., Shamiyeh, A., & Wayand, W. (1999). Morbidity following sentinel lymph node biopsy versus axillary lymph node dissection for patients with breast carcinoma. *Cancer, 88,* 608–614.

Schultz, I., Barholm, M., & Grondal, S. (1997). Delayed shoulder exercises in reducing seroma frequency after modified radical mastectomy: A prospective randomized study. *Annals of Surgical Oncology, 4,* 293–297.

Schwingl, P.J., Hulka, B.S., & Harlow, S.D. (1994). Risk factors for menopausal hot flashes. *Obstetrics and Gynecology, 84,* 29–34.

Sekine, H., Kobayashi, M., Honda, C., Aoki, M., Nakagawa, M., & Kanehira, C. (2000). Skin reactions after breast-conserving therapy and prediction of late complication using physiological functions. *Breast Cancer, 7,* 142–148.

Sener, S., Winchester, D., Martz, C., Feldman, J., Cavanaugh, J., Winchester, D., et al. (2001). Lymphedema after sentinel lymphadenectomy for breast carcinoma. *Cancer, 92,* 748–752.

Servelle, M. (1987). Surgical treatment of lymphedema: A report of 652 cases. *Surgery, 101,* 485–495.

Shamley, D.R., Barker, K., Simonite, V., & Beardshaw, A. (2005). Delayed versus immediate exercises following surgery for breast cancer: A systematic review. *Breast Cancer Research and Treatment, 90,* 263–271.

Shell, J., Stanutz, F., & Grimm, J. (1986). Comparison of moisture vapor permeable (MVP) dressing to conventional dressing for management of radiation skin reactions. *Oncology Nursing Forum, 13*(1), 11–16.

Sherwin, B.B. (2000). Mild cognitive impairment: Potential pharmacological treatment options. *Journal of the American Geriatrics Society, 48,* 431–441.

Shilling, V., Jenkins, V., Morris, R., Deutsch, D., & Bloomfield, D. (2005). The effects of adjuvant chemotherapy on cognition in women with breast cancer—preliminary results of an observational longitudinal study. *Breast, 14,* 142–150.

Simon, M.S., & Cody, R.L., (1992). Cellulitis after axillary node dissection for carcinoma of the breast. *American Journal of Medicine, 93,* 543–548.

Stanton, A., Levick, J., & Mortimer, P. (1996). Current puzzles presented by postmastectomy oedema (breast cancer related lymphoedema). *Vascular Medicine, 1,* 213–225.

Stearns, V., & Loprinzi, C.L. (2003). New therapeutic approaches for hot flashes in women. *Supportive Oncology, 1,* 11–21.

Stearns, V., Slack, R., Greep, N., Henry-Tilman, R., Osborne, M., Bunnell, C., et al. (2005). Paroxetine is an effective treatment for hot flashes: Results from a prospective randomized clinical trial. *Journal of Clinical Oncology, 23,* 6919–6930.

Stevens, P.E., Dibble, S.L., & Miaskowski, C. (1995). Prevalence, characteristics, and impact of postmastectomy pain syndrome: An investigation of women's experiences. *Pain, 61,* 61–68.

Stricker, C.T., Drake, D., Hoyer, K., & Mock, V. (2004). Evidence-based practice for fatigue management in adults with cancer: Exercise as an intervention. *Oncology Nursing Forum, 31,* 963–976.

Strunk, B., & Maher, K. (1993). Collaborative nurse management of multifactorial moist desquamation in a patient undergoing radiotherapy. *Journal of Enterostomal Nursing, 20,* 152–157.

Sugden, E.M., Rezvani, M., Harrison, J.M., & Hughes, L.K. (1998). Shoulder movement after the treatment of early stage breast cancer. *Clinical Oncology, 10,* 173–181.

Sverrisdottir, A., Fornander, T., Jacobsson, H., von Schoultz, E., & Rutqvist, L.E. (2004). Bone mineral density among premenopausal women with early breast cancer in a randomized trial of adjuvant endocrine therapy. *Journal of Clinical Oncology, 22,* 3694–3699.

Swenson, K.K., Nissen, M.J., Ceronsky, C., Swenson, L., Lee, M.W., & Tuttle, T.M. (2002). Comparison of side effects between sentinel lymph node and axillary lymph node dissection for breast cancer. *Annals of Surgical Oncology, 9,* 745–753.

Tannock, I.F., Ahles, T.A., Ganz, P.A., & van Dam, F.S. (2004). Cognitive impairment associated with chemotherapy for cancer: Report of a workshop. *Journal of Clinical Oncology, 22,* 2233–2239.

Tasmuth, T., von Smitten, K., Hietanen, P., Katja, M., & Kalso, E. (1995). Pain and other symptoms after different treatment modalities of breast cancer. *Annals of Oncology, 6,* 453–459.

Taylor, M.E., Perez, C.A., Halverson, K.J., Kuske, R.R., Philpott, G.W., Garcia, D.M., et al. (1995). Factors influencing cosmetic results after conservation therapy for breast cancer. *International Journal of Radiation Oncology, Biology, Physics, 31,* 753–764.

Turesson, I., Nyman, J., Holmberg, E., & Oden, A. (1996). Prognostic factors for acute and late skin reactions in radiotherapy patients. *International Journal of Radiation Oncology, Biology, Physics, 36,* 1065–1075.

Tuxen, M.K., & Werner, H.S. (1994). Neurotoxicity secondary to antineoplastic drugs. *Cancer Treatment Reviews, 20,* 191–214.

Twiss, J.J., Waltman, N., Ott, C.D., Gross, G.J., Lindsey, A.M., & Moore, T.E. (2001). Bone mineral density in postmenopausal breast cancer survivors. *Journal of the American Academy of Nurse Practitioners, 13,* 276–284.

van Dam, F.S., Schagen, S.B., Muller, M.J., Boogerd, W., Wall, E., Droogleever Fortuyn, M.E., et al. (1998). Impairment of cognitive function in women receiving adjuvant treatment for high-risk breast cancer: High-dose versus standard-dose chemotherapy. *Journal of the National Cancer Institute, 90,* 210–218.

Viale, P.H., & Yamamoto, D.S. (2003). Bisphosphonates: Expanded roles in the treatment of patients with cancer. *Clinical Journal of Oncology Nursing, 7,* 393–401.

Vogelzang, N., Breitbart, W., Cella, D., Curt, G., Groopman, J.E., Horning, S.J., et al. (1997). Patient, caregiver, and oncologist perceptions of cancer-related fatigue: Result of a tripart assessment survey. The Fatigue Coalition. *Seminars in Hematology, 34*(3 Suppl. 2), 4–12.

von Schoultz, E., & Rutqvist, L.E. (2005). Menopausal hormone therapy after breast cancer: The Stockholm randomized trial. *Journal of the National Cancer Institute, 97,* 533–535.

Waltman, N.L., Twiss, J.J., Ott, C.D., Gross, G.J., Lindsey, A.M., Moore, T.E., et al. (2003). Testing an intervention for preventing osteoporosis in postmenopausal breast cancer survivors. *Journal of Nursing Scholarship, 35,* 333–338.

Waltzman, R., Croot, C., Justice, G.R., Fesen, M.R., Charu, V., & Williams, D. (2005). Randomized comparison of epoetin alfa (40,000 U weekly) and darbepoetin alfa (200 µg every 2 weeks) in anemic patients with cancer receiving chemotherapy. *Oncologist, 10,* 642–650.

Warr, D.G., Hesketh, P.J., Gralla, R.J., Muss, H.B., Herrstedt, J., Eisenberg, P.D., et al. (2005). Efficacy and tolerability of aprepitant for the prevention of chemotherapy-induced nausea and vomiting in patients with breast cancer after emetogenic chemotherapy. *Journal of Clinical Oncology, 23,* 2822–2830.

Watson, C.P., & Evans, R.J. (1992). The postmastectomy pain syndrome and topical capsaicin: A randomized trial. *Pain, 51,* 375–379.

Wefel, J.S., Lenzi, R., Theriault, R., Buzdar, A.U., Cruickshank, S., & Meyers, C.A. (2004). "Chemobrain" in breast carcinoma. *Cancer, 101,* 466–475.

Wefel, J., Lenzi, R., Theriault, R.L., Davis, R.N., & Meyers, C.A. (2004). The cognitive sequelae of standard-dose adjuvant chemotherapy in women with breast carcinoma. *Cancer, 100,* 2292–2299.

Weinfurt, K.P., Wait, S.L., Boyko, W., & Schulman, K.A. (1998). Psychosocial quality of life in a phase III trial of letrozole [Abstract]. *Proceedings of the American Society of Clinical Oncology,* Abstract 417. Retrieved August 18, 2006, from http://www.asco.org

Weissleder, H., & Schuchhardt, C. (2001). *Lymphedema: Diagnosis and therapy* (3rd ed.). Cologne, Germany: Viavital Verlag.

Wells, M., Macmillan, M., Raab, G., MacBride, S., Bell, N., MacKinnon, K., et al. (2004). Does aqueous or sucralfate cream affect the severity of erythematous radiation skin reactions? A randomized controlled trial. *Radiotherapy and Oncology, 73,* 153–162.

Wengstrom, Y., Haggmark, C., Strander, H., & Forsberg, C. (2000). Perceived symptoms and quality of life in women with breast cancer receiving radiation therapy. *European Journal of Oncology Nursing, 4,* 78–90.

Whiteman, M.K., Staropoli, C.A., Langenberg, P.W., McCarter, R.J., Kjerulff, K.H., & Flaws, J.A. (2003). Smoking, body mass, and hot flashes in midlife women. *Obstetrics and Gynecology, 101,* 264–272.

Wickham, R. (2004). Nausea and vomiting. In C.H. Yarbro, M.H. Frogge, & M. Goodman (Eds.), *Cancer symptom management* (3rd ed., pp. 187–207). Sudbury, MA: Jones and Bartlett.

Wickline, M.M. (2004). Prevention and treatment of acute radiation dermatitis: A literature review. *Oncology Nursing Forum, 31,* 237–244.

Williams, M., Burk, M., Loprinzi, C., Hiel, M., Schomberg, P., Nearhood, K., et al. (1996). Phase III double-blind evaluation of an aloe vera gel as a prophylactic agent for radiation-induced skin toxicity. *International Journal of Radiation Oncology, Biology, Physics, 36,* 345–349.

Woo, B., Dibble, S.L., Piper, B.F., Keating, S.B., & Weiss, M.C. (1998). Differences in fatigue by treatment methods in women with breast cancer. *Oncology Nursing Forum, 25,* 915–920.

Wyon, Y., Wijma, K., Nedstrand, E., & Hammar, M. (2004). A comparison of acupuncture and oral estradiol treatment of vasomotor symptoms in postmenopausal women. *Climacteric, 7,* 153–164.

Yaffe, K., Krueger, K., Sarkar, S., Grady, D., Barrett-Connor, E., Cox, D.A., et al. (2001). Cognitive function in postmenopausal women treated with raloxifene. *New England Journal of Medicine, 344,* 1207–1213.

CHAPTER 9

Psychosocial Issues

Gail Osterman, PhD

Introduction

Although adjusting to the many physical changes associated with breast cancer and its treatment is a complex process, changes in emotional state, body image, and family role and adjustment to treatment side effects are psychosocial difficulties that also accompany a diagnosis of breast cancer. This chapter will identify areas of concern and explore ways that healthcare professionals can support women with breast cancer, their families, and significant others.

The diagnosis of breast cancer undoubtedly brings significant change and distress to both patients and their loved ones. Everyone reacts to the diagnosis differently. A diagnosis of breast cancer is a stressful event and often is accompanied with an increase in anxiety and depression (Payne, Hoffman, Theodoulou, Dosik, & Massier, 1999). Women diagnosed with breast cancer consistently score lower than the general female population on quality-of-life measures during their cancer diagnosis and treatment and for as long as a year following treatment (Schou, Ekeberg, Sandvik, Hjermstad, & Ruland, 2005). Not only is the diagnosis period stressful, but treatment and follow-up also have potential negative psychological consequences. Nurses need to be aware of the salient psychosocial aspects of diagnosis, treatment, and survival and implement appropriate strategies to assist patients and family members in coping. Figure 9-1 provides an overview of common psychosocial concerns in women diagnosed with breast cancer.

Overview

Estimates suggest that approximately 30% of women with a diagnosis of breast cancer show significant distress at some point during the illness and its treatment (Hewitt, Herdman, & Holland, 2004). A significant proportion of women will experience at least some degree of depression and anxiety

(Hewitt et al.). These symptoms may be brief adjustment reactions that decrease as patients receive more information about the diagnosis and treatment, or they may be present intermittently or long-term throughout the cancer continuum. The diagnosis is almost always a threat to patients' sense of security and order in life.

The psychological functioning of patients should be addressed throughout all phases of the cancer trajectory. Psychosocial health affects patients' quality of life as well as treatment outcomes. Potentially better disease status and longer survival have been documented in patients with fewer psychosocial disturbances (Aukst-Margetic, Jakovljevic, Margetic, Biscan, & Samija, 2005; Smith, Gomm, & Dickens, 2003; Spiegel, Bloom, Kraemer, & Gottheil, 1989).

The National Comprehensive Cancer Network (NCCN, 2005) guidelines that address psychosocial issues are titled

---

Figure 9-1. Psychosocial Concerns of Women Diagnosed With Breast Cancer

- Fear of recurrence
- Physical symptoms including fatigue, sleep disturbances, nausea, and pain
- Body image changes including those related to surgery, weight, skin, and hair
- Sexual dysfunction (e.g., painful intercourse, vaginal dryness, early menopause, decreased libido)
- Treatment-related anxieties
- Emotional distress (e.g., cognitive dysfunction, anxiety, depression, grief, helplessness, anger, low self-esteem)
- Persistent anxiety or intrusive distressing thoughts about body and illness
- Marital or partner communication issues
- Social isolation or difficulty communicating with friends
- Fears of vulnerability
- Difficulties completing duties associated with career or other roles
- Financial concerns
- Existential and related fears of death

"Distress Management." Interestingly, this terminology was chosen because it carries fewer stigmas than psychiatric, psychosocial, or emotional problems; it seems more "normal"; and it can be measured by simple self-report tools. For similar reasons, nurses may want to consider this strategy when addressing patients and their significant others.

Individuals may experience psychosocial distress as a result of cancer or its treatment. Psychosocial distress often is manifested as fears of recurrence or death, more generalized symptoms of worry, trouble sleeping, fatigue, and difficulty concentrating. According to NCCN (2005),

> Distress is a multifactorial unpleasant emotional experience of a psychological (cognitive, behavioral, emotional), social, and/or spiritual nature that may interfere with the ability to cope effectively with cancer, its physical symptoms, and its treatment. Distress extends along a continuum, ranging from common normal feelings of vulnerability, sadness, and fears to problems that can become disabling, such as depression, anxiety, panic, social isolation, and existential and spiritual crisis. (p. D1S-2)

Distress affects family life, employment, and psychosocial functioning.

Psychosocial Services Providers

Oncology caregivers should provide psychosocial services as part of total medical care. This responsibility initially falls to oncologists and oncology nurses. Often, referrals to specialists in psycho-oncology are indicated. This may include psychologists, social workers, pastoral counselors, and other professionals. Although such specialists often are limited, all women diagnosed with breast cancer should have a psychosocial assessment. Figure 9-2 provides an overview of healthcare providers who contribute to promoting psychosocial health in patients with cancer and their families.

Barriers to Providing and Accessing Psychosocial Care

Several barriers exist that prevent women from receiving adequate psychosocial care (Hewitt et al., 2004). Care has

---

Figure 9-2. Oncology Team Members Who Contribute to Psychosocial Care

- **Oncologists:** Oncologists direct patients' care. They may take responsibility for providing referrals for psychosocial care. Often oncologists will prescribe pharmacologic agents to help to manage psychological problems and other symptoms causing psychosocial distress.
- **Nurses:** Oncology nurses provide ongoing assessment and psychosocial support for patients undergoing active treatment as well as for long-term survivors. They may recommend interventions to facilitate psychosocial adjustment, and they also help to communicate concerns to other members of the oncology team.
- **Pharmacists:** Pharmacists not only fill prescriptions and dispense drugs, but they also are a great source of information. They educate healthcare professionals and patients about the expected effects and side effects of pharmacologic agents.
- **Dietitians:** Dietitians not only work with patients who are having difficulty eating but also help other patients to establish an appropriate dietary program. They can help long-term survivors to develop healthy habits.
- **Social workers:** Oncology social workers can have diverse job responsibilities. These may include helping individuals to find support groups, dealing directly with financial issues, providing guidance for how to deal with workplace issues, assisting with completing paperwork such as advance directives or living wills, providing direct support through counseling, finding ways to assist with transportation to office visits, and providing information on nutritional supplements, wigs, or prosthetics.
- **Psychologists:** Psychologists can help patients and families by talking with them and identifying specific psychosocial problems. Once these are identified, psychologists can help to develop a concrete plan for how to deal with psychosocial problems.
- **Psychiatrists:** Psychiatrists can be particularly helpful in assisting patients and families who have underlying mental illness concerns that may have existed prior to the diagnosis of cancer or have been exacerbated by the diagnosis and treatment. They can provide supportive therapy as well as prescribe medications for these disorders.
- **Patient educators:** Many institutions and practices have nurses who serve as patient educators. Their primary responsibility is to provide individual and group education on cancer and its treatment. They often work in information centers and help patients in selecting appropriate materials such as videos, pamphlets, Internet sites, and other educational tools. They may offer regular classes on cancer-related topics. They often provide individualized education and may facilitate support groups.
- **Genetics counselors:** Families with a hereditary susceptibility for developing cancer should be referred to genetics counselors or nurses with expertise in genetics to explore the risks and benefits of genetic testing for their particular family.
- **Homecare nurses:** Some patients may need assistance with healthcare needs at home, including wound care or infusion services. While in the home setting, homecare nurses often identify other psychosocial issues and can either manage these issues or refer them to other members of the healthcare team.
- **Occupational therapists:** Occupational therapists can help patients to regain, develop, or relearn skills needed for independent living. Many patients with breast cancer who have lymphedema utilize the services of these professionals.
- **Physical therapists:** Physical therapists often work with occupational therapists, and they help patients with learning exercises and instruct patients on ways to regain strength and mobility. They also may help with lymphedema services.
- **Chaplains:** Chaplains assist patients and families with the spiritual aspects of their care. They may pray with patients, discuss existential concerns, and provide supportive counseling. They may be based in the institution, or patients may know them from their own religious institution.

gradually shifted from the inpatient to outpatient setting. Many outpatient clinics lack a full complement of specialists in psychosocial care. Furthermore, insurance coverage for mental health services often is limited, and many women lack the financial means to afford such specialty care. Busy clinical settings also may discourage women from discussing psychosocial concerns, as they may have a stigma or be perceived as unnecessary extras. Figure 9-3 provides an overview of the barriers to assessing and promoting psychosocial care.

Figure 9-3. Barriers to Appropriate Use of Psychosocial Services

- Poor access to services because of a lack of readily available providers in some settings
- Healthcare providers' lack of awareness of community services
- Lack of communication between healthcare providers and patients about psychosocial concerns
- Poor health insurance coverage for psychosocial services
- Lack of financial resources at institutions for additional services such as psychosocial care
- Fragmentation among care providers
- Lack of a systematic method to routinely assess for psychosocial distress
- Lack of widespread adoption of clinical practice guidelines to promote psychosocial functioning
- General misconceptions about mental health care and psychological functioning
- Inadequate quality assurance and accountability for psychosocial care

---

Assessment of Psychosocial Functioning

The assessment of psychosocial distress is important because it is so prevalent. An estimated one-third to one-half of women diagnosed with breast cancer experience significant levels of distress (Hewitt et al., 2004). Predictors of increased stress include younger age at diagnosis, fewer social supports, and lower socioeconomic status. Figure 9-4 provides an overview of areas in which to facilitate psychosocial adaptation.

Younger Women

A diagnosis of breast cancer in women under the age of 40 can be particularly challenging and puts these women at increased risk for psychosocial distress. Studies repeatedly suggest that younger women with breast cancer are at greater risk for psychological distress (Ganz, Greendale, Peterson, Kahn, & Bower, 2003). If the diagnosis is made during a pregnancy or shortly after a delivery, the woman must not only confront the diagnosis but also must manage the demands of a family and infant. The threat of early menopause or infertility also is associated with increased psychological distress.

Furthermore, trying to juggle work and career development can be challenging for younger women.

Breast cancer has the potential to be devastating to the sexual function and self-esteem of premenopausal women (Sammarco, 2001). This may be related to ovarian failure, premature menopause, and significant hormonal disruption. They also may have more concerns about feminine self-image and intimacy. Protection of fertility is a significant concern that cannot be underestimated. Supportive spouses, friends, and children will ultimately build a better support system for patients.

Older Women

Women are living longer and, thus, over a lifetime are more likely to develop breast cancer. They are staying in the workforce longer, and a diagnosis of breast cancer can cause difficulty in maintaining financial and social independence. Some older women may be at increased risk for other physical function problems and chronic illnesses. They may or may not have a social support system, especially if they are widowed or divorced. Although they may experience less disruption of routines than younger women, they are at risk for psychosocial distress. Older women may perceive breast cancer as less threatening to their lives in the future, but they may be more vulnerable in terms of their physical health and functioning (Sammarco, 2001). The literature addresses problems in younger and older women. It may be appropriate to consider the impact of the diagnosis on women in their 50s to 70s, as well as in subsets of women (e.g., single women). This would require a more intensive review but probably is appropriate.

Figure 9-4. Suggested Measures to Facilitate Psychosocial Adaptation

- Clarify the diagnosis, treatment options, and side effects. Take time to ensure that patients understand each issue.
- Instruct that cancer has a trajectory and that needs will change over time. Assure patients and families that they will receive support during each phase as needed.
- Remind patients that psychosocial health is just as important as physical health. Instruct that this is why psychosocial assessment is conducted regularly.
- Acknowledge that distress is common; inform patients of expected points when distress might increase; and tell patients that they need to communicate about distress just as healthcare providers need to assess for distress.
- Suggest concrete recommendations for coping with distress, including journaling, speaking with a trained counselor (such as a psychologist, nurse, chaplain, social worker, etc.), or joining a support group.
- Coordinate resources, and make referrals as indicated.
- Manage symptoms promptly, and assess effectiveness of interventions.

Prior Psychosocial Functioning

Assessment of patients' past psychosocial history is beneficial. The diagnosis and treatment of breast cancer is stressful and could potentially exacerbate preexisting conditions that have been under control. For instance, a patient with a long-standing history of clinical depression may find that the diagnosis of breast cancer increases the depression, and she may require more intensive intervention. Assessment and understanding of past effective coping strategies may provide insight into how to manage the multiple stressors that accompany a diagnosis of breast cancer.

Assessment of Family Support

Supporting the patient also means supporting the family. Clinicians should assess the needs of the family at the time of diagnosis. Issues such as intimacy and sexuality, femininity, role changes, childcare needs, and ways to talk to partners or children about the diagnosis require assessment and often intervention.

Family and friends also play a critical role in patients' decisions regarding treatment. A patient may have a family member or friend who has been diagnosed with and treated for breast cancer, which could cause the newly diagnosed patient to assume she will have the same reactions. As part of the initial assessment, the healthcare team needs to determine whether the patient has any preconceived ideas based on reports from other patients, family members, or friends. This will provide an opportunity to dispel any misconceptions regarding the patient's diagnosis and provides an estimate of the baseline information that the woman and her family have about the diagnosis and its treatment.

Research suggests that the first year following the diagnosis is a critical time for women and their partners (Northouse, Templin, & Mood, 2001). During this time they need to adjust to the ramifications of having a potentially life-threatening diagnosis, recover and adjust to surgery and adjuvant treatment, cope with the side effects of therapy, and begin to establish a new normalcy and routine. When families have additional outside stressors, the disease is more likely to be perceived as threatening, and quality of life is decreased (Northouse et al.). Higher levels of support from a partner, family members, or friends are associated with the use of more positive coping strategies and indirectly contribute to improved mood. Adjustment shortly after the diagnosis is related to later levels of adjustment (Northouse et al.). For this reason, early assessment and intervention of potential problems are important.

The diagnosis of breast cancer in mothers with children living at home is disruptive to the routines in the home and especially to the accessibility and availability of mothers to children. Ultimately, this often results in negative effects on overall tension in the home and marriage (Kirsch, Brandt, &

Lewis, 2003). Cancer brings change to any family, whether it is a young couple, a couple with children, an older couple, single people, widowed people, or individuals living in nontraditional relationships. Healthcare providers need to assess the impact of the diagnosis and its subsequent changes in each specific situation. This includes an assessment of finances (including whether the patient can work during treatment), living arrangements (someone is available to assist the patient), and how daily activities will be managed (this can be especially important in families with children). A clear and thorough assessment may help to identify potential problems so that intervention can be delivered early.

Assessment Instruments

A multitude of instruments are available that have been used in the assessment of psychosocial distress for patients with breast cancer. Most instruments address issues of psychological functioning, physical functioning, social functioning, and symptoms and side effects. Many cancer-specific assessment tools are available to help to identify women who need more support throughout their treatment. One of the biggest challenges that health professionals face is finding an assessment tool that is brief and easy to administer that also rapidly identifies individuals and families who are at significant risk for psychosocial problems (Northouse et al., 2001). Figure 9-5 provides some examples of commonly used instruments.

A 1–10 scale is an easy way to assess patients' symptoms, and this can easily be communicated to the rest of the healthcare team (see Figure 9-6). This scale can be used at each appointment to track changes and allows for additional consultation as needed. A score of 5 or higher may alert the need for specific referrals to mental health professionals. The tool also is effective because it can be used repeatedly to assess improvements and new problems with distress. NCCN (2005) provides a detailed schema for managing distress. This tool can and should be used throughout the cancer trajectory. The accompanying problem list may be very helpful in identifying specific problems that merit further evaluation and intervention. Figure 9-7 examines the appropriate point of action to aid in psychosocial adjustment.

Psychosocial Concerns Across the Cancer Trajectory

Biopsy

The diagnostic period can be an extremely anxiety-provoking time for a woman. An estimated 10%–20% of breast biopsies are positive, which means that more than two million women will undergo some procedure to evaluate a breast change annually (Chappy, 2004). The psychosocial needs of

---

Figure 9-5. Selected Tools Used in the Psychosocial Assessment of Breast Cancer

- Brief Symptom Inventory (BSI): The BSI is a 53-item measure of psychological distress written at a sixth-grade reading level and requiring five to seven minutes to complete. Each item is referenced to the past seven days.
- Cancer Rehabilitation Evaluation System (CARES): CARES generates a report for both patients and healthcare professionals. There is a format for clinical and one for research. The clinical format allows patients to check a box if they desire help with a certain problem. It focuses on quality of life and related cancer-specific needs. Patients complete the instrument by rating problem statements on a scale of 0–4 as it applies to the previous month. It can include up to 193 items that focus on physical and psychosocial concerns, medical interactions with the care team, marital issues, and sexual issues.
- Distress Thermometer and Problem List from the National Comprehensive Cancer Network (NCCN) (see Figure 9-6): This tool is based on the NCCN guidelines for distress management in clinical practice. A 0–10 scale is used to measure a variety of psychosocial problems.
- European Organisation for Research and Treatment of Cancer (EORTC) Quality of Life Questionnaire: The EORTC questionnaire is used to assess quality of life in individuals with cancer participating in clinical trials. It considers physical symptoms, cognitive issues, fatigue, pain, nausea and vomiting, global health, and quality of life.
- Functional Assessment of Cancer Therapy–Breast (FACT-B): The FACT-B is a 46-item self-report scale that measures quality of life in the physical, social/family, emotional, and functional realms on a 5-point rating scale.
- Quality of Life Breast Cancer Instrument from City of Hope National Medical Center: Nineteen of the items are specific to breast cancer.
- Hospital Anxiety and Depression Scale (HADS): A brief tool that provides separate scores for anxiety and depression with suggested cutoff points to identify a possible mood disorder.
- The Medical Outcomes Study Short Form (SF-36): The SF-36 was designed for use in clinical practice, research health policy evaluations, and general surveys. It measures eight areas of functional status, well-being, and self-perceived health: physical functioning, social functioning, role limitations, mental health, energy and fatigue, pain, and general health perception.

Note. Based on information from Hewitt et al., 2004; National Comprehensive Cancer Network, 2005.

---

women in this phase of the cancer trajectory should not be overlooked. Finding a lump can be a frightening experience, as can an undefined or suspicious finding on a routine mammogram. This leads to additional appointments for more radiologic studies and often a biopsy. A period of days to a week or more can separate each phase of the diagnostic process. This can be a period of great anxiety and fear for women.

Women undergoing any type of biopsy may have escalated feelings of uncertainty and anxiety because of the potential diagnosis and its implications for relationships, mortality, and sexuality. Often this may be the first significant experience a woman has with health care or surgical procedures. Care during this time can be very fragmented, as a woman may be seen by radiologists, technicians, or surgeons. Specific psychosocial care services are very limited during this phase.

Waiting for the results of a pathologic diagnosis can be extremely difficult. It often takes nearly a week for a final report to become available, during which time women sometimes feel as though their lives are "on hold." Although many women eventually receive the good news that their biopsy was benign, a portion of women will receive a diagnosis of malignancy. Assisting women in finding a supportive environment and individuals during this phase is critical, especially when the diagnosis is a malignancy. Women who are inadequately informed as to what to expect during a biopsy usually have much higher levels of anxiety (Chappy, 2004). Stress can be increased with scheduling problems, long waits for appointments, and test results. All efforts should be made to reduce the time between the initial identification of the problem and the biopsy and to provide continuity of care with an identi-

fied provider who can answer questions and provide guidance along each step of the way. Comprehensive breast centers often have nurses who work in this capacity.

Reactions to the Diagnosis

Although women fear a diagnosis of breast cancer, the initial response when the diagnosis is confirmed and disclosed is often one of shock and disbelief (Hewitt et al., 2004), for them and their family or significant others. Although it is well publicized that a woman's lifetime risk of breast cancer is 1 in 8 (Morris, Wright, & Schlag, 2001), a breast cancer diagnosis at any point in a woman's life can be very stressful, very sudden, and unexpected. Without warning or choice, a woman is forced to abandon her current identified life to attend doctors' appointments and undergo tests that are unfamiliar and uncomfortable. Often, women feel as though they have lost control of their life during the days surrounding the initial diagnosis. Common reactions include denial, anger, fear, stress, anxiety, depression, sadness, guilt, and loneliness. Informing women that these are common reactions is the first step in facilitating adjustment to the diagnosis and its treatment.

Denial is a common reaction. The disbelief that the diagnosis has been made is actually psychologically protective, unless it persists for extended periods of time or impairs decision making regarding appropriate treatment. Short-term denial can be helpful because it gives patients time to enable their families and themselves to adjust to the diagnosis. Most patients work through the denial quickly and have some acceptance of the disease by the time treatment begins.

Figure 9-6. Distress Thermometer

SCREENING TOOLS FOR MEASURING DISTRESS

Instructions: First please circle the number (0-10) that best describes how much distress you have been experiencing in the past week including today.

Extreme distress 10

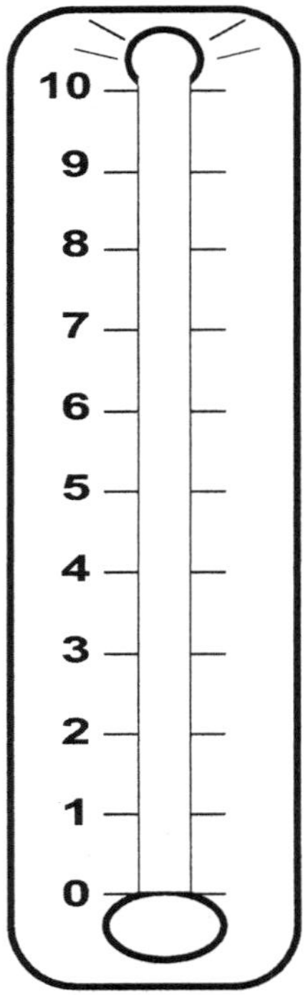

9

8

7

6

5

4

3

2

1

0 **No distress**

Second, please indicate if any of the following has been a problem for you in the past week including today. Be sure to check YES or NO for each.

YES NO **Practical Problems**
☐ ☐ Child care
☐ ☐ Housing
☐ ☐ Insurance/financial
☐ ☐ Transportation
☐ ☐ Work/school

Family Problems
☐ ☐ Dealing with children
☐ ☐ Dealing with partner

Emotional Problems
☐ ☐ Depression
☐ ☐ Fears
☐ ☐ Nervousness
☐ ☐ Sadness
☐ ☐ Worry
☐ ☐ Loss of interest in usual activities

☐ ☐ **Spiritual/religious concerns**

YES NO **Physical Problems**
☐ ☐ Appearance
☐ ☐ Bathing/dressing
☐ ☐ Breathing
☐ ☐ Changes in urination
☐ ☐ Constipation
☐ ☐ Diarrhea
☐ ☐ Eating
☐ ☐ Fatigue
☐ ☐ Feeling Swollen
☐ ☐ Fevers
☐ ☐ Getting around
☐ ☐ Indigestion
☐ ☐ Memory/concentration
☐ ☐ Mouth sores
☐ ☐ Nausea
☐ ☐ Nose dry/congested
☐ ☐ Pain
☐ ☐ Sexual
☐ ☐ Skin dry/itchy
☐ ☐ Sleep
☐ ☐ Tingling in hands/feet

Other Problems: _____
_____

Note. From "The NCCN (1.2007) Distress Management Guideline," in *The Complete Library of NCCN Clinical Practice Guidelines in Oncology* [CD-ROM], by National Comprehensive Cancer Network, June 2006, Jenkintown, PA.: Author. Copyright 2006 by the National Comprehensive Cancer Network. Reprinted with permission. To view the most recent and complete version of the guideline, visit www.nccn.org.

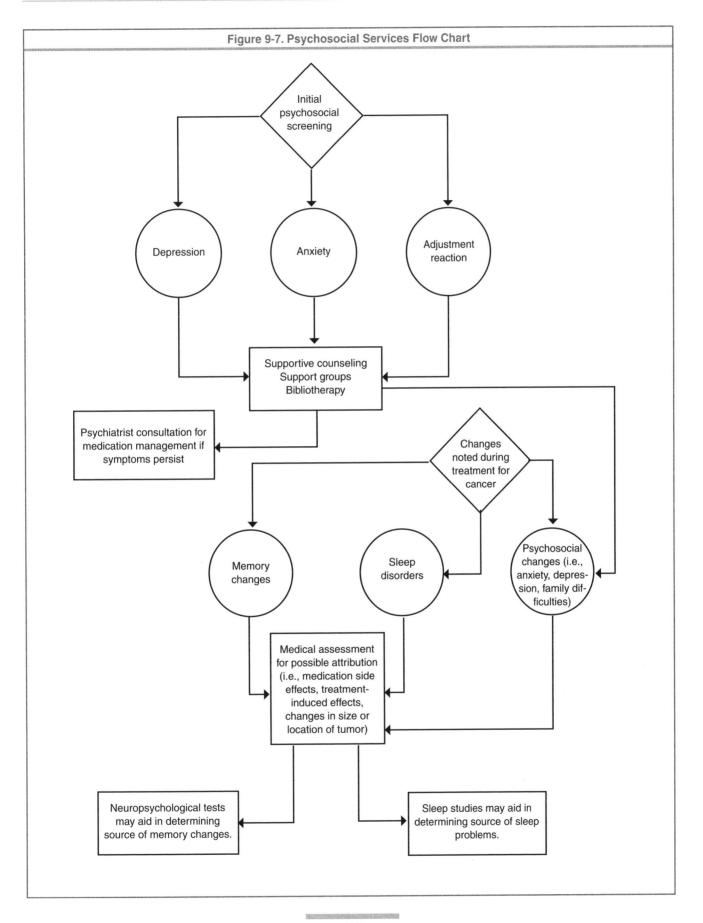

Figure 9-7. Psychosocial Services Flow Chart

Anger is another reaction that must be acknowledged and dealt with. Patients and families can be angry about the diagnosis and specifically with healthcare providers, family, friends, and sometimes an existential power. Encouraging individuals to discuss their feelings of anger can be an effective tool.

A wide range of fears and concerns can accompany the diagnosis of breast cancer. Patients and families most often are initially fearful of existential concerns and mortality. As the reality of the diagnosis surfaces, fears may shift toward experiencing pain, alopecia, nausea and vomiting, surgery, unknown healthcare procedures, and fatigue; managing day-to-day activities for the family; paying for the costs of treatment; and keeping a job. Patients with cancer also may have many fears and concerns about how to discuss the diagnosis with friends and others. Identification of specific fears and developing concrete strategies to manage each specific problem can be very effective in reducing stress.

Reactive depression commonly occurs when the diagnosis is initially made. Signs of depression include feelings of helplessness, hopelessness, and loss of interest in family, friends, and activities. Physical manifestations of depression might include loss of appetite, changes in energy level, or sleep disturbances. Depending on the seriousness of the depression and the length of obvious symptoms, short- or long-term intervention may be indicated. Women and their families need to be counseled that these interventions are not being delivered because the person is "weak" but rather to improve quality of life and facilitate tolerance of the treatment. Any suicidal thoughts require immediate intervention, and patients and families should be instructed on this point.

Guilt is another common reaction to the diagnosis of breast cancer. Some women feel guilt related to prior use of hormone replacement therapy or birth control pills. Others feel guilt if they believe they have a hereditary predisposition for developing breast cancer and fear they have passed the susceptibility gene on to a child. Others feel guilty because they perceive themselves to be a burden to others. Acknowledging that these feelings are common may be helpful, as well as encouraging patients to discuss them.

Information Seeking and Treatment Decision Making

Once the diagnosis of breast cancer has been made, the patient, family, and physicians will begin to discuss treatment. Most women are unprepared for the diagnosis and even less prepared for the array of medical consultants they will be scheduled to see in a relatively short period of time, as well as the number of treatment decisions they will have to make. Lives and work schedules usually are abruptly interrupted for not only the patients but also those supporting them during the decision-making and treatment process.

The first few days and weeks after the biopsy involve more diagnostic workups, which can be both a frightening and unfamiliar experience for patients. This is necessary to determine the stage of disease and other prognostic factors. This information can be technically complex. Many times, healthcare providers have difficulty explaining the details of the pathology reports, and patients can have significant difficulty understanding the findings. This can lead to more anxiety and distress for women with cancer and for those supporting them.

Following the discussion of the pathologic findings come the decisions regarding treatment. This can be a very overwhelming experience. Often, more than one treatment is discussed or suggested, which may require the patient to make choices about the best treatment(s) for her. Women frequently are asked to decide about the type of treatment (mastectomy with or without reconstruction or lumpectomy with radiation) and subsequent treatment (standard or investigational). Essentially, patients are asked to make important treatment decisions about which they usually have little knowledge and background and to choose a medical care team with which they are comfortable. Some patients find that this decision-making process restores a sense of control, whereas others find this choice very stressful. The ability to make informed decisions may be influenced by patients' educational level, stress level, family and social support systems, and previous experiences with the healthcare system. Women need to be reminded that although they must make a decision, they should not be too hasty, which can result in decisions that are later regretted (Hewitt et al., 2004). Patients can be encouraged to get a second opinion with another group of specialists to help to ensure that treatment decisions are appropriate.

Communication and patient education can be challenging because of the shock of the diagnosis. Shock and anxiety can limit one's ability to comprehend and register information (Kerr, Engel, Schlesinger-Raab, Sauer, & Holzel, 2003). Acceptance of the disease and its treatment comes at different rates for different individuals. Lack of information increases anxiety, and adequate information can provide individuals with some sense of control. Striking a balance is important.

Psychosocial distress also may be increased during this time because women may have to deal with multiple specialists. Although these providers ideally are seen as a team, often women must go from office to office or to different departments. Fragmentation of care can be an additional psychosocial burden (Hewitt et al., 2004).

Decisions regarding treatment lie with the patient but must be made based on information from the physician, nurse, and other resources. Some treatment alternatives are based on the size or location of the tumor, whereas other treatments may be suggested because of preexisting or comorbid conditions. With the decision to have surgery, patients then face the additional choice of lumpectomy versus mastectomy. This is a personal choice for women and may be based on fear, preconceived ideas about the surgery and body image changes, or financial concerns. Some women may fear recurrence of the breast cancer and feel they will have a better chance for survival if their entire breast or even both breasts are removed.

Additionally, body image plays a major role in treatment decisions. Some patients may choose a lumpectomy because of the perceived inability to handle the changes made by a mastectomy. Other women feel they will no longer "feel like a woman" without breasts. Some patients may agree to a mastectomy if immediate reconstruction can be done. This may be possible for some patients, but for others, there may be a medical reason to delay reconstruction, especially if postoperative chemotherapy and/or radiation therapy is needed. The treatment team, including the medical oncologist, radiation oncologist, surgeon, nurse, and patient, should discuss the reasons behind the delay.

A subset of women have a germ-line genetic predisposition for developing breast cancer, and these women may choose to undergo prophylactic surgery on the unaffected breast. The decision for a prophylactic mastectomy will reduce the chances of a second primary cancer occurring in the other breast and may improve cosmesis, especially in women with large breasts (see Chapter 2). The treatment team must discuss these issues and should explore the psychological consequences of patients' choices throughout the decision-making process.

Financial concerns also may play a role in the choice of treatment for patients with breast cancer. Financial assistance programs are available to help to defray the costs of some treatments (e.g., Partnership for Prescription Assistance [www.pparx.org]). Patients should be encouraged to discuss their financial concerns with the medical team to minimize anxiety about payment. Other support agencies are available to help patients in dealing with financial problems throughout treatment, such as the hospital's social work department, the American Cancer Society (www.cancer.org), or the American Association for Cancer Research (www.aacr.org).

Active Treatment

Once the treatment plan is determined, patients may feel some sense of relief, but then new fears and concerns related to the treatment usually surface. The shift toward outpatient and short-stay surgical procedures adds to the psychosocial distress for some families. Distress may be related to the presence of drains and dressings or to limited mobility because someone must be available to help with the management of the incision and household tasks. Careful assessment of the support system available to patients is necessary for successful care. Often, those who assist patients will have psychosocial concerns that also need to be addressed.

Following the initial adjustment to the diagnosis of cancer, patients begin the journey of treatment. Treatment may include any combination of surgery, chemotherapy, radiation therapy,

hormonal therapy, or close follow-up. Treatment results in a change in physical health, which also affects patients' psychosocial health. These include side effects from therapy, role changes, and body image alterations.

Depression and anxiety can increase as side effects worsen, which can intensify the physical symptoms. Depression can increase anxiety and pain, cause difficulty with concentration, and result in insomnia (Greene, Nail, Fieler, Dudgeon, & Jones, 1994; McDonald et al., 1999). This cycle (i.e., depression causing physical symptoms and physical symptoms causing more depression) often is difficult to identify and even harder to break. Psychosocial support can help to control some side effects, ultimately affecting patients' tolerance to treatment.

Long-Term Survivors

The end of treatment can be a time of mixed emotions. The stress associated with the transition often is underestimated. Patients may feel a sense of joy in completing treatment, but there also is the fear of leaving the close monitoring of the healthcare team. A sense of comfort comes from having chemotherapy or radiation therapy that will fight the cancer. When treatment is over, the sense of control over the cancer, in some patients, also is taken away. Talking with others who have completed treatment may help to normalize these feelings.

Patients also may have feelings of anxiety and depression about taking hormonal therapy after completion of surgery, chemotherapy, and/or radiation. The risk of future serious side effects frightens some women, ultimately affecting their adjustment to the end of treatment. Psychosocial support can help patients to identify their fears and find ways of discussing them with family, friends, and the healthcare team.

Many survivors also are unprepared for the lingering effects of therapy, including fatigue, cognitive dysfunction, and menstrual symptoms (Ganz et al., 2004). Researchers have found that general oncology clinicians often spend much time preparing patients for the acute toxicities of treatment (e.g., nausea, vomiting, fatigue, alopecia) and much less time on what to expect in the pattern of recovery and adjustment following active treatment. Although clinicians may tell patients that it takes as much time to recover as it did to complete the therapy, little is specifically known about how this recovery takes place.

Throughout the diagnosis and treatment period, it is common for a woman to identify herself as a patient with cancer. Other roles, such as wife, mother, or career woman, are put on hold, and cancer becomes the main focus. Although often difficult, it is important for patients with cancer to learn to integrate the cancer and related treatments into their lives. Some patients may find strength in groups where other women discuss how they returned to normal lives (i.e., their lives without cancer), whereas others may prefer individual counseling to help them to understand the meaning of the illness and return to a normal life. The ultimate goal is to understand the effects of the cancer on the individual and the best ways to move forward with life. For some, this may mean a change in career, whereas others may find they have a different perspective on life after having experienced a serious illness. They may be less bothered by everyday nuisances, or they may find themselves searching for new meaning in their lives.

Following the end of treatment, some women may find the possibility of a recurrence frightening and almost paralyzing. For some, this fear is manifested as an increased dependence on the healthcare team. Although the concerns may seem excessive to everyone other than the patient, a cancer survivor may consider every ache and pain to be related to a recurrence of the cancer. This may create unnecessary stress on both the patient and the healthcare team. Thewes, Butow, Girgis, and Pendlebury (2004) interviewed 18 breast cancer survivors and found that the majority of women reported a need to be reassured that late effects, such as aches and pains or fatigue, caused by past anticancer treatments were not a sign of recurrence.

The fear of recurrence also can affect a survivor's willingness to continue medical follow-up. These fears can be addressed in a support group setting or with individual psychosocial support. Many women find strength in having faced breast cancer and feel that their lives are stronger because of it.

Long-term survivorship can be influenced by healthy living habits following the diagnosis of and treatment for breast cancer. Exercise has been associated with higher quality of life at least 10 years after cancer diagnosis (Kendall, Mahue-Giangreco, Carpenter, Ganz, & Bernstein, 2005; Vallance, Courneya, Jones, & Reiman, 2005; van Weert et al., 2005) as well as decreasing long-term fatigue, which often is felt following treatment for cancer (Bower, 2005). Exercise also can have a positive effect on body image of breast cancer survivors and should be encouraged in patients throughout the cancer continuum (Blanchard et al., 2003).

Additionally, diet can have a positive impact on survivors of breast cancer. Women without a diagnosis of cancer often cater to their families' preference of food, whereas women with a diagnosis of breast cancer felt supported by their families in their choice to change to healthy eating habits following their diagnosis (Beagan & Chapman, 2004). Healthy eating habits also help in developing a positive body image, maintaining weight, decreasing fatigue, and increasing heart health.

Healthcare professionals should not underestimate the stressors and fears that often are present in long-term survivors. Although follow-up visits for these patients are not as complicated, these women and their families still require and benefit from careful psychosocial assessment and intervention. Figure 9-8 shows some helpful strategies to suggest to patients.

Recurrent/Advanced Disease

Although the overall prognosis for breast cancer is good, especially for those who have early-stage disease, an estimated 30%–40% of women will experience a recurrence of breast cancer (Hewitt et al., 2004). Recurrence is defined as the return of the disease after an initial course of treatment with a disease-free period. Although recurrence does not necessarily lead to terminal illness, patients with recurrent disease usually are much more aware of the reality of and potential mortality of their diagnosis. Often this event occurs years after the initial diagnosis. For many, it is considered a failure for both the patient and the treatment team. Because recurrence frequently is associated with clinical symptoms from the cancer, including increased pain, cough, headaches, or other changes, patients have a tangible constant reminder that their condition is serious and perhaps life-limiting. This can lead to enormous stress for both patients and families.

Recurrent disease may involve the same treatment as the initial cancer, a similar treatment, or something completely different. Women may feel overwhelmed by the treatment and their potential mortality. Recurrent disease is a distinctly different emotional event than the initial diagnosis (Mahon & Casperson, 1995). Women with recurrent breast cancer may have more anxiety about treatment because of previous experiences as well as more symptom distress, including fatigue and pain. Patients also may have anger, self-blame, and regret about prior treatment choices. Women may be less hopeful, as the first treatment did not completely eradicate the disease.

As the disease progresses, attention to symptom and pain relief becomes paramount. This phase of the illness also may be accompanied by spiritual and existential concerns. Patients encounter many fears in the terminal phases of disease, including fear of the unknown, pain, suffering, abandonment, loss of control, loss of identity, loss of body image, loss of loved ones, and loss of hope (Gorman, 2006). Acknowledgment of these fears and the fact that they are common reactions often is the first step in helping patients to cope with these overwhelming feelings. Open communication with family members and significant others may decrease some distress and offer an opportunity for closure not only for patients but also for those involved in their care.

Interventions to Promote Psychosocial Health

Bibliotherapy

Bibliotherapy is a form of therapy in which selected reading materials are used to help to identify and solve problems. The amount of information available regarding a diagnosis of breast cancer can be very overwhelming. Web sites, books,

---

> **Figure 9-8. Strategies and Interventions to Prepare Individuals and Families for Long-Term Survivorship**
>
> - Give patients and families a range of what to expect that could potentially happen in terms of prognosis, physical symptoms, emotional concerns, and sexual function.
> - Remind patients and significant others that they may never return to "normal" and that they may need to establish a new normalcy.
> - Specifically define what symptoms should promptly be reported for further evaluation.
> - Describe the anticipated follow-up schedule for office visits, scans, and laboratory work with the rationale for the proposed schedule.
> - Teach patients what tertiary prevention is and what specific tertiary screening measures will be recommended (i.e., colon screening, bone densitometry, gynecologic screening).
> - Develop a wellness plan including a specific strategy for exercise, diet, skin cancer prevention, and smoking cessation when indicated.
> - Remind patients and significant others that it is common to have "trigger" events that are upsetting such as the anniversary of diagnosis, the diagnosis of a loved one with a similar disease, or feelings of anxiety surrounding things that remind patients of unpleasant aspects of treatment.
> - Discuss that recovery from treatment is a gradual process and that it may take a year or more before full energy returns.
> - Assess for mental health problems. Manage depression and anxiety early. Remind patients and family members that it is common to have some feelings of depression, anxiety, or being overwhelmed even though treatment is completed. Discuss that treatments are available to manage these symptoms, and patients should bring these concerns to the attention of healthcare providers to explore the best means to improve this quality-of-life aspect.
> - Acknowledge that patients may need to adopt a new self-image in terms of energy, physical appearance, and sexuality. For many, staying active and exploring new hobbies and activities helps them to develop a new self-image.
> - Assess for financial problems. Survivors may be paying for the costs of care long after treatment is complete. If appropriate, remind patients that social services may be able to assist them.
> - Discuss the importance of maintaining continuous healthcare coverage. If the patient or family member carrying the insurance wants to switch jobs or something else occurs that would lead to a lapse in coverage, he or she should consider a referral to social services.
> - Patients and significant others may want to consider becoming an advocate for others with cancer or volunteering in some other way. Some individuals find benefit from continued participation in a support group.
> - Instruct patients to let their healthcare provider know if they are experiencing problems or changes with memory or concentration after chemotherapy, as sometimes there are strategies to decrease the impact of these problems.
> - Advise patients and their family members to consider learning more about genetic risk if the family history suggests hereditary susceptibility for developing the cancer and they have not yet received counseling about genetic testing.
> - Instruct survivors that they may need to plan what they want to disclose, how to disclose it, and how much to disclose. When meeting new people or dating, it can be awkward to know when to disclose that the individual has completed cancer treatment. Talking with other survivors can help patients to feel more comfortable with how and when to disclose.
> - Advise patients that they may still face challenges in the workplace related to follow-up care, energy levels, or other health-related concerns. Encourage patients to discuss these needs with their employer. If problems cannot be resolved, a referral to social services, local cancer advocacy services, or perhaps legal resources may be indicated.

pamphlets, and help lines are available to provide information about the diagnosis and treatment options and the use or misuse of complementary and alternative treatments. Although many of the resources available provide quality information, a wide range of medical misinformation and misrepresentation can be found in both the academic and popular press. For example, Bichakjian et al. (2002) conducted a study examining 74 of the most frequented medical Web sites on the topic of melanoma. The researchers critiqued the sites based on a 35-point checklist rating system that was developed using knowledge from the University of Michigan Multidisciplinary Melanoma Clinic. The authors found that strategies for the prevention of melanoma were poorly reported. Not only did the sites omit information on risk factors, prevention, and early detection, but also factual inaccuracies were noted in 14% of the Web sites. In another study, Berland et al. (2001) examined the quality of 25 health-information Web sites provided by one search engine. Thirty-four physicians examined the content for information on breast cancer, childhood asthma, depression, and obesity, in both English and Spanish languages. They found that less than one-fourth of the search engine's first pages of links led to relevant content (20% of the English-language Web sites and 12% of the Spanish-language Web sites). On average, 45% of the clinical elements on the English-language Web sites and 22% on the Spanish-language Web sites were more than minimally covered and completely accurate. In addition, 24% of the clinical elements on the English-language Web sites and 53% on the Spanish-language Web sites were not covered at all. These studies highlight that objective assessment of the accuracy and currentness of Web-accessed information is unavailable to those who peruse the resources, and ethics of advice given on the Web often are unexamined (Flowers-Coulson, Kushner, & Bankowski, 2000). Without this editorial control, online information may be published with a political or financial agenda rather than in the best interest of the patient. As a result, use of the Internet can be associated with negative consequences. These include medical misperceptions, unrealistic expectations, loss of confidence in conventional medicine, and possibly serious adverse effects from drugs procured by way of the Internet (Pereira, Bruera, Macmillan, & Kavanagh, 2000).

Consequently, with no peer-review processes or editorial mechanisms in place that allow Web-published material to undergo scientific scrutiny, patients are subject to information that may be wrong, sensationalized, or even dangerous (Pereira & Bruera, 1998).

Helping patients to identify appropriate sources of information regarding breast cancer should be a priority for healthcare professionals throughout the cancer trajectory. During the initial assessment, healthcare professionals should determine whether the patient wants a large amount of information or if only the essential information should be provided over time. Reliable resources are available through many Web sites to help patients in understanding breast cancer and the available treatment modalities (see Appendix 1).

Behavioral Techniques

Guided Imagery

Guided imagery is a technique that is used to help patients picture themselves in a relaxing environment. A common choice is a beach scene or a meadow with a stream flowing through. Patients are encouraged to relax their bodies. To encourage relaxation, a calm and soothing voice is used, and patients are led through an imaginary relaxing scene. Patients are encouraged to imagine the scene visually and how the scene smells or feels. They are given positive suggestions, such as allowing their bodies to relax and allowing the nausea to leave their bodies. They are encouraged to practice the skills of guided imagery on their own or with the help of an audio recording. Patients should be encouraged to identify the cues that trigger nausea and begin using guided imagery when needed. Guided imagery should not be used with patients who have a history of psychotic or dissociative disorders, as the risk of a psychotic episode can be increased during the imagery exercise. Examples of guided imagery scripts and an audio CD can be found in *Voice Massage: Scripts for Guided Imagery* (Edwards, 2002).

Progressive Muscle Relaxation

Progressive muscle relaxation therapy (PMRT) is a more active approach to relaxation. It is helpful for patients who need to gain a sense of control over their bodies. Patients are taught the difference between a tense or tight muscle and a relaxed muscle by tensing and relaxing muscle groups in a systematic way through the body. It is customary to begin relaxing the toes and then progressively tense and relax muscle groups throughout the body until reaching the head. The ability to identify stress in the form of muscle tension allows patients to reduce the tension through PMRT as needed. PMRT should not be used in patients who have pain that can be increased through muscle tension.

Hypnosis

Hypnosis also is used to alleviate some treatment-related side effects. Hypnosis helps patients to relax and creates an environment in which positive suggestions can be used to decrease side effects such as nausea and vomiting, offer pain relief, or increase appetite. Hypnosis uses similar relaxation strategies as discussed with guided imagery. Patients are instructed to relax, and suggestions are offered to deepen the relaxation to a particular state. In the suggestible state, positive suggestions can be applied to address the specific symptom. Because false or incorrect memories may be created during hypnosis, only trained professionals should perform hypnosis to minimize the potential for false memories that are believed to be true.

Supportive Measures for Specific Problems

Alopecia and Skin Changes

Hair loss, or alopecia, is a side effect that can cause great distress during treatment for breast cancer. Although some women embrace hair loss as a symbol of their fight against the disease, others may feel self-conscious. Alopecia can be a traumatic event, and preparing patients for this occurrence may help with the adjustment. Some patients want to keep their own hair for as long as possible, preferring that it falls out gradually. Other patients adjust better by cutting the hair short prior to the time they will begin to lose it. Both of these choices can help patients to gain a little control over what feels like—and basically is—an uncontrollable event.

Many options exist for hair covering, including wigs, scarves, and hats (see Figure 9-9). Patients may find it hard to see themselves without hair, and some women will wear a head covering even while alone (McGarvey, Baum, Pinderton, & Rogers, 2001). Many resources are available to help women with adjusting to the hair loss of cancer therapy as well as some of the other physical changes they may experience. "Look Good . . . Feel Better®" is a free program sponsored by the Cosmetic, Toiletry, and Fragrance Association Foundation in partnership with the American Cancer Society and the National Cosmetology Association. The program's Web site (www.lookgoodfeelbetter.org) has helpful tips for hair and makeup as well as a program finder for classes where women can learn hair and makeup tips while undergoing cancer treatment. The information is available in both English and Spanish, and specific information is available for teens. Another resource, *Facing the Mirror With Cancer* (Ovitz, 2004), can help patients to feel the best they can with their physical appearance.

In addition to hair loss, some patients also may experience skin changes from treatment. Radiation therapy can cause redness and irritation of the skin. Redness may occur early in the treatment, whereas dry or moist desquamation occurs nearer to the end of the scheduled treatment; both may continue following treatment. Another possible side effect of radiation therapy is hyperpigmentation, and the darker pigmentation

Figure 9-9. Head Coverings

Prior to beginning chemotherapy treatment, nurses should discuss with patients the options available for head coverings, including wigs, scarves, and hats.

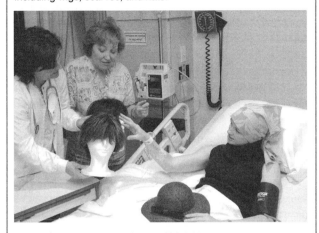

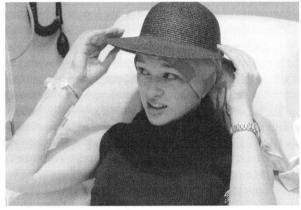

Note. Photos courtesy of Hoag Hospital. Used with permission.

may remain following treatment. Radiated skin is more sensitive to exposure to ultraviolet light, and skin protection must continue indefinitely. Hyperpigmentation also may occur following administration of some chemotherapeutic agents. Skin color should be expected to slowly return to normal following chemotherapy.

Weight Changes

For most people, food is a source of joy and comfort. However, for patients experiencing nausea, vomiting, and diarrhea, food can become a source of frustration. The question of "What did you eat today?" can be a problem among the patient, the family, and the healthcare team. The weight loss that occurs is a visual reminder of the stress of eating and the resulting changes in body image, which can contribute to feelings of anxiety and depression. Nutritional supplements are available to improve calorie and protein intake for patients

who are having a difficult time eating. The supplements come in many different forms, including powders, liquids, and semi-solids. A nutritional consultation may be helpful for women experiencing weight loss and difficulty eating.

Weight gain also can occur as a result of treatment for breast cancer and can have an impact on body image. Medications such as steroids used as part of a chemotherapy regimen can cause increased hunger and weight gain. An average gain of 5–14 pounds has been observed with the use of steroids, but a weight gain of up to 50 pounds has been reported with the use of hormonal therapy (Demark-Wahnefried, Rimer, & Winer, 1997). Extreme weight gains are more common in premenopausal women who have received a higher dosage of medication over a longer period of time or when multiagent treatments are used (Demark-Wahnefried et al.). At a time when the patient may already have difficulty with body image because of the diagnosis of cancer, weight gain may add more stress and prevent some women from agreeing to therapy.

Sexuality

Potential changes in sexuality must be addressed for women with breast cancer. Concerns about sexuality begin at the time of diagnosis. Many women connect sexuality with their breasts, and the removal of the breast or any part of a breast may affect their sexual identity. Women may feel uncomfortable initiating a discussion about sexuality at the time of diagnosis, a time when they feel the focus should be on the disease and treatment of the disease. In addition, discussing sexuality is frequently considered taboo. Following surgery for breast cancer, women may feel they do not want their partners to touch them in the same ways as prior to surgery based either on emotional concerns of touching the surgical area or because of altered sensations in the breast from the treatment. Women should be encouraged to communicate their needs and feelings to their partners to lessen discomfort physically and emotionally for both of them.

In addition to the issues surrounding body image, women also may experience sexual side effects based on their treatment. Distressing short-term effects of adjuvant chemotherapy include fatigue, alopecia, constipation, nausea, stomatitis, and weight gain. All of these side effects can contribute to altered sexual functioning because of decreased libido. Some changes that women may experience related to any combination of surgery, chemotherapy, and radiation therapy include vaginal dryness, altered libido, changes in menses and fertility, skin reactions, fatigue, and lymphedema.

Currently, most women without a diagnosis of breast cancer can expect to live at least one-third of their life in the postmenopausal state. For women treated aggressively for breast cancer, its duration can be significantly longer. Hot flashes may be more troublesome to younger women diagnosed with breast cancer (Schultz, Klein, Beck, Stava, & Sellin, 2005). An estimated 53%–89% of premenopausal women experience ovarian failure and premature menopause after receiving polyagent chemotherapy (Rogers & Kristjanson, 2002). The older the woman, the higher the risk. When menopause occurs quickly, the symptoms may be more profound, including increased and more severe mood swings, increased hot flashes, and vaginal dryness.

Vaginal dryness is an often overlooked concern. Use of hormone replacement therapy is controversial. Alternate therapies that should be suggested include the use of vaginal lubricants such as K-Y® Jelly (McNeil-PPC, Inc., Fort Washington, PA) or Replens® (Lil' Drug Store Products, Cedar Rapids, IA). Women should be informed that sexual dysfunction is common, and the first step in treatment is assessment and communication (Stead, 2003).

Psychosocial support may help women to cope with both the altered sexuality and body image. Instruction on how to communicate their needs and concerns to their partners can help to allay some anxiety. Once therapy has been completed, patients may continue to experience altered sexuality. Ongoing psychosocial counseling and support can help patients to learn ways to integrate the cancer and treatment effects into daily life.

Fertility

Although breast cancer most often is diagnosed in mid to later life, breast cancer also can be diagnosed in younger women. Some of the options offered to treat the cancer may affect patients' fertility. Many options are available to help these women with issues of infertility. Prior to a diagnosis of cancer, a woman who is at high risk for developing cancer of the breast or ovary may be offered genetic testing to assess her risk of developing cancer. At the time of the disclosure of her genetic results, she should be counseled regarding the options available to her, including earlier childbearing, egg harvesting, and storing fertilized embryos. Removal of the entire ovary for freezing is also a technique with a promising future for preserving fertility (Bedaiwy & Falcone, 2004). Following treatment, the embryos may be implanted into the woman, who may be able to carry a pregnancy to term. The type of tumor may affect patients' options for pregnancy, so complete knowledge of the tumor and the treatment that will be offered must be available prior to this discussion with patients. Estrogen and progesterone receptors may prevent women from carrying a pregnancy to term. Surrogacy and adoption are options that patients and their partners may need to consider if pregnancy is not possible.

The psychological consequences of infertility can be devastating to patients and may result in increased anxiety and depression. Younger women with breast cancer must cope not only with cancer at a young age but also with infertility, most likely caused by treatment for the breast cancer. Fertile Hope (www.fertilehope.org) is an organization designed to help patients with cancer to deal with fertility issues. It offers resources about options available prior to diagnosis, during treatment, and following treatment.

Body Image

After surgery and treatment for breast cancer, women may perceive their body as disfigured and feel that they have lost part of their feminine identity (Vos, Garssen, Visser, Duivenvoorden, & de Haes, 2004). Vos et al. reported that five years after treatment, 25%–75% of the women still had disturbances with their body image. This is probably related not only to the surgery and other treatments but also to individual coping styles and patients' perceived level of support.

Women need to be counseled about choices in breast restoration. This can include breast prosthetics or reconstructive surgery (see Chapter 5). This is important psychologically and physically. Psychologically, it helps women to feel better about themselves. Physically, weight replacement of the breast is important to prevent long-term shoulder and posture problems. Women should be encouraged to learn about all their options before making a choice. Women also should be reminded that one choice is not necessarily better than another. Women need to choose what is most comfortable for them and compatible with their lifestyle.

Pharmacologic Management

The exact prevalence of depression and other mental health problems in women with breast cancer is not fully understood. It may be as high as twice the incidence seen in the general population (Burgess et al., 2005). Suggested risk factors include younger age at diagnosis, previous problems with depression, and lack of adequate psychosocial support. Pharmacologic management may be used to alleviate some of the psychosocial effects of cancer and its treatment.

Antidepressants may help patients who feel extreme sadness, hopelessness, or a lack of interest in activities. Medications also may be used to help patients sleep, relax, and begin to cope with the diagnosis. As with any medication, potential side effects and interactions should be discussed that may occur with current medications and medical treatments. Common side effects of antidepressants and/or antianxiety medications include nausea, weight gain, sexual side effects, fatigue or insomnia, dry mouth, blurred vision, constipation, dizziness, mental slowing, and restlessness. A routine evaluation of the patient's response to these medications should be performed. See Table 9-1 for examples of commonly used antidepressants.

Family and Social Issues

Communication With Children

The American Cancer Society has useful tips to aid parents in talking to children in developmentally appropriate ways regarding cancer, and the Oncology Nursing Society offers

Table 9-1. Antidepressant Agents

Classification/Drug	Dose	Side Effects	Comments
SNRIs*, tricyclics (primary serotonin, mixed norepinephrine and serotonin uptake)			
Amitriptyline (generic only)	25–75 mg po every day up to 150–300 mg every day	High sedation, dry mouth, blurred vision, constipation, urinary hesitancy, confusion, orthostatic hypotension, seizures, weight gain, sexual disturbances	Time to steady state, 4–10 days; up to one month before beneficial effects are seen
Clomipramine (Anafranil®a)	25–75 mg po every day up to 150–240 mg every day	As above	Steady state 7–14 days
Doxepin (Sinequan®b)	25–75 mg po every day up to 150–300 mg every day	As above	Steady state 2–8 days; 2–3 weeks for maximum effect; available in capsule, elixir, and cream; used for chronic urticaria
Imipramine (Tofranil®a)	25–75 mg po every day up to 150–300 mg every day	Moderate sedation as above	Used for panic disorder; steady state 2–6 days
Trimipramine (Surmontil®c)	25–75 mg po every day up to 150–300 mg every day	As above	Steady state 2–6 days
SNRIs, tricyclics (secondary)			
Desipramine (Norpramin®d)	25–75 mg po every am	Slight sedation, bad taste, as above	Steady state 2–11 days; response in first week
Nortriptyline (Pamelor®a)	25–50 mg po every day up to 50–150 mg every day	As above	Steady state 4–19 days; available in elixir
Protriptyline (Vivactil®c)	15 mg po every am up to 15–60 mg every day	As above	Steady state 4–19 days
SNRIs, nontricyclic (third-generation heterocyclic) (serotonin and norepinephrine)			
Venlafaxine (Effexor®e)	75 mg po every day up to 150–225 mg/day in divided doses	Nausea, somnolence, sweating, dizziness, anxiety, sexual disturbances, hypertension	Available in extended release
MAO* inhibitors (serotonin, norepinephrine, dopamine)			
Phenazine (Nardil®b)	15 mg po tid up to 45–90 mg every day in divided doses	Headache, drowsiness, dry mouth, weight gain, postural hypotension, sexual disturbances, neuropathy	Give vitamin B$_6$ 50 mg po every day to avoid neuropathy; interacts with tyramine found in fermented foods and beverages; steady state 3–4 weeks
Tranylcypromine (Parnate®f)	10 mg po every am up to 10–40 mg/day in divided doses	As above	As above
SSRIs*			
Citalopram (Celexa®g)	20 mg po every day up to 60 mg po every day	Anxiety, insomnia, tremor, gastrointestinal symptoms, rashes, decreased libido, sexual dysfunction, slight sedation	–
Escitalopram (Lexapro®g)	10 mg po every day up to 20 mg po every day	As above	Available in elixir

(Continued on next page)

Table 9-1. Antidepressant Agents *(Continued)*			
Classification/Drug	**Dose**	**Side Effects**	**Comments**
SSRIs* *(Cont.)*			
Fluoxetine (Prozac[®h])	20 mg po every am up to 40 mg po every day	As above	Available in elixir
Fluvoxamine (Luvox[®i])	50 mg po every day up to 100–300 mg po in divided doses	As above	Avoid theophylline; increases caffeine half-life.
Sertraline (Zoloft[®b])	50 mg po every day up to 200 mg po every day	As above	–
Paroxetine (Paxil[®f])	20 mg po every day up to 50–200 mg po every day	As above	Available in elixir
NDRIs* (norepinephrine, some dopamine)			
Bupropion (Wellbutrin[®f])	100 mg po bid; after 4–7 days, increase to tid	Dizziness, dry mouth, sweating, tremor, aggravation of psychosis; potential seizures at high doses	Contraindicated with seizures, bulimia, anorexia; steady state 7–10 days
SARIs* (serotonin, 5HT$_2$ antagonists)			
Nefazodone (generic only)	100 mg po bid up to 300–600 mg every day in divided doses	Nausea, drowsiness, dizziness, insomnia, agitation	Avoid concurrent use with astemizole or cisapride.
Trazodone (Desyrel[®i])	50 mg po every day up to 400–600 mg every day in divided doses	As above; high sedation	–
Mirtazapine (Remeron[®k])	15 mg po at bedtime up to 45 mg daily	Agranulocytosis, dry mouth, increased appetite, somnolence	Oral disintegrating tablets available
Serotonin dopamine receptor antagonists			
Olanzapine (Zyprexa[®h])	5–10 mg every day up to 20 mg every day	Dry mouth, somnolence, insomnia	Oral disintegrating tablets available
Risperidone (Risperdal[®l])	1 mg po bid up to 16 mg a day	Insomnia, agitation, extrapyramidal symptoms	Oral disintegrating tablets available

*MAO—monoamine oxidase; NDRIs—norepinephrine-dopamine reuptake inhibitors; SARIs—serotonin antagonist and reuptake inhibitors; SNRIs—serotonin-norepinephrine reuptake inhibitors; SSRIs—selective serotonin reuptake inhibitors

[a] Mallinckrodt Inc., St. Louis, MO; [b] Pfizer Inc., New York, NY; [c] Odyssey Pharmaceuticals, Inc., Florham Park, NJ; [d] Aventis Pharmaceuticals Inc., Bridgewater, NJ; [e] Wyeth Pharmaceuticals Inc., Philadelphia, PA; [f] GlaxoSmithKline, Research Triangle Park, NC; [g] Forest Pharmaceuticals, Inc., St. Louis, MO; [h] Eli Lilly and Co., Indianapolis, IN; [i] Solvay Pharmaceuticals, Inc., Marietta, GA; [j] Bristol-Myers Squibb Co., Princeton, NJ; [k] Organon USA, Inc., Roseland, NJ; [l] Janssen Pharmaceutica Products, Titusville, NJ

Note. From *Clinical Manual for the Oncology Advanced Practice Nurse* (2nd ed., pp. 1187–1190), by D. Camp-Sorrell and R.A. Hawkins (Eds.), 2006, Pittsburgh, PA: Oncology Nursing Society. Copyright 2006 by the Oncology Nursing Society. Reprinted with permission.

resources for discussing a parent's diagnosis and treatment with children (Schmidt, 2003; Yaffe, 1998). Helping children to understand what is happening to their family can help them to adapt throughout the process (American Cancer Society, 2001). Young children may believe a parent's illness is a result of their behavior, and they are being punished. The child also may have questions about how people get cancer and how it is spread, or they may be curious about why their mom is losing her hair. It is important to create an environment where children are able to ask questions and receive age-appropriate answers. Women with breast cancer who are in need of further support in talking to their children should be encouraged to seek help from a trained professional. Support groups exist that target the psychological needs of young children, teenagers, and partners. Family roles can shift rapidly during cancer treatment, and children may need to take on caregiver roles. Each patient will need different types of family support, and encouraging open communication allows for decision making regarding how that support can be given.

Younger women with breast cancer who are caring for children may be particularly stressed with the diagnosis. This stress may have negative effects on parenting (Sigal, Perry, Robbins, Gagne, & Nassif, 2003). Important mediators of this stress include the severity of the illness, the mother's adjustment to the illness, the stability of family relationships, and the children's coping style. A child may perceive a depressed mood in the mother as emotional inaccessibility. Constraints from the illness and treatment also may make the mother physically inaccessible for periods of time. Furthermore, the stressors of the illness may narrow the parent's attention, ability, and threshold to parent and address behavioral issues in the child. This reduction in parental attention may negatively manifest itself in the child as disruptive behavior, or the child may become saddened because of the losses in the relationship with the mother. During periods of recurrence and advanced/terminal disease, mothers may believe that caring for their children is more important than disciplining them.

Families with childrearing concerns or children with concerns often benefit from services that are tailored to these needs. Mutual disclosure of fears, anxieties, and hopes among mothers, significant others, and children appears to have benefits for both patients and their families (Sigal et al., 2003).

Teenage children can have particular challenges and difficulty accepting and adjusting to the diagnosis of breast cancer in a mother. Verbalizing their feelings and concerns with their parents and significant others, and perhaps another trusted adult, may be very helpful.

Children and teens should be encouraged to go to school, complete homework, and continue to participate in extracurricular activities and sports. Parents may need to rely on the assistance of others from time to time to enable children to continue participating in these activities. If a woman is unable to attend an activity with a child, she should make every effort to find out about it when the child comes home. Often an event can be videotaped so the parent can share in the activity with the child at a later point. Helpful interventions include preparing the children for what is going to happen in the immediate future and what the more distant future holds. For some, relationships are strengthened by the challenges imposed by breast cancer and its treatment. Open communication with children and honest answers to emotionally laden questions, including questions about death, in age-appropriate terms are important. Parents may need coaching and assistance with these issues. Open communication helps parents to understand children's worries and thoughts and can lead to increased understanding. Support

should provide concrete strategies that are child appropriate and child oriented. Figure 9-10 provides specific suggestions for talking with children about cancer.

Figure 9-10. Tips for Parents on Talking With Children About Cancer

- Always be honest with children. If they ask a difficult question, think about it and then reply in an honest but as nonthreatening a way as possible.
- Assure children that they will be cared for no matter what happens during or as a result of treatment.
- Remind them that cancer is not universally fatal, and try to give them concrete examples of people they know and can relate to who are long-term survivors of the disease with good prognostic factors.
- Assure children of all ages that nothing they said, did, or thought could have led to the development of the cancer.
- Assure children that it is quite normal to be angry, scared, or sad when someone they love is diagnosed with cancer.
- Assure them that even though the appearance of their mother may change during treatment, they cannot "catch" the cancer.
- Recognize that it is sometimes helpful for children to participate in a support group with other children so that they realize they are not the only family experiencing a diagnosis of breast cancer.
- Help them to understand how and to what extent they should disclose information about what is happening in their family to others.
- Inform them that others may be reluctant to talk with them or, conversely, may seem like they are being overly kind and generous. Tell them this is a normal reaction, because they might not be sure of what to do or they may be really sad about the diagnosis as well.
- Be honest that home routines will probably be disrupted and that they may need to assume some extra responsibilities for a period of time and possibly permanently.
- Remind children that even if parents cannot attend a sports event or other activity, it does not mean that they are not interested. Remind them that it usually saddens parents as well when they have to miss those types of events. Try to send someone else.
- Remind children that they are still expected to keep up with studies and participate in extracurricular activities as before. The diagnosis is not an excuse to avoid studying.

Family Relationships

Relationships are tested and challenged throughout the diagnosis, treatment, and survival in breast cancer. Relationships already fraught with conflict may experience an exacerbation of problems with the diagnosis (Holmberg, Scott, Alexy, & Fife, 2001). Even caring, committed relationships will be stressed by the diagnosis. Emotional distance may surface because of the inability to discuss feelings about grief, loss and potential loss, significant changes in body images or a sense of loss of femininity, and partners wanting to protect the woman from other distressing situations or information.

Women without a partner, supportive friend(s), or family may have significant distress because of a lack of support.

Supporting Families During the Genetic Testing Process

In addition to coping with the diagnosis of breast cancer, many women must address a hereditary predisposition for developing cancer that puts daughters and sisters at significantly increased risk for developing cancer. Genetic testing for breast cancer is becoming increasingly available.

Families with a hereditary predisposition for developing breast and/or ovarian cancer should be referred to an expert in cancer genetics counseling and education. Many psychosocial ramifications are associated with testing that must be explored prior to ordering a test. Additional psychosocial needs often surface during and after the testing process. These women require services from a healthcare provider who takes and considers a detailed past medical and psychological history. Furthermore, these families need support about the meaning of results, the possibility of inconclusive or uninformative results, and how to share the results of genetic testing.

For those who test positive, an underlying fear often exists of when and where the cancer will develop. Decisions about prophylactic surgery are complex and very personal, especially in areas related to body image and premature menopause. Also, those who test positive may have feelings of guilt that other relatives may have inherited the susceptibility gene. Those who test negative for a known mutation may experience "survivor's guilt" in that they did not inherit the predisposition.

Financial, Employment, and Legal Concerns

All women, regardless of their socioeconomic situation, may eventually have financial, employment, and legal issues that are related to the diagnosis of breast cancer. Helping to address these issues often improves the quality of life for these women. The costs associated with breast cancer treatment can be staggering. In addition to healthcare costs for surgery, chemotherapy, and radiotherapy, treatment also carries many hidden costs. These include copayments for appointments, transportation and parking costs for treatment, time away from work for the patient and perhaps a significant other, increased childcare costs, and other unreimbursed charges. Unemployment or time away from work can result in an inability to meet regular living expenses. These costs can easily and quickly deplete savings. In many cases, agencies and social service resources are available that can assist families with these needs. Patients often are unaware of these resources. Ongoing assessment in this area is essential along with prompt referral when problems become evident.

Some women face multiple issues in the workplace, whereas others do not. Some women benefit from coaching and anticipatory preparation of what to expect when returning to work. Coworkers may not know how to approach a person who is newly diagnosed or returning to work after an absence. Sometimes employers may be unsure of how much a patient can or cannot do. They may not be aware of lingering fatigue, even after treatment is completed. Women with breast cancer need to anticipate what problems might occur and be prepared to address these issues. Women with breast cancer should be advised that it is illegal for employers to discriminate or treat them differently because of a cancer diagnosis. Some patients may need counseling about the Family and Medical Leave Act, which allows them to take unpaid leave to deal with medical problems.

In addition, women with breast cancer may need information about advance directives, wills and trusts, living wills, and durable power of attorney. Wills and trusts help to ensure that assets are distributed to patients' heirs and others as desired. A living will helps people to know what type of medical care patients desire if they become unable to make that decision or communicate their wishes. A durable power of attorney is the person appointed to make health and medical decisions for patients if they are unable to do so. The person who is appointed power of attorney makes financial decisions for another individual when he or she is unable to make them.

Therapeutic Strategies

A number of strategies exist that nurses can use to help to promote adjustment to the diagnosis of breast cancer and decrease distress throughout the cancer trajectory. The positive impact of these strategies on quality of life should not be underestimated. Patients need enough information to make good decisions. This means information that is culturally sensitive and at an appropriate level to be understood. Once a decision is made, healthcare providers need to support patients and families in the decision regardless of whether they personally agree with it.

Hope is important but may change throughout the cancer experience. Healthcare professionals need to continually help patients and families to identify hope in different situations. For newly diagnosed patients, this might mean hope that the therapy will be effective. For survivors, it might mean hope for a new normalcy in their life. For people in the terminal phases, it might mean hope for achieving good symptom management, finishing projects, or experiencing closure with loved ones.

Quality of life also is improved when problems are assessed and confronted directly. Nurses need to assess for symptoms that can be managed such as pain, psychosocial distress, or fatigue. Nurses must try to explain to patients why the symptom is occurring, whether it is a common one, and what concrete steps are going to be taken to decrease the negative effects of the symptom. When symptoms are decreased, quality of life usually improves.

Journaling is often an effective technique to decrease distress. It can help to identify symptoms that can be managed. It also can be used to identify positive things occurring in one's life. For some patients, it serves as a way to leave a legacy of what they experienced.

Often, referrals to a support group are appropriate. Support groups can help individuals to realize that many others share similar feelings and concerns. Before referring a patient to a support group, the healthcare professional should understand the focus of the support group, ground rules, biases of the facilitator, and how acute emotional distress is managed. If the group's philosophy is congruent with the healthcare team and the patient's value system, it may be a useful adjunct to improve quality of life. A specific type of support for patients with breast cancer is the American Cancer Society's "Reach to Recovery" program.

Cancer support groups are often an excellent place for the patient to receive education. When the educational component is delivered by a professional with expertise on the subject, it can be a very effective means to discuss issues related to cancer and cancer treatment. Support groups offer a way for people with cancer, and in many cases their significant others, to come together and talk with others facing similar problems and challenges.

A referral to a cancer information or resource center also can provide education and information. An RN who provides the education and support usually staffs an information center. Resource centers often distribute brochures, videos, educational models, wigs, head coverings, and temporary prostheses, which all help to facilitate psychosocial adjustment. The nurses in these centers can provide guidance on Internet searches and answer specific questions. Many institutions now offer these services, and healthcare providers should encourage and refer patients.

Conclusion

A diagnosis of breast cancer brings many psychosocial consequences. The diagnosis comes as a shock to most women and creates feelings of anxiety and depression. The treatments for breast cancer can be difficult, resulting in side effects and problems with adjustment. Although a diagnosis of breast cancer changes the life of anyone it touches, psychosocial support can help patients and their families throughout the journey.

NCCN (2005) noted that prompt and early intervention has many benefits in preventing and minimizing psychosocial distress. Ultimately, early intervention results in improved quality of life. Communication with family members, significant others, and healthcare providers is often significantly improved when distress is minimized. Finally, patients who have less distress may be more likely to complete a full course of therapy on time.

References

American Cancer Society. (2001, March 19). *Talking with children about cancer.* Retrieved September 5, 2006, from http://www.cancer.org/docroot/ESN/content/ESN_2_1x_Talking_with_Children_About_Cancer.asp?sitearea=ESN

Aukst-Margetic, B., Jakovljevic, M., Margetic, B., Biscan, M., & Samija, M. (2005). Religiosity, depression and pain in patients with breast cancer. *General Hospital Psychiatry, 27,* 250–255.

Beagan, B.L., & Chapman, G.E. (2004). Family influences on food choice: Context of surviving breast cancer. *Journal of Nutrition Education and Behavior, 36,* 320–326.

Bedaiwy, M., & Falcone, T. (2004). Ovarian tissue banking for cancer patients: Reduction of post-transplantation ischemic injury: Intact ovary freezing and transplantation. *Human Reproduction, 19,* 1242–1244.

Berland, G., Elliott, M., Morales, L., Algazy, J., Kravitz, R., Broder, M., et al. (2001). Health information on the Internet: Accessibility, quality, and readability in English and Spanish. *JAMA, 285,* 2612–2621.

Bichakjian, C., Schwartz, J., Wang, T., Hall, J., Johnson, T., & Biermann, J. (2002). Melanoma information on the Internet: Often incomplete—a public health opportunity? *Journal of Clinical Oncology, 20,* 134–141.

Blanchard, C., Denniston, M., Baker, F., Ainsworth, S., Courneya, K.S., Hann, D.M., et al. (2003). Do adults change their lifestyle behaviors after a cancer diagnosis? *American Journal of Health Behavior, 27,* 246–256.

Bower, J. (2005). Fatigue in cancer patients and survivors: Mechanisms and treatment. *Primary Psychiatry, 12*(5), 53–57.

Burgess, C., Cornelius, V., Love, S., Graham, J., Richards, M., & Ramirez, A. (2005). Depression and anxiety in women with early breast cancer: Five year observational cohort study. *BMJ, 330,* 702.

Chappy, S.L. (2004). Women's experience with breast biopsy. *AORN Journal, 80,* 885–901.

Demark-Wahnefried, W., Rimer, B., & Winer, E. (1997). Weight gain in women diagnosed with breast cancer. *Journal of the American Dietetic Association, 97,* 519–526.

Edwards, D.M. (2002). *Voice massage: Scripts for guided imagery.* Pittsburgh, PA: Oncology Nursing Society.

Flowers-Coulson, P., Kushner, M., & Bankowski, S. (2000). The information is out there, but is anyone getting it? Adolescent misconceptions about sexuality education and reproductive health and the use of the Internet to get answers. *Journal of Sex Education and Therapy, 25,* 178–188.

Ganz, P.A., Greendale, G.A., Peterson, L., Kahn, B., & Bower, J.E. (2003). Breast cancer in younger women: Reproductive and late health effects of treatment. *Journal of Clinical Oncology, 21,* 4184–4193.

Ganz, P.A., Kwan, L., Stanton, A.L., Krupnick, J.L., Rowland, J.H., Meyerowitz, B.E., et al. (2004). Quality of life at the end of primary treatment of breast cancer: First results from the Moving Beyond Cancer randomized trial. *Journal of the National Cancer Institute, 96,* 376–387.

Gorman, L.M. (2006). The psychosocial impact of cancer on the individual, family, and society. In R.M. Carroll-Johnson, L.M. Gorman, & N.J. Bush (Eds.), *Psychosocial nursing care along the cancer continuum* (2nd ed., pp. 3–23). Pittsburgh, PA: Oncology Nursing Society.

Greene, D., Nail, L., Fieler, V., Dudgeon, D., & Jones, L. (1994). A comparison of patient-reported side effects among three chemotherapy regimens for breast cancer. *Cancer Practice, 2,* 57–62.

Hewitt, M., Herdman, R., & Holland, J. (Eds.). (2004). *Meeting psychosocial needs of women with breast cancer.* Washington, DC: National Academies Press.

Holmberg, S.K., Scott, L.L., Alexy, W., & Fife, B.L. (2001). Relationship issues of women with breast cancer. *Cancer Nursing, 24,* 53–60.

Kendall, A., Mahue-Giangreco, M., Carpenter, C., Ganz, P., & Bernstein, L. (2005). Influence of exercise activity on quality of life in long-term breast cancer survivors. *Quality of Life Research, 14,* 361–371.

Kerr, J., Engel, J., Schlesinger-Raab, A., Sauer, H., & Holzel, D. (2003). Communication, quality of life and age: Results of a 5-year prospective study in breast cancer patients. *Annals of Oncology, 14,* 421–427.

Kirsch, S.E., Brandt, P.A., & Lewis, F.M. (2003). Making the most of the moment. When a child's mother has breast cancer. *Cancer Nursing, 26,* 47–54.

Mahon, S.M., & Casperson, D.S. (1995). Psychosocial concerns associated with recurrent cancer. *Cancer Practice, 3,* 372–380.

McDonald, M., Passik, S., Dugan, W., Rosenfeld, B., Theobald, D., & Edgerton, S. (1999). Nurses' recognition of depression in their patients with cancer. *Oncology Nursing Forum, 26,* 593–599.

McGarvey, E., Baum, L., Pinderton, R., & Rogers, L. (2001). Psychological sequelae and alopecia among women with cancer. *Cancer Practice, 9,* 283–289.

Morris, C., Wright, W., & Schlag, R. (2001). The risk of developing breast cancer within the next 5, 10, or 20 years of a woman's life. *American Journal of Preventive Medicine, 20,* 214–218.

National Comprehensive Cancer Network. (2005). *NCCN clinical practice guidelines in oncology: Distress management, version 1.2005.* Jenkintown, PA: Author.

Northouse, L., Templin, T., & Mood, D. (2001). Couple's adjustment to breast cancer during the first year following diagnosis. *Journal of Behavioral Medicine, 24,* 115–136.

Ovitz, L. (with Kabak, J.). (2004). *Facing the mirror with cancer.* Chicago: Belle Press.

Payne, D., Hoffman, R., Theodoulou, M., Dosik, M., & Massier, M.J. (1999). Screening for anxiety and depression in women with breast cancer. *Psychosomatics, 40,* 64–69.

Pereira, J., & Bruera, E. (1998). The Internet as a resource for palliative care and hospice: A review and proposals. *Journal of Pain and Symptom Management, 16,* 59–68.

Pereira, J., Bruera, E., Macmillan, K., & Kavanagh, S. (2000). Palliative cancer patients and their families on the Internet: Motivation and impact. *Journal of Palliative Care, 16,* 13–19.

Rogers, M., & Kristjanson, L.J. (2002). The impact of sexual functioning of chemotherapy-induced menopause in women with breast cancer. *Cancer Nursing, 25,* 57–65.

Sammarco, A. (2001). Psychosocial stages and quality of life of women with breast cancer. *Cancer Nursing, 24,* 272–277.

Schmidt, R.C. (2003). *My book about cancer.* Pittsburgh, PA: Oncology Nursing Society.

Schou, I., Ekeberg, O., Sandvik, L., Hjermstad, M., & Ruland, C. (2005). Multiple predictors or health-related quality of life in early stage breast cancer. Data from a year follow-up study compared with the general population. *Quality of Life Research, 14,* 1813–1823.

Schultz, P.N., Klein, M.J., Beck, M.L., Stava, C., & Sellin, R.V. (2005). Breast cancer: Relationship between menopausal symptoms, physiologic health effects of cancer treatment and physical constraints on quality of life in long-term survivors. *Journal of Clinical Nursing, 14,* 204–211.

Sigal, J.J., Perry, C., Robbins, J.M., Gagne, M., & Nassif, E. (2003). Maternal preoccupation and parenting and predictors of emotional and behavioral problems in children of women with breast cancer. *Journal of Clinical Oncology, 21,* 1155–1160.

Smith, E., Gomm, S., & Dickens, C. (2003). Assessing the independent contribution to quality of life from anxiety and depression in patients with advanced cancer. *Palliative Medicine, 17,* 509–513.

Spiegel, D., Bloom, J., Kraemer, H., & Gottheil, E. (1989). Effect of psychosocial treatment on survival of patients with metastatic breast cancer. *Lancet, 14,* 888–891.

Stead, M.L. (2003). Sexual dysfunction after treatment for gynaecologic and breast malignancies. *Current Opinion in Obstetrics and Gynecology, 15,* 57–61.

Thewes, B., Butow, P., Girgis, A., & Pendlebury, S. (2004). The psychosocial needs of breast cancer survivors: A qualitative study of the shared and unique needs of younger versus older survivors. *Psycho-Oncology, 13,* 177–189.

Vallance, J., Courneya, K., Jones, L., & Reiman, T. (2005). Differences in quality of life between non-Hodgkin's lymphoma survivors meeting and not meeting public health exercise guidelines. *Psycho-Oncology, 14,* 979–991.

van Weert, E., Hoekstra-Weebers, J., Grol, B., Otter, R., Arendzen, H., Postema, K., et al. (2005). A multidimensional cancer rehabilitation program for cancer survivors: Effectiveness on health-related quality of life. *Journal of Psychosomatic Research, 58,* 485–496.

Vos, P.J., Garssen, B., Visser, A.P., Duivenvoorden, H.J., & de Haes, H.C. (2004). Early stage breast cancer: Explaining level of psychosocial adjustment using structural equation modeling. *Journal of Behavioral Medicine, 27,* 557–580.

Yaffe, R.S. (1998). *Once upon a hopeful night.* Pittsburgh, PA: Oncology Nursing Society.

CHAPTER 10

Breast Cancer Research in the United States: Nursing Contributions 2000–2005

Ellen Giarelli, EdD, RN, CRNP

Introduction

What constitutes "nursing research"? It may be defined as research that is conducted by nurses using (or developing) nursing theories to advance nursing science or nursing practice. This definition, although pure, excludes a legion of nurses who collaborate on interdisciplinary teams, use established conceptual models from related sciences, conduct basic research in biobehavior, or contribute in ways that are peripheral but important. We may distinguish contributions along a continuum from basic scientist to bedside data collector.

Nurses participate in and contribute to research at all levels of involvement, from healthcare administration to symptom management and from theoretical modeling and basic bench research to bedside care. They are principal investigators, coinvestigators, and consultants. Research nurses are project coordinators, interventionists, managers, and data collectors. Nurses contribute unique expertise as members of investigative teams led by other scientists such as physicians, geneticists, sociologists, and psychologists. Although many nurse researchers aim to publish findings in journals that will reach the target audience, which is principally nurses, scientific findings also may be published in educational journals, medical journals, and journals from the behavioral and social sciences. When the answer to a research question might result either indirectly or directly in improving the human condition in general and health in particular, one may find the contributions of nurses. All of these aspects make up the nature of nursing research and by volume defy one's effort to create a comprehensive catalogue.

For decades, breast cancer research has captured the interests of nurses, and nurse scientists have distinguished themselves as pioneers in the study of symptom management and quality-of-life issues. Nurses who conduct research related to breast cancer publish their findings in oncology journals, and because their target audience is primarily oncology nurses, the majority of nursing research in the field of breast cancer can be found in oncology nursing journals. Because breast cancer

is a prevalent disease, research reports are found across the spectrum of publications.

For the purposes of this chapter, nursing research is specified as that which is conducted by nurses and is published in journals with an emphasis on oncology and nursing. This chapter describes the nature of nursing research related to breast cancer in the United States from 2000–2005. Oncology research is a rapidly changing field that responds quickly to advances in pharmacology and genomics. The short time period of 2000–2005 captures the most recent responses to these changes. The specificity of this chapter is used to contain the sheer volume of work, not to diminish or discount the significant contributions made by nurses practicing outside of the United States who publish their findings in international and U.S. journals. Descriptions include a summary of sources, number of articles, and geographic distributions. Findings from nursing studies are grouped into general categories of research. Specific findings or results from studies are not included, as these data are beyond the scope of the chapter.

Methodology

A variety of search engines were used to collect data for this sketch of breast cancer nursing research. Sources of data included MEDLINE® and CINAHL®. Search terms included *breast neoplasm, nursing, research,* and a variety of subcategories. An intensive search focused on the years 2000–2005 to produce information in three general categories: characteristics of the reports, characteristics of the team, and focus of the research. Characteristics of the reports included the number by year, names of the journals, and type of reports or methodology. Characteristics of the team included the institution and state in which the research was conducted and the composition of the team. The focus of the research identified the categories of topics and the number of reports by topic. For inclusion, the article must have been authored or coauthored by a nurse. In addition, a search of articles published prior to 2000 was conducted to add perspective and to place recent productivity in historical context.

Nursing Research in Breast Cancer

Literature Before 2000

Without doubt, nurses have been studying breast cancer in a variety of ways for as long as nurses have been caring for patients and families affected by the disease. In the past, the study of breast cancer was circumstantial—predominantly informal in design and substance. Nurses observed patient behaviors, conducted trials of nursing care, and reported findings. Although not published or even described as such, these behaviors illustrated aspects of the scientific method of problem solving, with steps of data collection, hypothesis testing, and dissemination of findings among peers. Over the past 45 years, nurses have worked in breast cancer research as subsidiary members of teams, such as data collectors and coordinators, or their research was entirely informal and a component of clinical practice.

A search of MEDLINE for *breast neoplasm* produced a count of 124,676 journal publications over 103 years. Between 1902 and 1999, there were 86,883 entries of articles on this topic. Between 2000 and 2005, the search produced 37,793 entries. This brief period of time (5 years, or approximately 5% of the time span) produced roughly 30% of all the publications in the entire century. This extraordinary proliferation of data and opinions makes breast cancer one of the leading topics of interest to investigators across disciplines. In addition, the search of CINAHL was for nursing-specific publications. This index began in 1960. The search yielded more than 11,158 nursing-specific publications on breast neoplasm between 1960 and 2005 and more than 6,642 between 2000 and 2005. Thus, more than 59% of all publications appeared in the last 5 of the 45 years that are catalogued in this index. Table 10-1 shows a breakdown of productivity.

The majority of the publications prior to 2000 were nonscientific. They included instructional papers such as continuing education programs on new medications, pathophysiology, and genetics; clinical case studies; opinion pieces; materials for patient education; and evaluation of patient education and screening programs. Although this does not represent an exhaustive search, it does provide a sense of how much attention is paid to the disease by the scientific community.

Characteristics of the Reports, 2000–2005

Over the past five to six years, there has been a steady production of articles concerning breast cancer. Productivity peaked in 2002 with a high of 72 articles, and the low was

Table 10-1. Frequency of Nursing Research Articles About Breast Cancer by Year of Publication

Year	Number of Articles
2000	61
2001	64
2002	72
2003	63
2004	46
2005	52

46 articles in 2004. Approximately 52 articles are credited to 2005, and approximately 360 articles were identified as authored by nurses and published between 2000 and 2005.

Six journals published the preponderance of manuscripts. They are listed in order of relative volume: *Oncology Nursing Forum (ONF), Clinical Journal of Oncology Nursing (CJON), Seminars in Oncology Nursing (SON), Cancer Nursing (CN), Cancer Practice (CP),* and *Journal of Cancer Education (JCE).* By far, the greatest percentage of published scientific manuscripts on breast cancer appeared in *ONF* and *CJON.* These two journals publish, as far as can be determined, almost exclusively the work of nurses (see Table 10-2). Both *CP* and *JCE* have a lower percentage of articles because these journals do not address cancer nursing in particular. One also may presume that because *ONF* and *CJON* have "nursing" in the title of the journal, non-nurse authors may dismiss these publications as hosts of their work.

Besides the six noted previously, 22 other publications were searched for nursing research on breast cancer. These journals are listed in Figure 10-1. A brief search of medical journals such as the *Journal of the American Medical Association,* the *New England Journal of Medicine, Cancer,* and *Cancer Investigation* yielded a small number of works that were written by nurses. It is possible, however, that a detailed analysis of individual articles also would yield nurse investigators and nursing research.

Table 10-2. Number of Articles About Breast Cancer in Major Nursing Journals That Focus on Oncology, 2000–2005

Publication	Number of Articles
Oncology Nursing Forum	83
Cancer Nursing	46
Clinical Journal of Oncology Nursing	39
Seminars in Oncology Nursing	14

Figure 10-1. Journals Included in Search History for Breast Cancer and Nursing Research in MEDLINE® and CINAHL®, 2000–2005

- *Advances in Nursing*
- *Cancer*
- *Cancer Nursing*
- *Cancer Practice*
- *Clinical Journal of Oncology Nursing*
- *Journal of Advanced Nursing*
- *Journal of the American Medical Association*
- *Journal of Cancer Education*
- *Journal of Clinical Oncology*
- *Journal of Clinical Nursing*
- *Journal of Holistic Nursing*
- *Journal of Nursing Scholarship*
- *Journal of Palliative Care*
- *MedSurg Nursing*
- *New England Journal of Medicine*
- *Nursing Clinics of North America*
- *Nursing Forum*
- *Nursing Inquiry*
- *Nursing Outlook*
- *Nursing Research*
- *Nursing Science Quarterly*
- *Oncology Nursing Forum*
- *Psycho-Oncology*
- *Qualitative Health Research*
- *Research in Nursing and Health*
- *Seminars in Oncology Nursing*
- *Social Science and Medicine*
- *Western Journal of Nursing Research*

The publications were evaluated for the kind of study conducted to determine whether the article was original scientific research or a nonresearch report such as a review of the literature, a clinical case study, or other nonempirical report. The majority of articles in *ONF, CN, CP,* and *JCE* were original reports. Study designs were descriptive, mixed methods, grounded theory, and phenomenology; single or multicenter clinical trials; some empirical case studies and evaluation research; and validation studies. *SON* published only reviews. In breast cancer research, *CN* published 75% reviews, and *CJON* published more than 80% reviews.

Characteristics of the Teams

Authors resided in nearly every state of the United States, but the preponderance of original research heralded from states with major research universities, such as Pennsylvania, Texas, California, Michigan, and Florida. Another large proportion originated from independent cancer centers such as the Memorial Sloan-Kettering Cancer Center (New York), the University of Texas M.D. Anderson Cancer Center (Texas), the H. Lee Moffitt Cancer Center and Research Institute (Florida), and the City of Hope National Medical Center (California). To a lesser degree, original research was attributed to authors practicing in the private sector, public or federal health agen-

cies (e.g., the National Cancer Institute), or sponsored by oncology divisions of pharmaceutical companies (e.g., Schering-Plough, Ortho Biotech) or nonprofit organizations (e.g., the American Cancer Society). Original research studies were more likely to be produced by investigators who practiced or taught at institutions that have a regulatory and administrative infrastructure, access to a diverse patient population, and a favorable intellectual climate to support nursing research. Most original reports were authored by multiple team members of two or more nurses with a doctoral-prepared nurse as first author. Nonscientific reports such as clinical case studies or review were typically authored by one to two nurses, and the first author was often a master's-level nurse.

Focus of Original Reports

Nurse researchers have conducted studies in many categories. Generally, the projects are complex and often address issues or key concepts that overlap. Nurse investigators have a penchant for conceptualizing research questions at the nexus of psychological, social, physical, and spiritual domains. For example, a study investigating the effect of exercise on patient fatigue might be categorized as self-care and also as symptom management. Examples of projects in multiple categories are that of Schneider, Prince-Paul, Allen, Silverman, and Talaba (2004), whose study of distraction as a means to control chemotherapy side effects falls under both complementary and alternative medicine (CAM) and symptom management. Survivorship, quality of life, and ethnic differences are the subjects of Dirksen's (2000) and Dirksen and Erickson's (2002) reports of Hispanic and non-Hispanic breast cancer survivors.

In an effort to group articles by focus area, the studies conducted between 2000 and 2005 were sorted by outcome measures for experimental/quasiexperimental designs and by patient-centered variables for descriptive and correlation designs. In addition, some nurses conducted research that did not have humans as subjects but rather used animal models. Eventually these studies might be translated to clinical practice. The 350 reports were divided among eight main topics: self-care and prevention; screening, early detection, and genetics; symptom management; functional status (quality of life); treatment; patient safety and side effects; palliation and end-of-life; and caregiver and family issues. Two other categories of publication are identified as bench research and CAM. Noticeable overlap occurs across categories. For example, an article about symptom management may well be categorized as one that addresses quality of life. Therefore, the publication title was used to indicate the focus of the research or review (see Table 10-3).

Self-Care and Prevention

The term *self-care* encompasses several categories of research that share an underlying philosophical assumption—

Table 10-3. Categories of Research Focus and Percent of Articles by Category, 2000–2005

Focus of Research	Percent
Screening, early detection, and genetics	24.3
Functional status/quality of life	18
Self-care and prevention	16.5
Symptom management	16.5
Treatment	13.2
Caregiver and family issues	4.8
Patient safety and side effects	3.5
Complementary and alternative medicine	2
Palliation and end of life	2
Bench research	< 1

that individuals should be involved in all or some aspects of their health care. The concept of self-care is the construct that is the basis of health-promoting activities (adhering to screening recommendations), such as self-monitoring (e.g., breast self-examination [BSE]). This category of nursing research distinguishes it from research in other disciplines. It first appeared in the health-related literature in 1971 as the seminal work of Orem (1971). Research in self-care has been applied across the life span for patients with breast cancer. Issues of self-care include self-surveillance activities such as BSE and any activities related to prevention and health promotion. Issues in this category also may include investigating the consequences of self-care behavior. These consequences might be increased patient satisfaction, decreased risk of complications, and enhanced recovery. Nurses have long been interested in improving the health of populations and individuals by encouraging health-promoting behaviors and enhancing patients' self-surveillance abilities. Self-care and prevention strategies empower patients.

This category of research accounted for 16.5% of the publications between 2000 and 2005. The highest percentage was 26% in 2000, and the lowest was 7.8% in 2003. This may be attributable to the shift in author attention to the related category of screening, early detection, and genetics. Nurse investigators may conceptualize participation in screening as a kind of health-promoting behavior.

Studies of BSE dominated the category of self-care and prevention. This category of research specifically addressed the training of patients to conduct BSE (Bragg Leight, Deirriggi, Hursh, Miller, & Leight, 2000), BSE in high-risk populations and racial minorities (Wood & Duffy, 2004; Wood, Duffy, Morris, & Carnes, 2002), and needs assessment for cultural groups (Chen & Bakken, 2004; Rashidi & Rajaram, 2000;

Wells, Bush, & Marshall, 2001). Gasalberti (2002) attempted to differently conceptualize the experience by identifying perceived barriers and health conception. Authors also have examined health promotion, such as Drake (2001), who investigated risk reduction in the relationship between physical activity and breast cancer prediction.

Screening, Early Detection, and Genetics

Cancer genetics opened up an important area of research for nurses. Previously, genetics research was relegated to the study of rare genetic disorders or identifying single gene disorders. Now researchers know that genetic alterations not only cause the specific diseases but also affect disease susceptibility, resistance, prognosis and progression, responses to illness, and responses to treatment. Advances in knowledge of the genetic nature of disease resulted in broadening of the legitimacy of different kinds of investigations. Research on issues related to predisposition testing and disease prevention strategies grew in prevalence and importance. Nurses have proved themselves to be well suited to explore these areas of genomics (i.e., the human response to disease). Issues related to this category included activities such as screening services, early identification using mammography, predisposition genetic testing, and pedigree analysis for genetic risk factors.

The highest percentage of articles was attributed to this category. When all years were combined, screening, early detection, and genetics accounted for 24.3% of the published reports, and these were produced in a steady stream across the years, with a low of 18% in 2000 and a peak of 31.1% in 2001. Predictably, many authors addressed screening using mammography. This method of screening was evaluated among ethnic and racial minority populations (Smith, Phillips, & Price, 2001) and rural populations (Coleman et al., 2003; Leslie et al., 2003).

With the start of the Human Genome Project in 2000 came a growing interest in the genetics of breast cancer and syndromes with clusters of breast cancer among affected people. While oncologists, biologists, and geneticists concentrated on the molecular and environmental determinants of breast cancer, nurse researchers were turning a critical eye to the experiences and the psychological distress associated with learning one's predisposition to the disease (Hutson, 2003) and living with elevated risk (Loescher, 2003). Nurse researchers holistically addressed the patients at risk in case studies (Kelly, 2003).

Symptom Management

Perhaps more than any other outcome, symptom management is under the purview of nurses. Researchers have long been interested in this category of nursing-sensitive outcomes because the outcomes flag a change in functioning and signify the reason for seeking health care (Dodd et al., 2001; Doran, 2003; McCorkle & Young, 1978). These studies interchangeably use the terms *symptom control* and *symptom management,* and most incorporate a method for symptom assessment or the experience of the symptom. The University of California, San Francisco Symptom Management Faculty Group (SMFG) ("A Model for Symptom Management," 1994) defined a symptom as the subjective experience of changes in biopsychosocial functioning, sensation, or cognition. Issues of symptom management revolve around three major areas of research: accurately naming the symptom, assessing its characteristics (single or multidimensional), and treating it. Early work in this area produced many excellent instruments from data collected from patients with cancer. One such instrument specific to breast cancer is the Breast Cancer Prevention Trial Symptom Checklist (Gantz, Day, Ware, Redmond, & Fisher, 1995; Gantz et al., 2000). Radiation therapy, chemotherapy, surgery, and combinations of treatment modalities for cancer generate multiple, serious adverse reactions. These are experienced as "symptoms" according to the definition proposed by the SMFG and therefore fall under the symptom management category.

Research and reviews on symptom management constitute 16.5% of the published reports, and, like articles in other categories, no single publication year or journal significantly surpassed the others in quantity. However, the number of articles in this category steadily increased over the five-year period from 13% in 2000 to 20.8% in 2005. This might reflect attention to the growing arsenal of medications available to mediate the effects of chemotherapy, which include nausea, vomiting, anorexia, fatigue, neutropenia, and, most recently, acne rash.

Reports on symptom management addressed the complex psychosocial dynamics of the cancer experience and symptom distress (Badger, Braden, & Mishel, 2001; Boehmke, 2004). Studies also have described the use of exercise therapy (Pickett et al., 2002; Schwartz, 2000) and treatment for early menopause (Knobf, 2001).

Functional Status (Quality of Life)

Functional status captures patients' perceptions of their day-to-day functioning and has been defined by nurse researchers in cancer care as the individual's actual performance of normal day-to-day activities (Cooley, 1998; Richmond, McCorkle, Tulman, & Fawcett, 1997). Functional status is viewed as a multidimensional construct that consists of behavioral, psychological, cognitive, and social components (Knight, 2000). Many terms have been used interchangeably in the literature, including function, functional ability, functional capacity, functional performance, health status, activities of daily living, and quality of life. Body image changes are included in this category. Although all these terms are interchangeable, the cancer care literature tends to focus on the term *quality of life* when describing the functional status of the patient. This is entirely appropriate and reflects sensitivity to the importance of patients' perceptions of disease. The tone captures the sympathetic attitude of oncology clinicians. The quality-of-life category might be subsumed by the symptom

management classification, but the sheer volume of work in this area warrants separate treatment.

Second only to screening and early detection, this category comprised 18% of published reports. Similar to symptom management, a steady increase in the number of articles occurred over time. As in other categories, articles addressing quality of life also may be categorized as reports of symptom management, palliation, side effects, and so on. Articles were placed in this category if the author specifically used the term *quality of life.*

Reports in this category described quality of life in terms of survivorship (Kessler, 2002), psychosocial adjustment (Dow & Lafferty, 2000), and social support (Sammarco, 2001). Nurse authors were able to express empathy and a higher understanding of the experiences of patients in reports such as Manning-Walsh's (2005) study of spiritual struggle and Ponto et al.'s (2003) article titled "Stories of Breast Cancer Through Art." These works capture the depth and breadth of the personal impact of cancer and the effect on the human condition.

Treatment

A separate category was included that described novel or new treatments for patients with cancer. Like others, this category may include original research, but most often these articles were instructional and summarized essential information for the clinician. These reports, although not typically original research, constituted a collection of information vital to responsible and expert clinical practice. It remains the principal method for disseminating results from medical, pharmacologic, and bench research. Such articles often described nursing management considerations with chemotherapeutic agents that were newly released or showed promise in clinical trials (Burke, 2005; Davison, 2005; Frankel, 2000; Harwood, 2004; Lynn, 2002; Wampler, Hamolsky, Hamel, Melisko, & Topp, 2005). This category of publication comprised 13.2% of reports, which appeared primarily in practice journals such as *CJON*. This type of article is essential to cancer nursing and lessens the divide between research and practice.

Patient Safety and Side Effects

Current antineoplastic approaches often include intense multimodality therapies, which improve survival. However, these treatments have the potential for creating a variety of physiologic adverse late effects that may result in late morbidity and for which careful surveillance is needed for early detection and appropriate treatment. Young children appear to be especially vulnerable to such late effects. This category is dedicated to those articles that focus on post-treatment safety issues, such as side effects and late effects.

Nurses have demonstrated interest in managing the side effects of cancer treatments, such as anorexia, alopecia, and nausea associated with chemotherapy (Williams & Schreier, 2004). Several articles described the care of cancer survivors with osteoporosis (Lindsey et al., 2002; Waltman et al., 2003). There were far fewer that addressed technical issues such as safety considerations when handling chemotherapy agents (Griffin, 2003). This kind of report tended to be a review. Some studies tested interventions for side effects (Baron et al., 2000). The average number of reports in the patient safety and side effects category was 3.5%. This was far fewer than expected but understandable because topics may overlap with symptom management and quality of life.

Palliation and End-of-Life

Professionals caring for frail older adults observe the general shift in location of care from hospital to home as patients and families wish to stay close to that which they know and care about. Studies on palliation and end of life addressed the physical, emotional, and spiritual suffering of patients with end-stage breast cancer. The optimal care for patients with chronic and progressive illnesses requires all members of the multidisciplinary team to be proficient in the assessment and relief of suffering in the environment in which patients choose to live their final days. This type of whole-person care for patients whose diseases are not responsive to curative treatment is also called *palliative care.* Physicians and other caregivers must concentrate on targeting pain and other discomforting symptoms in each patient and provide relief through appropriate pharmacologic and nonpharmacologic treatments. Beyond physical care, professionals providing palliation also are responsible for communicating with patients and their families, informing them of treatments, and providing expectations for their illness or condition. Moreover, working with end-of-life patients brings unique ethical concerns and dilemmas associated with pain management and termination of treatment.

This category did not yield as many articles as expected based on the importance of this subject to nurses, patients, and families. Only 2% of the reports pertained to palliation and end-of-life. The volume of articles in every other category surpassed this figure. This rate is inconsistent with the intention to place greatest effort where need is greatest. Patients with cancer will die, and families will struggle with the spiritual and psychological punishment of watching a loved one suffer. One may suspect that research on end-of-life care and palliation is a victim of investigator denial and avoidance, similar to how the topic of death and dying is avoided in polite conversation. Much more and varied research is needed in this area to follow the works of Lackan, Freeman, and Goodwin (2003) on hospice care and Strauss (2000) on accessing "last hope" clinical trials.

Caregiver, Family, and Survivorship Issues

Cancer survivors are those individuals who have been diagnosed with cancer and lived after treatment. These patients may be cured or in a state of remission. There may be more than one way to define issues related to "survivorship."

Another more abstract way to define a cancer survivor is in the context of the family. Cancer is now conceptualized as an illness that affects not only the patient but all those who are close to and care for the patient. In one sense, these people are survivors of the cancer experience. This definition was used for articles published about the experiences of spouses and children of people who either have cancer or who have succumbed to the disease. Northouse et al. (2002) addressed the phenomenon of care for the whole family during the cancer experience.

Several articles addressed the needs and experiences of spouses of women with breast cancer. In particular, Hilton, Crawford, and Tarko (2000) examined men's perspectives on family coping when the wife had breast cancer. Another article described the supportive care needs of spouses of women with cancer (Petrie, Logan, & DeGrasse, 2001). A few studies, such as Davis Kirsch, Brandt, and Lewis (2003), have addressed the experiences of children of women with breast cancer, but more are needed now that genetic testing is available for high-risk families.

Approximately 4.8% of the articles were on caregiver and family issues. This was the only category that showed a drop in volume from 9.8 to 0 from 2000 to 2005. This change does not mean that nurse scientists are no longer interested in the experiences of family members nor that they believe all questions have been answered. It does, however, indicate that nurses should refresh their attention to the cancer experiences of whole families. This attention may take on a new perspective and appeal if framed within the context of genetics and lifelong surveillance for high-risk patient cohorts.

Special Category: Bench Research

This category of research included biologic, physiologic, and animal studies such as experiments carried out in the laboratory ("bench"). Bench studies might include stem cell research, cell isolation and culturing, and gene therapy. This category also may include preclinical studies that involve animal models. Preclinical experiments are those carried out in animal models as opposed to clinical or patient-based studies. Nurses rarely engage in this type of research, and if done, one might find the studies published in non-nursing journals by investigators who have postdoctoral experience in sciences and who later became RNs. An example of this kind of research is the study by Wood, Maher, Bunton, and Resar (2000), in which the lead author had conducted several years of postdoctoral work in virology before receiving a bachelor's in nursing. Many non-nursing journals do not include the credentials of authors. Rather, unless stated otherwise, it is assumed that the lead author is doctoral-prepared. Without firsthand knowledge, the institutional affiliation may provide the only clue to the authors' credentials. Other than the articles previously described, no nursing research was found in this category.

Special Category: Complementary and Alternative Medicine

Conventional medicine is medicine that is practiced by holders of medical doctor degrees or doctor of osteopathy degrees and by allied health professionals, such as physical therapists, psychologists, and RNs. Other terms for conventional medicine include allopathy; Western, mainstream, orthodox, and regular medicine; and biomedicine. Some conventional medical practitioners are also practitioners of CAM.

CAM, as defined by the National Center for Complementary and Alternative Medicine (NCCAM, 2005), is a group of diverse medical and healthcare systems, practices, and products that are not currently considered to be part of conventional medicine. Other terms for CAM include unconventional, nonconventional, unproven, and irregular medicine or health care. Although some scientific evidence exists regarding some CAM therapies, for most, key questions have yet to be answered, such as whether these therapies are safe and whether they work for the diseases or medical conditions for which they are used. The list of what is considered to be CAM changes continually, as those therapies that are proved to be safe and effective become adopted into conventional health care and as new approaches to health care emerge. For example, some uses of dietary supplements have been incorporated into conventional medicine. Scientists have found that folic acid prevents certain birth defects and that a regimen of vitamins and zinc can slow the progression of an eye disease called age-related macular degeneration (NCCAM, 2005). Other examples of CAM are therapeutic touch, music and movement therapy, and massage therapy.

Complementary medicine is different than alternative medicine. Complementary medicine is used together with conventional medicine. Examples of the use of complementary therapy are aromatherapy, imagery, and progressive relaxation to help to lessen patients' discomfort following medical treatments such as surgery. Conversely, alternative medicine is used in place of conventional medicine. An example of an alternative therapy is using a special diet to treat cancer instead of undergoing surgery, radiation, or chemotherapy that has been recommended by a conventional doctor.

Despite the recent attention to this topic in public discourse, only 2% of reports are in this category. Some, like that of Decker (2001), are instructive. Others take a bolder tack and attempt to test the effect of various CAM therapies on patient outcomes. For example, guided imagery was the focus of a clinical trial (Kwekkeboom, 2001). Other investigators developed a research program that explored patterns of CAM use among patients with breast cancer (Lengacher, Bennett, Kipp, Berarducci, & Cox, 2003; Lengacher et al., 2002). Based on anecdotal evidence and patient report, this area should receive more attention in the future.

Any changes in the focus of the research across the years are most likely due to the influence of medical advances in cancer care. Nurses are expert "responders" and quickly react to changes in their practice environments. For example, a rise in the publication of articles regarding treatment and side effects followed the release of the results from the clinical trial of tamoxifen and raloxifene. One area of research that is not represented is the study of oncology nurses and practice settings. Research in this area could contribute to nurses' understanding of and ability to advance the interests of nurses caring for patients with breast cancer.

Critique of Impact of Nursing Research on Cancer Care

The sheer volume of literature generated by nurses is proxy for the impact on cancer care. Although many of the original, empirical studies have been reductionistic, such that they explore discrete variables, they still retain a quality unique to a humanistic profession. The studies take into account the real-world experiences of people. In this regard, nurse researchers have demonstrated scientific expertise that is unique and thoroughly consistent with the professional code of ethics and professional practice. As long as research and publication are encouraged, oncology nurses will continue to improve cancer care. Consequently, nurses who seek out and read the literature will benefit from these efforts.

The great majority of readers of some nursing journals are nurses. This may be especially true for journals that include the word *nurse* in the title. A non-nurse may discount such a publication solely based on professional group membership. It is somewhat unfortunate for patients and families that nursing research is published almost exclusively in nursing journals. Physicians, social workers, and other providers of health services for patients with cancer and their families could benefit from the work of nurses. An open-minded physician will overlook the name of the publication and focus on the subject of the research when conducting a literature review on MEDLINE. A tactic that has greater chance of ensuring broad dissemination of nurses' research is the publication or reprinting of such studies in interdisciplinary journals. The apparent disadvantage of this approach is that findings will be less readily available to practicing nurses who rely on literature in their profession for clinical updates, new ideas, and evidence-based practice implications.

One area of research not noted in the literature is the meta-analysis of nursing studies of breast cancer. This absence is most conspicuous, and the research is sorely missed. Nurse researchers must periodically summarize findings from nursing studies to construct a coherent, "fluid" whole. The synthesis of findings can be used by clinicians, other nurse researchers, and professionals to uncover gaps in the science and inform topic selection for additional studies. Synthesis of findings also should be used to determine how and when evidence can affect practice. It appears that cancer nurse researchers—as teams or as individuals—work in isolation. Most often, the teams refer to their own work when developing research agendas and additional studies.

The profession needs a larger view, one that comes from stepping back, perusing the research environment, and describing in the largest sense how the work interconnects. This view is attainable and will clarify the heritage and future mission of research in cancer nursing. It could inform nurses' discussion of when evidence should and must affect practice.

Limitations

This chapter was conceived to be a summary and to provide a sense of what work has been done. The summary is not exhaustive but merely representative. Some journals do not list authors' credentials or the home department of their institutions. Thus, some nurse-authored publications probably were missed because the background and preparation of the author could not be ascertained. In addition, publications on studies of several kinds of cancer, including breast cancer, were not included in the search. Therefore, the absolute number of articles that could have been included is higher, and the presumed impact of nursing research on cancer care is a modest guess.

Conclusion

Surely, placing the credential "RN" after a name indicates that person is a nurse. But, is this statutory definition sufficient to capture the nature of nursing? It is entirely appropriate to assign the moniker of *nurse* to someone who, without the benefit of formal education, ministers to the sick. Which definition of nurse is assigned to the person who conducts research? Is a nurse who conducts research necessarily a nurse researcher? If the answer to this question is maybe, then the debate should continue as to what constitutes nursing research. Nursing has struggled for the past century with the blurring of professional boundaries as members acquired multiple degrees, as responsibilities were parsed out and new roles carved for physical therapists, respiratory therapists, counselors, physician assistants, and so on.

Some comments surface when nurses talk about their profession and what seems to be valued most by patients and physicians. Nurses "do it all"; they "care for the whole person"; they "see the big picture"; and they are "humanistic in all senses of the word." Nurse researchers might be those who refer to a conceptual or theoretical framework to maintain the "big picture." They consider the problem in some social context. Nurse researchers also address some aspect of the care of people. Transforming these comments to criteria may help to distinguish "nurse researchers" from nurses who do research and to distinguish nursing research as separate, special, and distinct from all other disciplines.

References

A model for symptom management. The University of California, San Francisco School of Nursing Symptom Management Faculty Group. (1994). *Image: The Journal of Nursing Scholarship, 26,* 272–276.

Badger, T.A., Braden, C.J., & Mishel, M.H. (2001). Depression burden, self-help interventions, and side effects experience in women receiving treatment for breast cancer. *Oncology Nursing Forum, 28,* 567–574.

Baron, R.H., Kelvin, J.F., Bookbinder, M., Cramer, L., Borgen, P.I., & Thaler, H.T. (2000). Patients' sensations after breast cancer surgery: A pilot study. *Cancer Practice, 8,* 215–222.

Boehmke, M.M. (2004). Measurement of symptom distress in women with early-stage breast cancer. *Cancer Nursing, 27,* 144–152.

Bragg Leight, S., Deirriggi, P., Hursh, D., Miller, D., & Leight, V. (2000). The effect of structured training on breast self-examination search behaviors as measured using biomedical instrumentation. *Nursing Research, 49,* 283–289.

Burke, C. (2005). Endometrial cancer and tamoxifen. *Clinical Journal of Oncology Nursing, 9,* 247–249.

Chen, W.T., & Bakken, S. (2004). Breast cancer knowledge assessment in female Chinese immigrants in New York. *Cancer Nursing, 27,* 407–412.

Coleman, E.A., Lord, J., Heard, J., Coon, S., Cantrell, M., Mohrmann, C., et al. (2003). The Delta project: Increasing breast cancer screening among rural minority and older women by targeting rural healthcare providers. *Oncology Nursing Forum, 30,* 669–677.

Cooley, M.E. (1998). Quality of life in persons with non-small cell lung cancer: A concept analysis. *Cancer Nursing, 21,* 151–161.

Davis Kirsch, S.E., Brandt, P.A., & Lewis, F.M. (2003). Making the most of the moment: When a child's mother has breast cancer. *Cancer Nursing, 26,* 47–54.

Davison, D. (2005). Novel breast-imaging methods. *Clinical Journal of Oncology Nursing, 9,* 255–256.

Decker, G. (2001). Patients are talking about Iscador (mistletoe). *Clinical Journal of Oncology Nursing, 5,* 183–184.

Dirksen, S.R. (2000). Predicting well-being among breast cancer survivors. *Journal of Advanced Nursing, 32,* 937–943.

Dirksen, S.R., & Erickson, J.R. (2002). Well-being in Hispanic and non-Hispanic white survivors of breast cancer. *Oncology Nursing Forum, 29,* 820–826.

Dodd, M., Janson, S., Facione, N., Fawcett, J., Froelicher, E.S., Humphreys, J., et al. (2001). Advancing the science of symptom management. *Journal of Advanced Nursing, 33,* 668–676.

Doran, D.M. (Ed.). (2003). *Nursing-sensitive outcomes: State of the science.* Sudbury, MA: Jones and Bartlett.

Dow, K.H., & Lafferty, P. (2000). Quality of life, survivorship, and psychosocial adjustment of young women with breast cancer after breast-conserving surgery and radiation therapy. *Oncology Nursing Forum, 27,* 1555–1564.

Drake, D.A. (2001). A longitudinal study of physical activity and breast cancer prediction. *Cancer Nursing, 24,* 371–377.

Frankel, C. (2000). Nursing management considerations with trastuzumab (Herceptin). *Seminars in Oncology Nursing, 16*(4 Suppl. 1), 23–28.

Gantz, P.A., Day, R., Ware, J.E., Redmond, C., & Fisher, B. (1995). Baseline quality of life assessment in the National Surgical Adjuvant Breast and Bowel Project. *Journal of the National Cancer Institute, 87,* 1372–1382.

Gantz, P.A., Greendale, G.A., Peterson, L., Zibecchi, L., Kahn, B., & Belin, T.R. (2000). Managing menopausal symptoms in breast cancer survivors: Results of a randomized controlled trial. *Journal of the National Cancer Institute, 92,* 1054–1064.

Gasalberti, G. (2002). Early detection of breast cancer by self-examination: The influence of perceived barriers and health conception. *Oncology Nursing Forum, 29,* 1341–1347.

Griffin, E. (2003). Safety considerations and safe handling of oral chemotherapy agents. *Clinical Journal of Oncology Nursing, 7*(Suppl. 6), 25–29.

Harwood, K.V. (2004). Advances in endocrine therapy for breast cancer: Considering efficacy, safety, and quality of life. *Clinical Journal of Oncology Nursing, 8,* 629–637.

Hilton, B.A., Crawford, J.A., & Tarko, M.A. (2000). Men's perspectives on individual and family coping with their wives' breast cancer and chemotherapy. *Western Journal of Nursing Research, 22,* 438–459.

Hutson, S.P. (2003). Attitudes and psychological impact of genetic testing, genetic counseling, and breast cancer risk assessment among women at increased risk. *Oncology Nursing Forum, 30,* 241–246.

Kelly, P. (2003). Hereditary breast cancer considering Cowden's syndrome: A case study. *Cancer Nursing, 26,* 370–375.

Kessler, T.A. (2002). Contextual variables, emotional state, and current and expected quality of life in breast cancer survivors. *Oncology Nursing Forum, 29,* 1109–1116.

Knight, M.M. (2000). Cognitive ability and functional status. *Journal of Advanced Nursing, 31,* 1459–1468.

Knobf, M.T. (2001). The menopausal symptom experience in young mid-life women with breast cancer. *Cancer Nursing, 24,* 201–210.

Kwekkeboom, K.L. (2001). Outcome expectancy and success with cognitive-behavioral interventions: The case for guided imagery. *Oncology Nursing Forum, 28,* 1125–1132.

Lackan, N.A., Freeman, J.L., & Goodwin, J.S. (2003). Hospice use by older women dying with breast cancer between 1991 and 1996. *Journal of Palliative Care, 19,* 49–53.

Lengacher, C.A., Bennett, M.P., Kipp, K.E., Berarducci, A., & Cox, C.E. (2003). Design and testing of the use of complementary and alternative therapies survey in women with breast cancer. *Oncology Nursing Forum, 30,* 811–821.

Lengacher, C.A., Bennett, M.P., Kipp, K.E., Keller, R., LaVance, M.S., Smith, L.S., et al. (2002). Frequency of use of complementary and alternative medicine in women with breast cancer. *Oncology Nursing Forum, 29,* 1445–1452.

Leslie, N.S., Deiriggi, P., Gross, S., DuRant, E., Smith, C., & Veshnesky, J.G. (2003). Knowledge, attitudes and practices surrounding breast cancer screening in educated Appalachian women. *Oncology Nursing Forum, 30,* 659–667.

Lindsey, A.M., Gross, G., Twiss, J., Waltman, N., Ott, C., & Moore, T.E. (2002). Postmenopausal survivors of breast cancer at risk for osteoporosis: Nutritional intake and body size. *Cancer Nursing, 25,* 50–56.

Loescher, L.J. (2003). Cancer worry in women with hereditary risk factors for breast cancer. *Oncology Nursing Forum, 30,* 767–772.

Lynn, J. (2002). Estrogen receptor downregulators: New advances in managing advanced breast cancer. *Cancer Nursing, 25*(Suppl. 2), 2S–5S.

Manning-Walsh, J. (2005). Spiritual struggle: Effect on quality of life and life satisfaction in women with breast cancer. *Journal of Holistic Nursing, 23,* 120–140.

McCorkle, R., & Young, K. (1978). Development of a symptom distress scale. *Cancer Nursing, 5,* 373–378.

National Center for Complementary and Alternative Medicine. (2005). *What is complementary and alternative medicine?* Retrieved November 1, 2005, from http://nccam.nih.gov/health/whatiscam/#sup2#sup2

Northouse, L.L., Walker, J., Schafenacker, A., Mood, D., Mellon, S., Galvin, E., et al. (2002). A family-based program of care for women with recurrent breast cancer and their family members. *Oncology Nursing Forum, 29,* 1411–1419.

Orem, D. (1971). *Nursing: Concepts of practice.* New York: McGraw-Hill.

Petrie, W., Logan, J., & DeGrasse, C. (2001). Research review of the supportive care needs of spouses of women with breast cancer. *Oncology Nursing Forum, 28,* 1601–1607.

Pickett, M., Mock, V., Ropka, M.E., Cameron, L., Coleman, M., & Podewils, L. (2002). Adherence to moderate-intensity exercise during breast cancer therapy. *Cancer Practice, 10,* 284–292.

Ponto, J.A., Frost, M.H., Thompson, R., Allers, T., Reed-Will, T., Zahasky, K., et al. (2003). Stories of breast cancer through art. *Oncology Nursing Forum, 30,* 1007–1013.

Rashidi, A., & Rajaram, S.S. (2000). Middle Eastern Asian Islamic women and breast self-examination: Needs assessment. *Cancer Nursing, 23,* 64–70.

Richmond, T., McCorkle, R., Tulman, L., & Fawcett, J. (1997). Measuring function. In M. Frank-Stromborg & S.J. Olsen (Eds.), *Instruments for clinical health-care research* (2nd ed., pp. 75–85). Sudbury, MA: Jones and Bartlett.

Sammarco, A. (2001). Perceived social support, uncertainty, and quality of life of younger breast cancer survivors. *Cancer Nursing, 24,* 212–219.

Schneider, S.M., Prince-Paul, M., Allen, M.J., Silverman, P., & Talaba, D. (2004). Virtual reality as a distraction intervention for women receiving chemotherapy. *Oncology Nursing Forum, 31,* 81–88.

Schwartz, A.L. (2000). Exercise and weight gain in breast cancer patients receiving chemotherapy. *Cancer Practice, 8,* 231–237.

Smith, E.D., Phillips, J.M., & Price, M.M. (2001). Screening and early detection among racial and ethnic minority women [Review]. *Seminars in Oncology Nursing, 17,* 159–170.

Strauss, B. (2000). Best hope or last hope: Access to phase III clinical trials of Her-2/neu for advanced stage breast cancer patients. *Journal of Advanced Nursing, 31,* 259–266.

Waltman, N., Twiss, J.J., Ott, C.D., Gross, G., Lindsey, A.M., Moore, T.E., et al. (2003). Testing an intervention for preventing osteoporosis in postmenopausal breast cancer survivors. *Journal of Nursing Scholarship, 35,* 333–338.

Wampler, M.A., Hamolsky, D., Hamel, K., Melisko, M., & Topp, K.S. (2005). Case report: Painful peripheral neuropathy following treatment with Docetaxel for breast cancer. *Clinical Journal of Oncology Nursing, 9,* 189–193.

Wells, J.N., Bush, H.A., & Marshall, D. (2001). Psychometric evaluation of Breast Health Behavior Questionnaire: Spanish version. *Cancer Nursing, 24,* 320–327.

Williams, S.A., & Schreier, A.M. (2004). The effect of education in managing side effects in women receiving chemotherapy for treatment of breast cancer [Online exclusive]. *Oncology Nursing Forum, 31,* E16–E23.

Wood, L.J., Maher, J.F., Bunton, T.E., & Resar, L.M.S. (2000). The oncogenic properties of the HMG-I gene family. *Cancer Research, 60,* 4256–4261.

Wood, R.Y., & Duffy, M.E. (2004). Video breast health kits: Testing a cancer education innovation in older high-risk populations. *Journal of Cancer Education, 19,* 98–102.

Wood, R.Y., Duffy, M.E., Morris, S.J., & Carnes, J.E. (2002). The effect of an educational intervention on promoting breast self-examination in older African-American and Caucasian women. *Oncology Nursing Forum, 29,* 1081–1090.

Appendices

Appendix 1. Resources Related to Breast Cancer

General Information

American Cancer Society (ACS)
National Home Office, 1599 Clifton Road, Atlanta, GA 30329
Phone: 800-ACS-2345
Web site: www.cancer.org
The ACS provides authoritative information on breast cancer prevention, early detection, treatment, side effects, symptom management, and coping.

CancerSource.com
280 Summer Street, Ninth Floor, Boston, MA 02210
Phone: 617-399-4485
Web site: www.cancersource.com
CancerSource.com is dedicated to providing up-to-date cancer information, symptom management, and resources for people who have cancer, those who care for them, and healthcare professionals.

MedlinePlus
U.S. National Library of Medicine, 8600 Rockville Pike, Bethesda, MD 20894
Phone: 888-FIND-NLM
Web site: www.nlm.nih.gov/medlineplus/breastcancer.html
This Web site provides a compendium of authoritative information from a multitude of reliable resources on topics related to breast cancer and its treatment.

National Cancer Institute (NCI)
6116 Executive Boulevard, Room 3036A, Bethesda, MD 20892
Phone: 800-4-CANCER
Web site: www.cancer.gov
Cancer Information Service: http://cis.nci.nih.gov
NCI provides comprehensive information on cancer treatment, screening, prevention, supportive care, complementary and alternative treatments, and clinical trials.

People Living with Cancer
American Society of Clinical Oncology, 1900 Duke Street, Suite 200, Alexandria, VA 22314
Phone: 703-797-1914
Web site: www.plwc.org
This patient information Web site of the American Society of Clinical Oncology is designed to help patients with decision making, symptom management, coping, and clinical trials.

Reach to Recovery
Phone: 800-ACS-2345
Available through www.cancer.org
ACS sponsors the Reach to Recovery program, through which trained volunteers provide information and support to patients with cancer and those close to them either face-to-face or over the phone.

Susan G. Komen for the Cure
5005 LBJ Freeway, Suite 250, Dallas, TX 75244
Phone: 972-855-1600, Helpline: 800-I'M-AWARE®
Web site: www.komen.org
This is a national organization that provides information regarding breast cancer prevention, early detection, treatment, and symptom management, along with support services.

SusanLoveMD.org
P.O. Box 846, Pacific Palisades, CA 90272
Phone: 310-230-1712
Web site: www.susanlove.org
This Web site provides up-to-date information on breast cancer news, treatments, side effects, symptom management, and support.

The Wellness Community (TWC)
National Headquarters, 919 18th Street, NW, Suite 54, Washington, DC 20006
Phone: 202-659-9709, Toll-free: 888-793-WELL
Web site: www.thewellnesscommunity.org
TWC is an international nonprofit organization dedicated to providing support, education, and hope for all people affected by cancer at no cost. There are 21 Wellness Communities in the United States.

Y-ME National Breast Cancer Organization
212 W. Van Buren, Suite 1000, Chicago, IL 60607
Phone: 312-986-8338, 24-hour hotline: 800-221-2141
Web site: www.y-me.org
Y-ME is a national organization that provides support and information regarding breast cancer to survivors and families about early detection, prevention, treatment, and symptom management. Single copies of booklets and brochures can be ordered free of charge in both English and Spanish by completing an order form online or by calling 800-221-2141. Many of the pamphlets are available in printable form directly from the Web site.

(Continued on next page)

Appendix 1. Resources Related to Breast Cancer *(Continued)*

Genetics/Screening/Prevention

Facing Our Risk of Cancer Empowered (FORCE)
16057 Tampa Palms Boulevard W, PMB #373, Tampa, FL 33647
Phone: 954-255-8732
Web site: www.facingourrisk.org/index.php
FORCE is a nonprofit organization for women with increased risk of cancer due to family history and genetic status and for members of families in which a BRCA mutation may be present.

GeneTests
9725 Third Avenue NE, Suite 602, Seattle, WA 98115
Fax: 206-221-4679
Web site: www.genetests.org
GeneTests provides current, reviewed information on genetic testing and its use in diagnosis and management, as well as information on genetic counseling. It also promotes the appropriate use of genetic services in patient care and personal decision making. Funded by the National Institutes of Health, GeneTests provides scientific and review information on genetic conditions, patient resources, and laboratory testing.

International Society of Nurses in Genetics (ISONG)
461 Cochran Road, Box 246, Pittsburgh, PA 15228
Phone: 412-344-1414
Web site: www.isong.org
ISONG is an international nursing specialty organization dedicated to promoting the scientific and professional growth of nurses in human genetics and genomics worldwide.

Lymphedema

Lymphatic Research Foundation (LRF)
100 Forest Drive, East Hills, NY 11548
Phone: 516-625-9675
Web site: www.lymphaticresearch.org
LRF is an organization that was developed to advance research of the lymphatic system and to increase public and private funding for lymphatic research.

Lymphology Association of North America (LANA)
P.O. Box 466, Wilmette, IL 60091
Phone: 773-756-8971
Web site: www.clt-lana.org
LANA is an organization developed to promote standards for management of people with lymphedema. The organization also sponsors a certification exam for lymphedema specialists.

National Lymphedema Network (NLN)
Latham Square, 1611 Telegraph Avenue, Suite 1111, Oakland, CA 94612
Phone: 510-208-3200, Toll-free: 800-541-3259
Web site: www.lymphnet.org
The NLN is an internationally recognized organization whose goals are to provide education and guidance to healthcare professionals, the public, and patients with lymphedema.

Research

American Association for Cancer Research (AACR)
615 Chestnut Street, 17th Floor, Philadelphia, PA 19106
Phone: 215-440-9300, Toll-free: 866-423-3965
Web site: www.aacr.org
AACR focuses on information about advances in the causes, diagnosis, treatment, and prevention of cancer through publishing journals; conducting conferences, workshops, and meetings; and promoting awareness of cancer research.

Clinicaltrials.gov
National Institutes of Health, 900 Rockville Pike, Bethesda, MD 20892
Phone: 301-496-4000
Web site: www.clinicaltrials.gov
This resource is a National Institutes of Health–sponsored Web site that provides regularly updated information regarding federally and privately funded clinical research.

(Continued on next page)

Appendix 1. Resources Related to Breast Cancer *(Continued)*

Survivorship

Lance Armstrong Foundation (LAF)
P.O. Box 161150, Austin, TX 78716
Phone: 512-236-8820
Web site: www.livestrong.org
Founded in 1997 by cancer survivor and champion cyclist Lance Armstrong, LAF provides the practical information and tools that people living with cancer need. The organization's mission is to inspire and empower people with cancer through education, advocacy, and public health and research programs. LIVESTRONG™ Survivor*Care* offers assistance to all cancer survivors, including the person diagnosed, caregivers, family members, and friends through education, qualified referrals, and counseling services. Case managers are available by phone at 866-235-7205, Monday through Friday from 9 am to 5 pm EST, or through an e-mail form on the Web site. A Cancer Clinical Trial Matching Service also is available through the Web site or by calling 800-620-6167, Monday through Friday from 7 am to 5:30 pm CST.

Young Survival Coalition (YSC)
61 Broadway, Suite 2235, New York, NY 10006
Phone: 646-257-3000
Web site: www.youngsurvival.org
YSC is the only international nonprofit network of breast cancer survivors and supporters dedicated to the concerns and issues that are unique to young women with breast cancer. Through action, advocacy, and awareness, YSC seeks to educate the medical, research, breast cancer, and legislative communities and persuade them to address breast cancer in women age 40 and under. YSC also serves as a point of contact for young women living with breast cancer.

Symptom Management

CancerSymptoms.org
Oncology Nursing Society, 125 Enterprise Drive, Pittsburgh, PA 15275
Phone: 866-257-4ONS
Web site: www.cancersymptoms.org
This site, sponsored by the Oncology Nursing Society, provides symptom management for common side effects of cancer treatment, including fatigue, hormonal issues, pain, and cognitive changes.

Chemocare.com, Scott Hamilton CARES Initiative
Cleveland Clinic Taussig Cancer Center, 9500 Euclid Avenue, Cleveland, OH 44195
Phone: 800-440-4140 Ext. 53082
Web site: www.chemocare.com
A program of the Scott Hamilton CARES initiative, Chemocare. com is a source for information on chemotherapy side effects and drug information.

Fertile Hope
P.O. Box 624, New York, NY 10014
Phone: 888-994-HOPE
Web site: www.fertilehope.org
Founded in October 2001, Fertile Hope is a national nonprofit organization dedicated to providing reproductive information, support, and hope to patients with cancer whose medical treatments present the risk of infertility.

Gilda's Club Worldwide
322 Eighth Avenue, Suite 1402, New York, NY 10001
Phone: 888-GILDA-4-U
Web site: www.gildasclub.org
Gilda's Club focuses on addressing the emotional and social issues of patients with cancer and anyone touched by the disease. It seeks to provide supportive communities for patients with cancer and their friends and families at locations throughout the world.

Look Good . . . Feel Better (LGFB)
Phone: 800-395-LOOK
Web site: www.lookgoodfeelbetter.org
LGFB is a free national public service program supported by corporate donors to help women to offset appearance-related changes from cancer treatment.

NIH Osteoporosis and Related Bone Diseases National Resource Center
2 AMS Circle, Bethesda, MD 20892
Phone: 800-624-BONE
Web site: www.niams.nih.gov/bone
The Osteoporosis and Related Bone Diseases National Resource Center is an NIH department dedicated to increasing awareness, knowledge, and understanding of the prevention, early detection, and treatment of osteoporosis.

Appendix 2. Oncology Nursing Society Position on Breast Cancer Screening

Breast cancer is a significant public health problem. Although all women are at risk for developing breast cancer, the risk is greater in women as they grow older, especially after the age of 40, and in women with a hereditary predisposition for developing breast cancer. Breast cancer treatment is usually less aggressive and better tolerated when the disease is detected early. Currently, the three primary tools used for the early detection of breast cancer are breast self-examination (BSE), clinical breast examination (CBE) by a healthcare provider, and mammography (National Comprehensive Cancer Network [NCCN], 2005).

Systematic monthly BSE has been recommended since 1933; however, more than 30 nonrandomized trials have produced conflicting results about the efficacy, sensitivity, and specificity of the practice (Austoker, 2003; Havey, Miller, Baines, & Corey, 1997). The effectiveness of BSE is largely dependent on the skill of the woman practicing BSE, and the consensus is that BSE should be used in combination with other breast cancer screening modalities (NCCN, 2005).

Sensitivity for CBE has been reported to range from 40%–69%, and its specificity ranges from 88%–99% (Humphrey, Helfand, Chan, & Woolf, 2002). Trials in which CBE is combined with mammography have demonstrated a mortality reduction of 14%–29% (Humphrey et al.). Like BSE, the sensitivity and usefulness of CBE is related, in part, to the skill of the healthcare provider performing the examination. When CBE is performed prior to mammography, it may be useful in identifying an area of suspicion that might not be readily visible on mammography or provide guidance in selecting additional imaging techniques (Smith, 2003).

The primary evidence for supporting mammography comes from seven large randomized clinical trials that show a statistically significant mortality reduction from breast cancer in women aged 40–69 years who underwent regular mammography screening (Smith et al., 2003). Overall, the trials suggested a 24% mortality reduction associated with mammography use. The sensitivity for annual mammography ranges from 71%–96%, with lower sensitivity seen in younger women who tend to have dense breasts, and specificity ranges from 94%–97% (Humphrey et al., 2002).

It Is the Position of ONS That
- Oncology nurses should review the scientific basis for each breast screening modality and interpret the data for women. Educational materials need to be culturally competent and appropriate for the literacy and educational level of each woman.
- Risk assessment is a component of regular health care and integral to the cancer screening process. Although general guidelines exist for offering cancer screening tests, they often must be modified based on the presence of significant risk factors. Recommendations for breast cancer screening should be made only after a woman's risk is assessed and interpreted.
- The benefits, risks, and potential limitations of BSE, CBE, and mammography need to be discussed with each woman and tailored to her risk factor assessment.
- Women at higher-than-average risk for breast cancer should be referred to a healthcare provider with expertise in breast cancer risk assessment and cancer genetics for guidance about the appropriate age and frequency for screening.
- Women should have access to comprehensive breast cancer screening.
- Every woman, after having a comprehensive breast cancer risk assessment, has the right to make an informed decision about breast cancer screening.
- Women should be instructed on the strengths and limitations of BSE and be allowed to make a choice about their BSE practice. All women should be offered the opportunity to learn proper BSE technique beginning at age 20. Nurses should use instruction regarding BSE to heighten awareness about the early detection of breast cancer because it provides an opportunity to further educate women about comprehensive early cancer detection and prevention strategies.
- CBE should be performed by a healthcare provider with training and expertise on an annual basis to all women beginning at age 20.
- Women should begin regular, annual mammography starting at age 40. Mammography equipment should be dedicated to breast examinations and meet federal, state, and professional standards for quality and safety. Films should be interpreted by radiologists with expertise in reading mammograms.
- Oncology nurses need to support legislation that improves access to breast cancer screening.
- Oncology nurses should obtain ongoing continuing education to enhance knowledge and skills, implement risk assessment strategies, and identify factors that promote breast cancer screening.
- Oncology nurses need to conduct and support further and ongoing research on the prevention and early detection of breast cancer.

References
Austoker, J. (2003). Breast self-examination: Does not prevent deaths due to breast cancer, but breast awareness is still important. *BMJ, 326,* 1–2.
Havey, B.J., Miller, A., Baines, C., & Corey, P.N. (1997). Effect of breast self-examination techniques on the risk of death from breast cancer. *Canadian Medical Association Journal, 157,* 1205–1212.
Humphrey, L.L., Helfand, M., Chan, B., & Woolf, S.H. (2002). Breast cancer screening: A summary of the evidence for the U.S. Preventive Services Task Force. *Annals of Internal Medicine, 137*(5 Pt. 1), E347–E367.
National Comprehensive Cancer Network. (2005). *Breast cancer screening and diagnosis guidelines version 1.2005.* Retrieved February 2, 2006, from http://www.nccn.org/professionals/physician_gls/PDF/breast-screening.pdf
Smith, R.A. (2003). An overview of mammography: Benefits and limitations. *Journal of the National Comprehensive Cancer Network, 1,* 264–271.
Smith, R.A., Saslow, D., Sawyer, K.A., Burke, W., Costanza, M.E., Evans, W.P., et al. (2003). American Cancer Society guidelines for breast cancer screening: Update 2003. *CA: A Cancer Journal for Clinicians, 53,* 141–169.

Approved by the ONS Board of Directors 3/06.

Appendix 3. Oncology Nursing Society Position on Cancer Predisposition Genetic Testing and Risk Assessment Counseling

The ability to identify individuals who are at increased risk for developing cancer because of an inherited altered (mutated) cancer predisposition gene is possible through cancer predisposition genetic testing. However, while providing the capability to target high-risk individuals who might benefit from specific strategies for medical management, genetic testing also raises ethical, legal, and social issues associated with revealing a person's genetic makeup.

It Is the Position of ONS That

- Risk assessment counseling and cancer predisposition genetic testing are components of comprehensive cancer care and should be available despite the cost to the healthcare system.
- All healthcare providers offering these services to patients and family members must have educational preparation in both human genetic principles and oncology.
- Cancer predisposition genetic testing requires informed consent and must include pre- and post-test counseling and follow-up by qualified individuals (e.g., advanced practice oncology nurses, oncologists with specialized education in hereditary cancer genetics, certified genetic counselors with specialized training in oncology).
- Ethical principles of beneficence, nonmaleficence, respect for autonomy, and justice must form the foundation for counseling services, guide the development of standards of care in cancer genetic counseling, and be included in criteria used to identify potential problems arising from cancer predisposition genetic testing and the counseling process.
- Comprehensive cancer genetic counseling must occur in a manner consistent with individual cultural and healthcare beliefs.
- Efforts must be made to include family members in the counseling process and to seek ways to address barriers to genetic testing and risk assessment in diverse populations.
- Legislation that provides protection from genetic discrimination in both employment and insurance arenas and reimbursement for and access to genetic counseling, cancer predisposition genetic testing services, and appropriate medical management must be implemented and monitored.
- Ongoing educational resources for healthcare providers, individuals at increased risk, and the lay public must be developed, evaluated, and disseminated.
- A research plan related to all aspects of cancer genetics, including the efficacy of programs for prevention and early detection, the psychological impact of cancer predisposition genetic testing, and long-term outcomes of testing and risk management strategies, must be developed and evaluated.
- Efforts to improve the standardization and regulation of laboratories that provide cancer predisposition genetic testing must be evaluated and monitored.

Bibliography

Lowrey, K.M. (2004). Legal and ethical issues in cancer genetics nursing. *Seminars in Oncology Nursing, 20,* 203–208.

Mahon, S.M. (1998). Cancer risk assessment: Conceptual considerations for clinical practice. *Oncology Nursing Forum, 25,* 1535–1547.

Tranin, A.S., Masny, A., & Jenkins, J. (Eds.). (2003). *Genetics in oncology practice: Cancer risk assessment.* Pittsburgh, PA: Oncology Nursing Society.

Approved by the ONS Board of Directors, 8/97; revised 8/00, 7/02, 10/04.

Appendix 4. Association of Rehabilitation Nurses (ARN) and
Oncology Nursing Society Position on Rehabilitation of People With Cancer

More than 1,284,000 Americans were diagnosed with invasive cancer in 2002 (American Cancer Society, 2002). The number of cancer survivors increases each year because of advances in early detection and innovative treatments. Cancer is a chronic disease with concurrent physical, functional, psychological, and spiritual sequelae. These sequelae are best addressed through a comprehensive oncology rehabilitation program. The focus of the program must be collaborative and interdisciplinary, whether based in acute, subacute, or home care.

It Is the Position of ARN and ONS That
- Oncology rehabilitation care is part of quality cancer care, which is a right for all citizens.
- Oncology rehabilitation is an option for all patients at any stage of cancer.
- Oncology rehabilitation incorporates the individual with cancer and the family as fully informed partners and decision makers.
- Oncology rehabilitation includes timely access to and reimbursement for a coordinated, comprehensive, interdisciplinary approach.
- Oncology rehabilitation is coordinated and delivered by competent rehabilitative cancer care providers.
- Accountability and coordination of quality oncology rehabilitation care is best accomplished by registered nurses who have been educated and certified in oncology or rehabilitation specialities.

Background
ARN and ONS believe the oncology rehabilitation registered nurse's role in the interdisciplinary team is pivotal in creating an environment conducive to quality patient care. "The goal of rehabilitation nursing is to assist the individual with disability and chronic illness in the restoration and maintenance of maximal health" (ARN, 1998, p. 5). It is imperative that ongoing research and education in rehabilitation be funded to find ways to improve care. With ongoing collaboration and interdisciplinary efforts, cancer rehabilitation will maximize both the quantity and quality of each individual's life for the present and in the future.

References
American Cancer Society. (2002). *Cancer facts and figures, 2002.* Atlanta, GA: Author.
Association of Rehabilitation Nurses. (1998). *Certified rehabilitation registered nurse: Certification information handbook.* Glenview, IL: Author.

ONS Board of Directors approved October 1999; revised March 2003.
ARN Board of Directors approved October 1999; revised March 2003.

Appendix 5. Oncology Nursing Society Position on Prevention and Early Detection of Cancer in the United States

In the United States, more than 1,280,000 new cancers are diagnosed in individuals across the life span each year. The lifetime risk of developing cancer in the United States is 43% for men and 38% for women. Cancer is the second leading cause of death in the United States, with one in every four deaths caused by cancer. Cancer is the leading cause of death in individuals 40–79 years of age (Jemal, Thomas, Murray, & Thun, 2002). Consequently, cancer is a major public health problem in the United States. Adopting healthier lifestyles and avoiding carcinogen exposure could prevent many cancers. According to the American Cancer Society (ACS), institution of prevention measures and early detection of cancer are two of the most important and effective strategies for reaching important public health goals of saving lives lost from cancer, diminishing suffering from cancer, and eliminating cancer as a major health problem.

It Is the Position of ONS That
Professional Education
- Oncology nurses, at both the generalist and advanced practice levels, must have educational preparation in the behavioral, biologic, educational, and economic principles of cancer prevention and early detection.
- Continuing education and specialized educational programs must be developed and provided to practicing nurses to facilitate integration of cancer prevention and early detection into clinical practice.
- Oncology specialty certification examinations and nursing licensure examinations should include evaluation of knowledge related to cancer prevention and detection practices in the general population.

Public Education
- All oncology nurses are well suited to provide education to the general public about prevention measures and general population screening guidelines for the early detection of cancer.
- Oncology nurses also are well suited to provide the necessary information and education to facilitate client decision making about participation in cancer prevention and control clinical trials.
- Oncology nurses must strive to provide comprehensive cancer prevention education and early detection services in a manner consistent with the cultural background and healthcare beliefs of individuals and families. Educational materials should be used that are targeted to the appropriate level of literacy and are culturally sensitive.
- Oncology nurses must be involved in the development of educational resources that have a focus on wellness, including the prevention and early detection of cancer in at-risk populations.
- Education programs must be developed and provided on the primary prevention of cancer (e.g., smoking cessation programs, nutritional counseling, avoidance of exposure to ultraviolet light) beginning in childhood and throughout the life span to encourage people to adopt healthy lifestyles.

Cancer Prevention and Detection Services
- Oncology nurses need to develop, implement, and evaluate measures to ensure that individuals and families have access to education about cancer prevention and appropriate cancer screening.
- Advanced practice oncology nurses can obtain, document, and interpret cancer risk assessments; recommend appropriate cancer early detection and prevention strategies to individuals and families; and arrange or provide comprehensive cancer screening services based on the individual's level of risk. These practices must be consistent with guidelines defined by the appropriate state's nurse practice act, educational preparation, and role scope, along with standards of oncology nursing practice.
- As genetic technology evolves and knowledge of cancer genetics expands, healthcare providers must respond by informing patients, families, and the public about the implications of these developments for cancer prevention, early detection, and treatment. Nurses providing comprehensive cancer genetic counseling must be advanced practice oncology nurses with specialized education in hereditary cancer genetics.
- Individuals who have survived a cancer diagnosis also should receive age-appropriate cancer screening for other cancers.
- Programs that are focused on delivering services for the early detection of individual cancers (e.g., breast, prostate) also should ensure that patients receive education and are referred for screening for other common cancers. An immediate opportunity exists to implement this approach in men and women who are covered by Medicare and already eligible for reimbursement of the respective screening tests for breast, cervical, colorectal, and prostate cancers.
- Individuals should be assessed for eligibility for chemoprevention trials based on personal level of risk and referred for consideration at the appropriate clinical site.
- Individuals should be fully informed of their options for managing their personal risks for developing cancer and should understand the limitations, benefits, and risks of each strategy.

Research
- Oncology nurses need to conduct research to further assess the efficacy of cancer prevention and early detection programs, the psychological impact of cancer prevention and detection strategies, and promotion of participation in prevention and early detection activities.
- Research related to cancer prevention and detection strategies must be integrated into practice.

(Continued on next page)

Appendix 5. Oncology Nursing Society Position on Prevention and Early Detection of Cancer in the United States *(Continued)*

Health Policy
- The development and evaluation of cancer prevention and detection health policy should be based on current cancer control research and involve multidisciplinary academicians and clinicians (including oncology nurses) and the public.
- Payors must be encouraged to provide coverage for prevention measures, counseling on prevention strategies, nutrition, and smoking cessation and for early detection and screening services based on individual risk levels.
- The ability to identify individuals who are at increased risk for developing cancer because of inherited altered (mutated) cancer predisposition genes is possible through cancer predisposition genetic testing. Risk assessment counseling and cancer predisposition genetic testing are components of comprehensive cancer care, and payors should cover them.
- Payors should cover clinical trials evaluating cancer prevention and detection strategies and chemoprevention.

Background
Primary cancer prevention refers to the prevention of cancer through health promotion and risk reduction. This includes carcinogen avoidance and, more recently, the use of chemoprevention agents and consideration of prophylactic surgeries in individuals at high risk for developing cancer, such as those with genetic predispositions. Secondary cancer prevention refers to the early detection and treatment of subclinical disease or early disease in people without signs or symptoms of cancer. Early detection is defined as the application of a test to detect a potential cancer in individuals who have no signs or symptoms of the cancer. Cancer screening refers to looking for cancer in a population at risk for a particular cancer. Cancer screening and early detection are forms of secondary cancer prevention aimed at detecting cancer early, when it is most treatable in asymptomatic people. Tertiary cancer prevention refers to the prevention and early detection of second primary cancers in individuals who have been diagnosed with cancer. This includes the application of specific tests to detect cancer and the use of chemoprevention agents to prevent the development of additional cancers.

Cancer continues to be a significant health problem in the United States. Everyone is at risk for developing cancer. Many cancers could be prevented by avoidance of carcinogens and mutagens. ACS estimated that 171,000 cancer deaths result annually from tobacco use, and 19,000 deaths are related to excessive alcohol use (Jemal et al., 2002). An additional 185,000 cancer deaths are attributed to diet, nutrition, and other lifestyle factors and are probably preventable. Many of the 1.3 million skin cancers diagnosed annually could be prevented or controlled if people decreased their exposure to ultraviolet light. These facts underscore the importance of educating the public about the importance of a healthy lifestyle and strategies that can be instituted for the prevention of cancer. Public policy should support programs that provide education to the public about cancer prevention measures. Public education about the importance of cancer prevention measures and recommended cancer screening guidelines is an important component of oncology nursing practice and should occur both across the life span and the continuum of cancer care.

Cancer morbidity and mortality could be reduced further by the early detection of cancer in asymptomatic individuals. Cancers of the breast, colon, rectum, cervix, prostate, testis, oral cavity, and skin can be detected early, when treatment is more likely to be effective. These cancers alone account for about one half of all cancer cases diagnosed annually in the United States. The ACS (2001) estimated that the current five-year relative survival rate for these cancers is about 80%. If all Americans participated in regular cancer screening, this rate could increase to 95%. Payors must include coverage of cancer screening services to achieve this goal.

References
American Cancer Society. (2001). *Cancer facts and figures, 2001.* Atlanta, GA: Author.
Jemal, A., Thomas, A., Murray, T., & Thun, M. (2002). Cancer statistics, 2002. *CA: A Cancer Journal for Clinicians, 52,* 23–47.

Additional Resources
- Carroll-Johnson, R.M. (Ed.). (2000). Cancer prevention and early detection: Oncology nursing's next frontier. *Oncology Nursing Forum, 27*(Suppl. 9), 1–61.
- Jennings-Dozier, K., & Mahon, S.M. (Eds.) (2002). *Cancer prevention, detection, and control: A nursing perspective.* Pittsburgh, PA: Oncology Nursing Society.
- National Cancer Institute, www.nci.nih.gov

Approved by the ONS Board of Directors, April 2001; revised August 2002.
The Board of Directors acknowledges the collective wisdom, contributions, and recommendations of these ONS members with recognized experience in the prevention and detection of cancer: Suzanne M. Mahon, RN, DNSc, AOCN®, assistant clinical professor in the Division of Hematology and Oncology at Saint Louis University in Missouri; and Lois J. Loescher, PhD, RN, cancer prevention fellow at Arizona Cancer Center at the University of Arizona in Tucson. The Board also acknowledges the contributions of Kathleen Jennings-Dozier, PhD, MPH, RN, CS, former associate professor at MCP Hahnemann University College of Nursing and Health Professions in Philadelphia, PA, who died from cancer in May 2002.

Index

The letter f *after a page number indicates that relevant content appears in a figure; the letter* t, *in a table.*